Osteoporosis

BEST PRACTICE & RESEARCH COMPENDIUM

Edited by

Cyrus Cooper MA, DM, FRCP, FFPH, FMedSci

Professor of Rheumatology and Director, MRC Epidemiology Resource Centre,
University of Southampton, Southampton General Hospital, Southampton, UK

and

Anthony D. Woolf BSc, MBBS, FRCP

Professor of Rheumatology, Department of Rheumatology, Royal Cornwall Hospital, Truro, UK

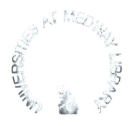

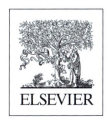

ELSEVIER

EDINBURGH LONDON NEW YORK OXFORD
PHILADELPHIA ST LOUIS SYDNEY TORONTO 2006

ELSEVIER

ISBN-13: 978-0-08-044685-1
ISBN-10: 0-08-044685-X

British Library Cataloguing in Publication Data
A catalogue record for this book is available from the British Library.

Library of Congress Cataloging in Publication Data
A catalog record for this book is available from the Library of Congress.

Note
Knowledge and best practice in this field are constantly changing. As new research and experience broaden our knowledge, changes in practice, treatment and drug therapy may become necessary or appropriate. Readers are advised to check the most current information provided (i) on procedures featured or (ii) by the manufacturer of each product to be administered, to verify the recommended dose or formula, the method and duration of administration, and contraindications. It is the responsibility of the practitioner, relying on their own experience and knowledge of the patient, to make diagnoses, to determine dosages and the best treatment for each individual patient, and to take all appropriate safety precautions. To the fullest extent of the law, neither the Publisher nor the Editors assumes any liability for any injury and/or damage to persons or property arising out or related to any use of the material contained in this book.

The Publisher

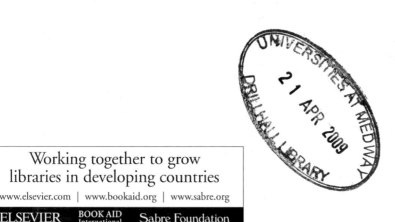

Printed in Spain.

your source for books, journals and multimedia in the health sciences

www.elsevierhealth.com

The Publisher's policy is to use **paper manufactured from sustainable forests**

Contents

Contributors

Jonathan D. Adachi MD, FRCPC
Professor, Department of Medicine
St. Joseph's Healthcare – McMaster
University
Hamilton, Ontario
Canada

Kristina Åkesson MD, PhD
Associate Professor
Lund University
Department of Orthopaedics
Malmö University Hospital
Malmö, Sweden

Shreyasee Amin MDCM, FRCP(C),
MPH
Assistant Professor
Division of Rheumatology
Mayo Clinic College of Medicine
Rochester, Minnesota
USA

Rolando Cimaz MD
Fondazione Policlinico Mangiagalli
Milano, Italy, and
Université Claude Bernard
Lyon, France

Jackie A. Clowes MBChB, MRCP, PhD
ARC Clinical Scientist
Assistant Professor of Medicine
Endocrine Research Unit
Mayo Clinic College of Medicine
Rochester, Minnesota
USA

Cyrus Cooper MA, DM, FRCP, FFPH,
FMedSci
Professor of Rheumatology and Director
MRC Epidemiology Resource Centre
University of Southampton
Southampton General Hospital
Southampton, UK

Alison M. Duncan PhD, RD
Assistant Professor
Department of Human Health and
Nutritional Sciences
University of Guelph
Guelph, Ontario
Canada

Richard Eastell MD, FRCP, FRCPI,
FRCPath, FMedSci
Professor of Bone Metabolism
University of Sheffield
Clinical Sciences Centre
Northern General Hospital
Sheffield, UK

Peter R. Ebeling MD, FRACP
Chair of Medicine
Head of Endocrinology
Department of Medicine/Western
Hospital
University of Melbourne
Footscray, Victoria, Australia

Rachael L. Fleurence PhD
Research Scientist
The MEDTAP Institute at UBC
Bethesda, Maryland
USA

Roger M. Francis MB, ChB, FRCP
Professor of Geriatric Medicine
University of Newcastle upon Tyne
Newcastle, UK

Dr. Claus-C. Glüer
Professor of Medical Physics
Arbeitsgruppe Medizinische Physik
Klinik für Diagnostische Radiologie
Universitätsklinikum Schleswig-Holstein
Campus Kiel, Kiel, Germany

Cynthia P. Iglesias MSc
Department of Health Sciences
University of York
Heslington
York, UK

M. Kassim Javaid MRCP, PhD
Clinical Fellow
MRC Epidemiology Resource Centre
Southampton General Hospital
Southampton, UK

Olof Johnell MD, PhD
Professor
Department of Orthopaedics
UMAS
Malmö, Sweden

Kelsey M. Jordan MBChB, MRCP
Rheumatology Department
Princess Royal Hospital
Brighton and Sussex University Hospitals
Haywards Heath
West Sussex, UK

Mindy S. Kurzer PhD
Professor
Department of Food Science and
Nutrition
University of Minnesota
St Paul, Minnesota
USA

Chris E. D. H. De Laet MD, PhD
Senior Expert
Belgian Healthcare Knowledge Centre
Wetstraat, Brussel
Belgium

Edith M. C. Lau MD, FRCP, FFPHM,
MSc, MBBS
Hong Kong Orthopaedic and
Osteoporosis Center for Treatment and
Research
Hong Kong, China

Paul Lips MD, PhD
VU University Medical Center
Department of Endocrinology
Amsterdam, The Netherlands

Christine Manette MD
Department of Gynaecology and
Obstetrics
University of Liège
Liège, Belgium

Ira Pande MD, PhD, FRCP
Consultant Rheumatology and
Honorary Lecturer
Nottingham University Hospitals NHS
Trust
Nottingham, UK

William R. Phipps MD
Associate Professor
Department of Obstetrics and
Gynecology
University of Rochester
Rochester, New York
USA

Huibert A. P. Pols MD, PhD
Professor of Medicine
Department of Internal Medicine
Erasmus Medical Center
Rotterdam, The Netherlands

David W. Purdie MD, FRCP Ed
Edinburgh Osteoporosis Centre
1 Wemyss Place
Edinburgh, UK

Jean-Yves Reginster MD, PhD
Unité d'Exploration du Métabolisme de
l'Os et du Cartilage
CHU-Centre Ville +9
Liège, Belgium

Ian R. Reid MD, FRACP
Professor of Medicine
Faculty of Medical and Health Sciences
University of Auckland
Auckland, New Zealand

Clifford J. Rosen MD
Director, Maine Center for Osteoporosis
Research and Education
St Joseph Hospital
Bangor, Maine
USA

MaryFran Sowers PhD
Professor of Epidemiology
University of Michigan
Ann Arbor, Michigan
USA

David J. Torgerson PhD
Director, York Trials Unit
Department of Health Sciences
University of York
Heslington
York, UK

Natasja M. van Schoor PhD
EMGO Institute
VU University Medical Center
Amsterdam, The Netherlands

Tricia K. W. Woo MD, MSc, FRCPC
Assistant Professor
Department of Medicine
St Peter's Hospital – McMaster University
Hamilton, Ontario
Canada

Osteoporosis is a disease whose time has come. It is estimated that around one in two women and one in five men are at risk of developing an osteoporotic fracture throughout their lifetimes and enormous strides have been made in our understanding of the causation, pathophysiology, diagnosis, prevention and treatment of this disorder. This volume brings together updated reviews addressing these issues and provides an anthology on the subject which will be of great value to clinicians, policy makers and scientists alike.

Key sections address innovations in risk assessment, the use of bone densitometry and biochemical markers; osteoporosis in men and among patients on glucocorticoids; as well as advances in pharmacotherapy such as PTH analogues and strontium. It is to be hoped that translation of these research findings into coherent preventive and therapeutic strategies will lead to a reduction in the morbidity, mortality and economic costs of this common chronic age-related disorder.

Anthony D. Woolf
Cyrus Cooper
January 2006

Chapter 1
Epidemiology of osteoporosis

Kelsey M. Jordan and Cyrus Cooper

DEFINITION OF OSTEOPOROSIS

Osteoporosis has been defined by a Consensus Development Conference as 'a systemic skeletal disorder characterized by low bone mass and microarchitectural deterioration of bone tissue, with a consequent increase in bone fragility and susceptibility to fracture'.[1] Historically, involutional bone loss was recognized 150 years ago by Sir Astley Cooper, who observed its association with hip fracture. The term 'osteoporosis', however, was first used in medical circles in the nineteenth century by German and French physicians when describing the histological appearance of osteoporotic bone.

Clinically, osteoporosis is recognized by the occurrence of characteristic low trauma fractures, so that any meaningful definition of osteoporosis must account for the risk of fracture. Using fracture as a diagnostic criterion is advantageous, as it is a discrete event that can easily be formulated into a diagnostic algorithm. The obvious disadvantage is that diagnosis will be delayed in a disorder, where prevention is an important end goal. This reasoning has led to the use of bone mineral densitometry as a means of defining osteoporosis and as a tool to non-invasively assess bone mass in an attempt to predict fracture. Low bone mineral density (BMD) is one of the strongest risk factors for fracture and is, in this context, analogous to high blood pressure or an elevated serum cholesterol. The risk of fracture increases as bone mass falls, just as the risk of stroke increases with rising blood pressure.

BONE DENSITY AND FRACTURE

There is a well-established relationship between bone mineral density (BMD) and the ability of bone to withstand trauma, such that 75–90% of the variance in bone strength is related to BMD.[2] Other factors, including bone geometry, microarchitecture and size, also influence bone strength. Dual X-ray absorptiometry (DXA) provides a safe, convenient means to measure BMD accurately, reproducibly and with minimal radiation exposure. Using this technique, studies have shown that BMD has a normal population distribution in subjects of all ages and in both sexes. Fracture risk increases 1.5–3-fold for each standard deviation fall in BMD.[3] Thus, a woman at the age of menopause whose hip BMD is 1 standard deviation below average will have a 30% greater remaining lifetime risk of fracture.

The World Health Organization has proposed that both BMD and fracture be combined in a stratified definition of osteoporosis.[4] Four categories were recommended:

- Normal – a value for BMD that is not more than 1 SD below the young adult mean value.
- Osteopoenia – a value for BMD that lies between 1 and 2.5 SD below the young adult mean value.
- Osteoporosis – a value for BMD that is more than 2.5 SD below the young adult mean value.
- Severe (or established) osteoporosis – a value for BMD more than 2.5 SD below the young adult mean value in the presence of one or more fragility fractures.

There is an appreciable overlap in the BMD distribution of normal and fracture populations. Thus, in the case of vertebral fracture, a lumbar spine BMD that is 2 standard deviations below the young adult mean has sensitivity and specificity for fracture of only around 60%.[5] Likewise, a 50-year-old woman with a radial BMD equal to that of the young adult mean has a 15% lifetime risk of hip fracture compared with a 25% lifetime risk for a woman of the same age whose BMD falls 2.5 standard deviations below the young adult mean.[6] This means that the criteria we use are useful in population-based measurements but less useful in assessing individual risk.

PRACTICE POINTS

- BMD is a good tool to help stratify those at risk of osteoporosis.
- Lifetime risk of fracture increases with a fall in BMD substantially.

INCIDENCE, PREVALENCE AND GEOGRAPHIC VARIATION IN OSTEOPOROTIC FRACTURE

Fracture incidence in the community is bimodal, with peaks in youth and in the elderly. In youth, fractures of the long bones predominate; these usually follow substantial trauma and the incidence is greater in young men than in young women. Above the age of 35 years, overall fracture incidence rises steeply in women so that female rates become twice those of men.

With advancing age a greater proportion of women will have a low bone mass. In a population-based estimate in Rochester, Minnesota, it was estimated that by age 80 years, 27% of women are osteopoenic and 70% are osteoporotic at the hip, lumbar spine or distal forearm (Table 1.1). Further, it has been estimated that, in the USA, 16.8 million (54%) post-menopausal white women are osteopoenic and 9.4 million (30%) are osteoporotic.[7]

From the perspective of fracture, it is estimated that around 40% of all US white women and 13% of US white men aged 50 years will experience at least one clinically apparent fragility fracture in their lifetime.[7] The Markov model on which these estimates are based predicts that 35% of women will have a vertebral fracture, 18% a hip fracture and 17% a Colles fracture.[8] Hip fracture will be recurrent in 14% of women and 25% will have multiple vertebral fractures. Taking into account sites other than the hip, spine and distal forearm, the lifetime risk of fracture in women over 50 years may be as high as 70%. Figure 1.1 demonstrates the incidence of hip, non-vertebral and wrist fractures by age in women and men. A recent study looked at the 10-year risk of osteoporotic fracture according to age, sex and relative risk. It was noted that screening women in order that intervention can be directed to them, at the age of 65 years and targeting 25% of the population, could save up to 23% of all fractures in these women over the following 10-year period.[9]

Fracture rates are higher in the United States and Scandinavia than in Britain and Central Europe. Estimates for the British population are about 20% lower.

Table 1.1. Proportion of Rochester, Minnesota women with BMD more than 2.5 standard deviations below the mean for young normal women.

Age group (years)	Proportion by site (%)			
	Lumbar spine	Either hip	Mid-radius	Spine, hip or mid-radius
50–59	7.6	3.9	3.7	14.8
60–69	11.8	8.0	11.8	21.6
70–79	25.0	24.5	23.1	38.5
≥80	32.0	47.5	50.0	70.0
Total	16.5	16.2	17.4	30.3

Reproduced with permission from Melton LJ III. *J Bone Miner Res* 1995; **10**: 175–177.[7]

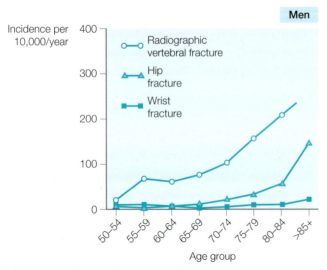
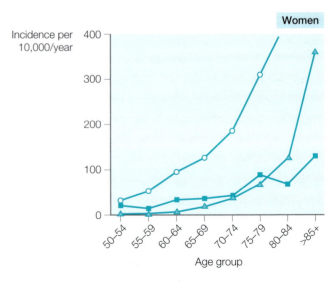

Figure 1.1. Incidence of osteoporotic fractures.

Hip fracture

Hip fracture is the most serious consequence of osteoporosis. It is most closely linked to bone mineral density as compared with other types of fracture. Costs associated with hip fracture are high and there is more disability than with any other type of osteoporotic fracture. Hip fracture rates increase exponentially with age in both sexes with rates of 2 per 100,000 person-years in women aged less than 35 years up to 3032 per 100,000 person-years in women aged 85 years and older; in men the rates are 4 and 1909 respectively.[10] In a UK-based study, hip fracture rates derived from the General Practice Research Database during the period 1988–1998 were 17 per 10,000 person-years for women and 5.3 per 10,000 person years in men[11] (Table 1.2). Approximately half as many fractures are seen in men in the elderly age groups in most studies. This is due to a combination of women losing more bone as they age and a tendency to fall more often. Women also live longer than men and therefore hip fractures are more commonly seen. Nearly three-quarters of all hip fractures occur in women. The lifetime risk of a hip fracture from age 50 years onwards has been estimated at 17% for white women as compared with only 6% for white men in the USA.[12]

There is a marked geographic and ethnic variation in the incidence of hip fracture worldwide.

Age-adjusted incidence rates are higher among white women in Scandinavia than in women of comparable age in North America or Oceania.[13] Similar variation is seen in the USA, higher rates being seen in the south-east as compared with the north or west of the USA.[14] In the USA, the age-adjusted rate in white women increases with decreasing latitude, socio-economic deprivation, decreased January sunlight, decreasing water hardness, the proportion of the population drinking fluoridated water and the percentage of land in agricultural use. Regional variation did not correspond with obesity, cigarette smoking, alcohol consumption or Scandinavian heritage.[15]

Fracture rates are lower in Asian and Black populations.[16] This variation cannot be explained by race-specific variation in bone density.[17] The number of hip fractures seen in Asian populations is rising; it has been estimated that by the year 2050 more than half of all hip fractures worldwide will occur in Asia.[18] The projected number worldwide will be 6.3 million, with 3.2 million in Asia.

There are several populations, including the Maoris in New Zealand[19] and the Bantus in South Africa,[20] in which the incidence of fracture in men is equal to or greater than that seen in women. The explanation for this is unknown, but neither population exhibits the dramatic rise in age seen in the West.

Table 1.2. Estimated risks of fractures at various ages.

	Current age (years)	Any fractures (%)	Radius/ulna (%)	Femur/hip (%)	Vertebra (%)
Lifetime risk					
Women	50	53.2	16.6	11.4	3.1
	60	45.5	14.0	11.6	2.9
	70	36.9	10.4	12.1	2.6
	80	28.6	6.9	12.3	1.9
Men	50	20.7	2.9	3.1	1.2
	60	14.7	2.0	3.1	1.1
	70	11.4	1.4	3.3	1.0
	80	9.6	1.1	3.7	0.8
10-year risk					
Women	50	9.8	3.2	0.3	0.3
	60	13.3	4.9	1.1	0.6
	70	17.0	5.6	3.4	1.3
	80	21.7	5.5	8.7	1.6
Men	50	7.1	1.1	0.2	0.2
	60	5.7	0.9	0.4	0.3
	70	6.2	0.9	1.4	0.5
	80	8.0	0.9	2.9	0.7

Source: Van Staa TP et al. *Bone* 2001; **29**: 517–522.[11]

Table 1.3. Observed and expected survival (%) following a fracture among men and women aged ≥65 years.

	Radius/ulna		Femur/hip		Vertebra	
	Observed	Expected	Observed	Expected	Observed	Expected
Women						
3 months	98.2	98.6	85.6	97.7	94.3	98.4
12 months	94.0	94.4	74.9	91.1	86.5	93.6
5 years	75.5	73.8	41.7	60.9	56.5	69.6
Men						
3 months	97.3	98.0	77.7	97.3	87.8	97.9
12 months	89.6	92.4	63.3	90.0	74.3	91.8
5 years	62.8	66.4	32.2	58.2	42.1	64.4

Source: Van Staa TP et al. *Bone* 2001; **29**: 517–522.[11]

Hip fracture is associated with a high increase in both morbidity and mortality. Five-year survival post-hip fracture is 82% of that expected, with most of the deaths occurring within the first 6 months post-fracture.[21]

Vertebral fracture

Compared with hip fracture, the epidemiology of vertebral fracture is less well characterized. This is predominantly due to the lack of universally accepted diagnostic criteria of what defines an osteoporotic vertebral fracture. Also, substantial proportions of vertebral fractures are asymptomatic and therefore escape clinical detection. The development of definitions based on vertebral morphometry with fixed cut-off values, which have increased specificity, have allowed for more reliable work in the field.[22] The association between pain and morphometric deformity is stronger when using more rigorous criteria for diagnosis (a reduction in ratio of 4 standard deviations), with 80% of these cases seeking medical attention. Severe vertebral deformities have a predilection for the thoracolumbar junction (T10–L1), whereas milder deformities are seen more uniformly throughout the rest of the thoracolumbar spine. It is estimated that only one-third of vertebral fractures come to clinical attention,[23] with less than 10% necessitating admission to hospital.

The incidence of vertebral fracture increases with age in both sexes. Most studies indicate that the prevalence of vertebral fracture in men is similar to or even greater than those seen in women to age 50 or 60 years.[24,25] The age-adjusted prevalence rate of radiological fracture has been estimated at between 8% and 25% in women over 50 years, depending on the definition used.[24,26,27]

Prevalence of vertebral fracture has been more similar across regions than that seen for hip fracture. Vertebral fracture is as frequent in Asian as white women.[28,29] Vertebral fracture also appears to be less common in African-American[30] and Hispanic[31] populations.

A history of vertebral fracture, even an asymptomatic fracture, increases the likelihood of further fracture by at least four-fold.[32] This is independent of bone density, so that vertebral fractures that arise with minimum trauma signal an underlying bone fragility that is not measured by bone densitometry. Such fractures are regarded as clinical evidence for the diagnosis of osteoporosis.

Vertebral fractures are associated with a similar increase in mortality at 5 years as seen with hip fracture (Table 1.3). This increase, however, is gradual over the 5-year period, unlike hip fracture, where it is highest in the first 6 months following fracture.[21]

Distal forearm fracture

Wrist fractures are the most common fractures sustained in perimenopausal women.[11] More wrist fractures occur outdoors when compared with other fractures and a winter peak in incidence is seen,[33] particularly in icy weather.

There is a greater female preponderance with an age-adjusted women:men ratio of 4:1, with 85% of fractures occurring in women.[34] The incidence in men is relatively constant between 20 and 80 years of age,[13] in contrast to women, where there is a rapid rise after the menopause, which plateaus around age 65 years. The reason for the plateau may be due to age-related decreases in the speed and strength of extending the arm to protect other parts of the body during falls, and also the cessation of the rapid trabecular bone loss that occurs following the menopause.

The geographical variation tends to mimic that seen in hip fracture. There is some evidence to suggest that distal forearm fracture is much less frequent in Asian[35] and Black[36] populations when compared to Caucasians.

There is no excess mortality in patients who sustain a distal forearm fracture.[21] There is, however, data suggesting that although less than 1% of patients become dependent as a result of this type of fracture, only 50% of subjects report a good functional outcome at 6 months.[37]

Other fractures

Most other sorts of fractures have also been associated with low bone density. These include the proximal humerus, pelvis, proximal tibia and distal femur. These fractures increase with age in elderly women and also to a lesser extent in elderly men.[13]

PRACTICE POINTS

- Hip and vertebral fracture are associated with an increased mortality (Table 1.3).
- There are regional and geographic variations in fracture incidence and prevalence.
- Different osteoporotic fractures occur at different ages.

RISK FACTORS FOR OSTEOPOROSIS

Detailed understanding of the risk factors for osteoporosis are important for several reasons:

1. They may help us understand the pathophysiology of the disorder.
2. They contribute to the clinical treatment of individual patients.
3. They may help in the design of preventative strategies against fracture.

Risk factors for osteoporotic fracture can be grouped into different categories: those that influence the risk of falling and the responses to trauma; those that influence the accretion and loss of bone mineral density throughout the life course; and influences on skeletal strength independent of bone mineral density. Table 1.4 summarizes the risk factors for osteoporosis and fracture.

Table 1.4. Risk factors for osteoporosis and fracture.

Age

Female sex

Body mass index

Maternal family history of hip fracture

Prior fragility fractures

Low bone mineral density

Low birth weight

Genetic factors

Sex hormones
   Premature menopause
   Primary or secondary amenorrhoea
   Primary and secondary hypogonadism in men

Disease states
   Thyrotoxicosis, Cushing's disease, hyperparathyroidism
   Stroke
   Inflammatory arthritides

Drugs
   Corticosteroids
   Anticonvulsants
   Heparin

Smoking

Alcohol

Dietary calcium and vitamin D deficiency

Intrauterine and early postnatal programming

There is now good evidence to support the hypothesis that the growth trajectory may be programmed in utero or during very early postnatal life, and that environmental factors at this stage in development may influence peak bone mass and later bone loss, and thus the later risk of osteoporosis. Programming is the term used to describe persisting changes in structure and function caused by environmental stimuli during critical periods of early development.[38] The embryo does not contain a description of the person to whom it will give rise; rather, it contains in its genes a generative programme for making a person.[39] Different tissues of the body grow during different periods of rapid cell division, so-called critical periods. Brief periods of undernutrition during intrauterine life can permanently reduce the numbers of cells in particular organs. This is one of the mechanisms by which undernutrition may permanently programme the body. It is not in question that the human body can be programmed by undernutrition; rickets serves as a demonstration that undernutrition at a critical stage of early life leads to persisting changes in structure.

Studies in both Britain and Sweden have provided evidence that weight in infancy is a determinant of bone mass in adulthood. In one study, 153 women born in Bath were followed up at age 21 years.[40] There was a statistically significant relationship between weight at 1 year and bone mineral content at 21 years; the relationship was independent of BMI, diet and lifestyle. Similar findings were seen in a Swedish cohort of boys and girls aged 15 years.[41] These relationships were seen to persist into later life, as demonstrated by a study of 189 women and 224 men aged 63–73 years born in Hertfordshire. Bone mineral density at the hip and spine showed a 12–15% difference between those in the lowest third of the distribution for weight at 1 year compared with those in the highest third.[42] Again, these results remained after adjusting for lifestyle and dietary risk factors.

Further evidence for osteoporosis programming can be demonstrated by a study of 144 neonates whose mothers had their characteristics assessed at 18 and 28 weeks gestation. Neonatal bone mineral content was positively correlated with birth weight, birth length and placental weight. Maternal smoking and maternal physical activity were, however, negatively associated. This implies that maternal nutrition can modify foetal nutrient supply and subsequent bone accretion. If these effects are maintained through adolescence to the attainment of peak bone mass, they will have far-reaching consequences in terms of future fracture risk.

Genetic factors

There also appear to be genetic influences on bone density and fracture. Family studies have shown clustering of low spine BMD among first-degree relatives of osteoporotic parents and among the daughters of osteoporotic mothers.[43] A family history of osteoporotic fracture predicts low bone mass in men and women,[44] and is an independent predictor of fracture at the same site (relative risk 1.5–3.0).[45] This relationship appears strongest for a maternal history of hip fracture.

Twin studies have suggested that around 50% of the variance in BMD might be genetic[46] and current data suggest that several genes are involved, each with a relatively modest effect. Candidates include the vitamin D receptor gene[47] and the collagen type I alpha-1 (COLIA1) gene.[48] Others are being investigated.

Sex hormones

An acceleration in bone loss is well recognized in post-menopausal women, particularly during the first decade after cessation of ovarian function. Women who undergo premature menopause before the age of 45 years are at the highest risk of low bone mass and fracture. Conversely, a greater number of fertile years from menarche to menopause is associated with a reduced risk of fracture. In the EVOS study, late menarche correlated with increased risk of vertebral deformity, whilst late menopause, hormone replacement therapy and the oral contraceptive pill were found to be protective.[49]

Low bone density is also a feature seen in men with primary hypogonadism. Causes of secondary amenorrhoea – for instance, chronic disease, anorexia or excessive exercise – can also result in an increased risk of osteoporosis.

Diseases

Cases of secondary osteoporosis include thyrotoxicosis, Cushing's disease, hyperparathyroidism and male hypogonadism, as well as stroke and the inflammatory arthritides.

Drug therapy

Chronic utilization of corticosteroids, heparin and anticonvulsants result in accelerated bone loss. Thiazide diuretics may have a protective effect.

Smoking

Smoking is well defined as a risk factor for osteoporosis. There is an inverse relationship with bone mineral density. A meta-analysis concluded that although there was no demonstrable difference in bone density between the smoker and non-smoker at age 50 years, there was a subsequent loss of 2% in bone mass at every 10-year interval for the smoker. By age 80 years, there was a 6% difference between the two groups.[50] There is an independent effect of smoking on the risk of hip fracture.

Alcohol

Studies amongst alcohol misusers have shown that they have lower bone mass and also a greater rate of bone loss. Alcohol has a direct toxic effect on osteoblast activity, and is associated with a lower body mass index, chronic liver disease, smoking and poor nutrition. Falls are also more common in this group of patients.

In moderation, however, alcohol may have a protective effect on bone.[51]

Physical activity

Bone adapts according to the physical load and stresses exerted upon it. Physical activity during the first three decades of life may increase peak bone mass and reduce future osteoporotic fractures. A review of physical activity and hip fracture showed a strong association with physical activity in leisure and a weaker association with respect to activity at work. The association was present from childhood to adult age and consistent across geographical regions, USA, Asia, Australia and Europe. It was estimated that to be physically active reduced the risk of later hip fracture by up to 50%. It was noted that even daily chores, such as climbing stairs, were also protective.[52]

Dietary calcium and vitamin D

Good dietary intake of calcium in childhood results in enhanced bone mineral density in young women. Vitamin D levels are well known to correlate directly with bone mineral density. Low levels of circulating vitamin D are prevalent in elderly populations.

Weight

Low body weight is negatively correlated with peak bone mass. Low body mass index and weight are also strongly correlated with fracture risk as compared with higher adiposity, which is protective against the risk of both hip and vertebral fractures.

Falls

Falls increase the likelihood of fracture. Risk factors for this include poor eyesight, a previous history of falls and gait or balance problems.

PRACTICE POINTS

- There are multifactorial risk factors involved in increasing the risk of osteoporosis.
- Many risk factors can easily be targeted in childhood and early adulthood to reduce the risk of future fracture.

SUMMARY

Osteoporosis is becoming an escalating problem worldwide due to an increase in life expectancy and therefore in the ageing population. It therefore constitutes a huge burden in terms of morbidity, mortality and cost. The total cost of osteoporotic fractures to the UK healthcare system is in the region of £17 billion per annum. Fortunately, osteoporosis is a preventable disease with well-recognized risk factors. An understanding of the epidemiology of osteoporotic fracture can help identify those at greatest risk, and permit appropriate targeting of treatment for prevention of fracture.

RESEARCH AGENDA

- Further studies aimed at delineating the important risk factors in prediction of fracture and bone mineral density.
- Further epidemiological studies in non-white populations.
- Studies on the most cost-effective means of targeting at-risk populations who may have asymptomatic fractures.

REFERENCES

1. Consensus Development Conference. Diagnosis, prophylaxis and treatment of osteoporosis. *Am J Med* 1993; **94**: 646–650.

2. Lauritzen JB. Hip fractures: incidence, risk factors, energy absorption and prevention. *Bone* 1996; **18**: S65–75.

3. Marshall D, Johnell O & Wedel H. Meta-analysis of how well measures of bone density predicts occurrence of osteoporotic fractures. *BMJ* 1996; **312**: 1254–1259.

4. World Health Organization. Assessment of fracture risk and its application to screening for postmenopausal women. *WHO Technical Report Series 843*. Geneva: WHO, 1994.

5. Overgaard K, Hansen MA, Riis BJ et al. Discriminatory ability of bone mass measurements (SPA and DEXA) for fractures in elderly postmenopausal women. *Calcif Tissue Int* 1992; **50**: 30–35.

6. Suman V, Atkinson EJ, O'Fallon WM et al. A nonogram for predicting lifetime hip fracture risk from radius bone mineral density and age. *Bone* 1993; **14**: 834–846.

7. Melton LJ III. How many women have osteoporosis now? *J Bone Miner Res* 1995; **10**: 175–177.

8. Chrischilles EA, Butler CD, Davis CS et al. A model of lifetime osteoporosis impact. *Arch Intern Med* 1991; **151**: 1005–1010.

9. Kanis JA, Johnell O, Oden A et al. Ten-year risk of osteoporotic fracture and the effect of risk factors on screening strategies. *Bone* 2002; **30**: 251–258.

10. Cooper C, Melton LJ III. Epidemiology of osteoporosis. *Trends Endocrinol Metab* 1992; **314**: 224–229.

11. Van Staa TP, Dennison EM, Leufkens HGM et al. Epidemiology of fractures in England and Wales. *Bone* 2001; **29**: 517–522.

12. Melton LJ III. Who has osteoporosis? A conflict between clinical and public health perspectives. *J Bone Miner Res* 2000; **15**: 2309–2314.

13. Melton LJ III & Cooper C. Magnitude and impact of osteoporosis and fracture. In: Marcus R, Feldman D & Kelsey J, eds. *Osteoporosis*, 2nd edn, Vol. 1. San Diego: Academic Press, 2001; 557–567.

14. Jacobsen SJ, Goldberg J, Miles TP et al. Regional variation in the incidence of hip fracture: US white women aged 65 years or older. *JAMA* 1990; **264**: 500–502.

15. Melton LJ III. Epidemiology of age related fracture. In: Avion LV, ed. *The Osteoporosis Syndrome: Detection, Prevention and Treatment*. New York: Wiley-Liss, 1993; 17–18.

16. Melton LJ III. Differing patterns of osteoporosis around the world. In: Chestnut CH III, ed. *New Dimensions in Osteoporosis in the 1990s, Asia Pacific Conference Series No. 125*. Hong Kong: Excerpta Medica, 1991; 13–18.

17. Marquez MA, Melton LJ III, Muhs JM et al. Bone density in an immigrant population from Southeast Asia. *Osteoporosis Int* 2001; **12**: 595–604.

18. Cooper C, Campion G & Melton LJ III. Hip fracture in the elderly: a worldwide projection. *Osteoporosis Int* 1992; **2**: 285–289.

19. Stott S & Gray DH. The incidence of femoral neck fracture in New Zealand. *NZ Med J* 1980; **91**: 6–9.

20. Solomon L. Osteoporosis and fracture of the femoral neck in the South African Bantu. *J Bone Joint Surg (Br)* 1968; **50B**: 2–13.

21. Cooper C, Atkinson EJ, Jacobsen SJ et al. Population-based study of survival following osteoporotic fracture. *Am J Epidemiol* 1993; **137**: 1001–1005.

22. McCloskey EV, Spector TD, Eyres KS et al. The assessment of vertebral deformity: A method for use in population studies and clinical trials. *Osteoporosis Int* 1993; **3**: 138–147.

23. Cooper C, Atkinson EJ, O'Fallon WM et al. Incidence of clinically diagnosed vertebral fractures: a population-based study in Rochester, Minnesota, 1985–1989. *J Bone Miner Res* 1992; **7**: 221–227.

24. O'Neill TW, Felsenberg D, Varlow J et al. The prevalence of vertebral deformity in European men and women: the European Vertebral Osteoporosis Study. *J Bone Miner Res* 1996; **11**: 1010–1018.

25. Davies KM, Stegman MR, Heaney RP et al. Prevalence and severity of vertebral fracture: the Saunders County Bone Study. *Osteoporosis Int* 1996; **6**: 160–165.

26. Spector TD, McCloskey EV, Doyle DV et al. Prevalence of vertebral fracture in women and the relationship with bone density and symptoms: The Chingford Study. *J Bone Miner Res* 1993; **7**: 817–822.

27. Melton LJ III, Lane AW, Cooper C et al. Prevalence and increase of vertebral deformities. *Osteoporosis Int* 1993; **3**: 113–119.

28. Ross PD, Fujiwara S, Huang C et al. Vertebral fracture prevalence in Hiroshima compared with Caucasians or Japanese in the US. *Int J Epidemiol* 1995; **24**: 1171–1177.

29. Lau EMC, Chan HHL, Woo J et al. Normal ranges for vertebral height and prevalence of vertebral fracture in Hong Kong Chinese: a comparison with American Caucasians. *J Bone Miner Res* 1996; **11**: 1364–1368.

30. Jacobsen SJ, Cooper C, Gottlieb MS et al. Hospitalisation with vertebral fracture among the aged: a national population-based study, 1986–1989. *Epidemiology* 1992; **3**: 515–518.

31. Bauer RL & Deyo RA. Low risk of vertebral fracture in Mexican American women. *Arch Intern Med* 1987; **147**: 1437–1439.

32. The European Prospective Osteoporosis Study Group. Incidence of vertebral fractures in Europe: results from the European prospective osteoporosis study (EPOS). *J Bone Miner Res* 2002; **17**: 716–724.

33. Jacobsen SJ, Sargent DJ, Atkinson EJ et al. Contribution of weather to the seasonality of distal forearm fractures: a population based study in Rochester, Minnesota. *Osteoporosis Int* 1999; **9**: 254–259.

34. Owen RA, Melton LJ III, Johnson KA et al. Incidence of Colles' fractures in a North American community. *Am J Public Health* 1982; **72**: 605–607.

35. Hagiro H, Yamamoto K, Teshima R et al. The incidence of fracture of the proximal femur and the distal radius in Tottori prefecture, Japan. *Arch Orthop Trauma Surg* 1989; **109**: 43–44.

36. Griffin MR, Ray WA, Fought RL et al. Black–white difference in fracture rates. *Am J Epidemiol* 1992; **136**: 1378–1385.

37. Kaukonen JP, Karaharju EO, Porras M et al. Functional recovery after fractures of the distal forearm. *Ann Chir Gynaecol* 1988; **77**: 27–31.

38. Barker DJP. Programming the baby. In: Barker DJP, ed. *Mothers, Babies and Disease in Later Life*. London: BMJ, 1994; 14–36.

39. Barker DJP. The Wellcome Foundation Lecture, 1994. The fetal origins of adult disease. *Proc R Soc Lond Ser B, Biol Sci* 1995; **262**: 37–43.

40. Cooper C, Cawley MID, Bhalla A et al. Childhood growth, physical activity and peak bone mass in women. *J Bone Miner Res* 1995; **10**: 940–947.

41. Duppe H, Cooper C, Gardsell P et al. The relationship between childhood growth, bone mass and muscle strength in male and female adolescents. *Calcif Tissue Int* 1997; **60**: 405–409.

42. Cooper C, Fall C, Egger P et al. Growth in infancy and bone mass in later life. *Ann Rheum Dis* 1997; **56**: 17–21.

43. Seeman E, Hopper JL, Bach LA et al. Reduced bone mass in daughters of women with osteoporosis. *N Engl J Med* 1989; **320**: 554–558.

44. Kelly PJ, Eisman JA & Sandbrook PN. Interaction of genetic and environmental influences on peak bone density. *Osteoporosis Int* 1990; **1**: 56–60.

45. Fox KM, Cummings SR & Threets K. Family history and risk of osteoporotic fracture. *J Bone Miner Res* 1994; **9**(Suppl. 1): S153.

46. Slemenda CW, Christian JC, Williams CJ et al. Genetic determinants of bone mass in adult women: a re-evaluation of the twin model and the potential importance of gene interaction on heritability estimates. *J Bone Miner Res* 1991; **6**: 561–567.

47. Morrison NA, Yeoman R, Kelly PJ et al. Contribution of trans-acting factor alleles to normal physiological variability: Vitamin D receptor gene polymorphisms and circulating osteocalcin. *Proc Natl Acad Sci USA* 1992; **89**: 6665–6669.

48. Uitterlinden AG, Burger H, Huang Q et al. Relation of alleles of the collagen type I alpha1 gene to bone density and the risk of osteoporotic fractures in postmenopausal women. *N Engl J Med* 1998; **338**: 1016–1021.

49. O'Neill TW, Silman AJ, Naves-Diaz M et al. Influence of hormonal and reproductive factors on the risk of vertebral deformity in European women. European Vertebral Osteoporosis Group. *Osteoporosis Int* 1997; **7**: 72–78.

50. Law MR & Hackshaw AK. A meta-analysis of cigarette smoking, bone mineral density, and risk of hip fracture: recognition of a major effect. *BMJ* 1997; **315**: 841–846.

51. Seeman E. The effects of tobacco and alcohol use on bone. In: Marcus R, Feldman D & Kelsey J, eds. *Osteoporosis*. San Diego: Academic Press, 1996; 577–597.

52. Joakimsen RM, Magnus JH & Fonnebo V. Physical activity and predisposition for hip fractures: a review. *Osteoporosis Int* 1997; **7**: 503–513.

Chapter 2

Fractures in the elderly: epidemiology and demography

Edith M. C. Lau, Huibert A. P. Pols and Chris E. D. H. De Laet

INTRODUCTION

Osteoporosis can be defined as a 'systematic skeletal disease characterized by low bone mass, and microarchitectural deterioration of bony tissue, with a consequent increase in bone fragility and susceptibility to fractures'.[1] As fragility fractures are the main health consequence of osteoporosis, an understanding of their epidemiology is vital in the development of clinical and public health policy for osteoporosis.

FRACTURE EPIDEMIOLOGY

There is no universal definition of osteoporotic fractures. It seems logical to consider low-energy fractures as being osteoporotic, for osteoporotic individuals are more likely to fracture than their normal counterparts.[2] By this definition, fractures of the hip, vertebra and forearm can be considered to be osteoporotic fractures. They share common epidemiological features: the incidences are higher in women than in men, increase exponentially with age and occur at sites with a large proportion of trabecular bone.[3]

Hip fracture
Geographical pattern

There is pronounced geographical variation in the incidence of hip fracture, with rates being highest in Caucasians living in North Europe, followed by Caucasians living in North America. The rates are intermediate in urbanized parts of Asia (Hong Kong) and low in mainland China and Turkey[4] (Figures 2.1 and 2.2).

The incidence of hip fracture also varies between subjects of the same origin, but living in different parts of the same continents. In Europe, the incidences of hip fracture vary more than seven-fold from one country to another.[5] The incidence in Sweden is highest, the relative incidence compared with that of the USA being 1.3 in women and 1.7 in men.[6] In Finland, the rate is comparable to that of the USA for women but slightly

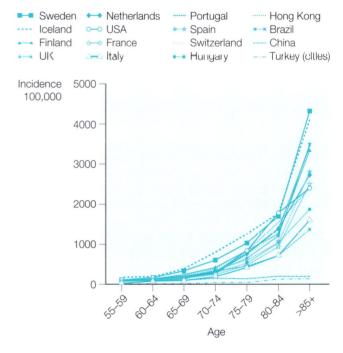

Figure 2.1. One-year cumulative incidence of hip fracture in women per 100,000 in several countries.

higher in men. In the UK, the Netherlands and Germany, the incidence is very similar to that observed in the USA. For southern European countries, the incidence is much lower, that in France, Greece and Spain being about 70% of that in the USA, while in Italy and Portugal the incidence is as low as 50% of that in the USA.

There is some evidence that the incidence of hip fracture is raising rapidly in developing Asian countries. For instance, in Hong Kong, a highly urbanized city in China, the incidence of hip fracture has increased by 200% in the last three decades.[7] A recent multinational study conducted in four Asian countries

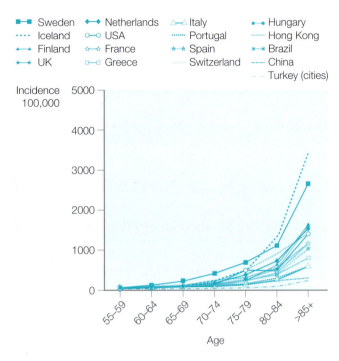

Sweden · **Netherlands** · Italy · Hungary
Iceland · USA · Portugal · Hong Kong
Finland · France · Spain · Brazil
UK · Greece · Switzerland · China
Turkey (cities)

Figure 2.2. One-year cumulative incidence of hip fracture in men per 100,000 in several countries.

showed the incidence of hip fracture to be directly proportional to economic development. The adjusted rates in Hong Kong and Singapore were almost identical to American Caucasians (at 19 per 10,000), while the rates in Thailand and Malaysia were two-thirds and one-half of the Hong Kong rate respectively.[8] With rapid economic development and ageing of the population, hip fracture will be a major health problem in Asia.

Indeed, Cooper et al.[9] had projected that, by the year 2050, more than half of all hip fractures in the world would occur in Asia. The projected number of fractures will be 6.3 million, with 3.2 million in Asia.

The variation in the incidence of hip fracture between countries applies to both women and men. In both Europe[4] and Asia,[8] countries with high incidence of hip fracture in women also display high incidence in men.

Secular trends

Recent research has suggested that the incidence of hip fracture has experienced either a levelling off or a slight downturn in North America and Europe. In Malmö, Sweden, Gullberg et al.[10] described a levelling off of hip fracture incidence during the mid 1980s. Nungu et al.[11] reported that the age-adjusted incidence of hip fracture remained at around 6/1000 population in Uppsala, Sweden in the same period.

In the Canton of Vaud, Switzerland, Jéquier et al.[12] found a slight increase in hip fracture incidence in Swiss men, but not in women, from 1986 to 1991. In Siena, Italy, the incidence of hip fracture increased slightly in men, but not in women, from 1980 to 1991.[13]

The time trends for hip fracture in the UK from 1968 to 1986 were studied by Spector et al.[14] using data from the Hospital Inpatient Enquiry. The standardized admission rates for hip fracture increased tremendously from 1968 to 1980 in both sexes, after which the rates levelled off. A more recent study by Evans et al.[15] confirmed these results.

Similar trends have been observed in North America. Melton et al. reported a downturn in hip fracture incidence in Rochester, Minnesota, between 1984 and 1987.[16] It is not known if such changes are due to health education, lifestyle changes or cohort effects. Assuming no increase in hip fracture incidence, the number of hip fracture patients will continue to rise in all continents, as a result of population ageing.

Gender ratio

The global female-to-male ratio for the absolute number of hip fractures is around 3.5:1 in most countries, but this high female-to-male ratio is largely due to demography. When the incidence rates are compared, the female-to-male ratio is between 1.6:1 and 2:1 in most Western countries. Only in Sweden and Finland have lower ratios (1.3:1 and 1.4:1 respectively) been reported. The Turkish data were again strikingly different, with a female-to-male ratio of about 1:1 in Istanbul and Ankara, and a reversal of the ratio (around 0.4) in rural areas, especially in older participants. A reversal of the female-to-male ratio has also been observed in China (Beijing).

The reason for both the huge geographical variation in hip fracture incidence and the reversal of the gender ratio in some countries is largely unknown. It is probably due to a combination of genetic, lifestyle and environmental factors, and is clearly a topic for future research.

Future trends

A consideration of the age structure of populations and estimates of the secular trend permits the size of the problem of hip fracture to be estimated for the future.[9] For example, in 2000, approximately 1.4 million hip fractures occurred worldwide among men and women. As mentioned, this will increase to over 6 million by the year 2050. A more conservative estimate predicted the number of hip fractures to be 2.6 million by 2025.[17]

Vertebral fracture

Epidemiological studies on vertebral fractures are hampered by the lack of universally accepted criteria for the definition of vertebral fracture. Moreover, a substantial proportion of vertebral deformities are clinically silent.

Geographical pattern

According to radiographic studies, 19–26% of post-menopausal women have a vertebral deformity.[18–21] Vertebral fractures are as frequent in Asians as in white women.[22,23] However, vertebral fractures are less common in African-American[24] and Hispanic[25] populations.

The incidence of new vertebral fracture has been estimated to be around three times that of hip fracture, with a female-to-male ratio of 2:1.[26]

Temporal trends

The temporal trends for vertebral fracture are not as well studied as for hip fracture, and the results are mixed. According to Bengnèr et al.,[27] the prevalence of vertebral fracture increased in Sweden between the periods 1950–1952 and 1982–1983.

Nevertheless, the temporal trend was found to be stable in Rochester, USA, from 1950 to 1989.[28]

Distal forearm fracture

The change in incidence with age for distal forearm fracture is different from fractures of the hip and vertebra. Study results from the Mayo clinic suggested that incidence rates increased linearly from age 40 to 65 years and then stabilized.[29] However, in men, the incidence remained relatively constant between 20 and 80 years. The female-to-male ratio for forearm fracture was 4:1. This ratio was much larger than the 2:1 ratio found for vertebral and hip fracture.

The international pattern for forearm fracture is not well delineated. There is some evidence to suggest that forearm fracture is much less frequent in Asian[30] and Black[31] populations than in Caucasians.

SOCIO-ECONOMIC IMPACT OF OSTEOPOROSIS

Mortality

The mortality attributable to osteoporosis results largely from hip fractures. Hip fracture causes a 12–20% reduction in expected survival.[32] Hospital-based studies showed that the mortality rate was higher in men, older patients and in non-white populations.[33] Such observations can be explained by the difference in the prevalence of co-morbidity in population subgroups.[34]

Morbidity and quality of life

Osteoporotic fractures cause varying degrees of morbidity. Colles' fractures have only short-term consequences, while hip fracture causes much disability. Many hip fracture patients become permanently disabled. Up to one-third of hip fracture patients become totally dependent, necessitating institutionalization.[34]

The morbidity caused by vertebral fracture varies with the frequency of fractures. Multiple fractures typically cause the most pain and disability. Ettinger et al.[35,36] demonstrated that vertebral fracture caused significant back pain, disability and height loss in Americans.

The effects of vertebral fracture on back pain and low morale have been consistently demonstrated in Chinese men and women.[37]

COSTS OF OSTEOPOROSIS

Studies in various countries have shown that the costs of osteoporosis are very substantial. Hip fracture is a major cause of hospital admission in the elderly. The acute care cost associated with hip fracture is tremendous in all developed countries. In the USA, the direct cost of hip fractures was around US$13.8 billion in 1995.[38] In the UK, the direct cost of hip fracture was £942 million in 1998.[39] The predicted annual treatment costs in Australia for atraumatic fractures occurring in subjects ≥60 years was A$779 million (or approximately A$44 million per million of population per annum).[40] The majority of direct cost (95%) were incurred by hospitalized patients and related to hospital and rehabilitation costs.[40] In 1996, the acute hospital care cost of hip fracture per annum amounted to 1% of the total hospital budget, or US$17 million, for Hong Kong with a population of 6 million (Lau, unpublished data).

In the USA, the average nursing home care cost for each hip fracture patient was as much as US$3875 in 1995.[38] This approximates to 28% of the total cost for hip fracture. As death due to hip fracture occurs mainly in the elderly, the indirect cost due to reduced productivity is much lower than for other chronic disorders, such as ischaemic heart disease, stroke or breast cancer. However, the direct cost is comparable.

SUMMARY AND RESEARCH AGENDA

The incidence of hip fractures is well documented in most countries, increasing exponentially with age up to about 1% per year for women at age 80 in Western countries. There is, however, a large geographical variation in the incidence of hip fracture, a very low incidence rate being reported in China and Turkey. Nevertheless, there is some evidence that the incidence may be rising in Asian countries. The reason for this variation is largely unknown, and more research is needed in this area.

In most areas of the world, hip fractures occur more frequently in women than in men, the typical female-to-male ratio for the occurrence of hip fracture being between 1.6:1 and 2:1. A large increase in the number of hip fractures worldwide is expected as a result of the ageing of the population. A better understanding of the causes of the geographical difference, as well as of the reversal of the female-to-male ratio in some countries, could help to unravel the aetiological pathways and possibly lead to more effective prevention strategies. Without such intervention, it is expected that over 6 million hip fractures a year will occur by the year 2050, an increase from 1.7 million in 1990.

Information on the occurrence of other fractures is scarcer, and more research worldwide is needed. For vertebral fractures the main problem is that there is no universally accepted definition. Consequently, the reported incidence rates vary greatly, as shown by an overview of four studies. Agreement on a definition of vertebral fracture should be high on the research agenda.

For the other fractures, a modest increase with age is observed and this increase is slightly steeper in women. It is unclear whether all these fractures are related to osteoporosis and therefore whether intervention to prevent osteoporosis would reduce these fractures. As the burden of osteoporotic fractures in the immediate and distant future will rest in Asia, research into the epidemiology, aetiology and prevention of this condition in this continent would be of tremendous importance.

<table>
<tr><td>

PRACTICE POINTS

- There are large geographical variations in the incidence of hip fracture in various countries, with the rates being highest in northern Europe and lowest in rural Asia.

- The global number of hip fractures has been projected to rise exponentially in the future.

- The female-to-male ratio for hip fractures varies from as low as 1:1 in Turkey to 2:1 in Europe and the USA.

- The prevalence of vertebral fractures varies from 19% to 26% in post-menopausal women, and the incidence of new vertebral fractures could be three times that of hip fractures.

</td><td>

RESEARCH AGENDA

- Cohort studies to document the incidence of osteoporotic fractures in Asia and international variations in osteoporotic fractures are required.

- The changes in the epidemiology of osteoporotic fractures should be carefully monitored.

- Intervention studies on how to control the global epidemic of osteoporosis are indicated.

</td></tr>
</table>

REFERENCES

1. Anonymous. Consensus development conference: diagnosis, prophylaxis and treatment of osteoporosis. *Am J Med* 1993; **94**: 646–650.

2. Sanders KM, Pasco JA, Ugoni AM et al. The exclusion of high trauma fractures may underestimate the prevalence of bone fragility fractures in the community. The GEELONG osteoporosis study. *J Bone Miner Res* 1998; **13**: 1337–1342.

3. Melton LJ III. Epidemiology of fractures. In: Riggs BL & Melton LJ III, eds. *Osteoporosis: Etiology, Diagnosis and Management.* New York: Raven Press, 1995; 225–248.

4. De Laet CEDH & Pols HAD. Fracture in the elderly: epidemiology and demography. *Baillière's Clin Endocrinol Metab* 2000; **14**(2): 171–179.

5. Ellfors I, Allander E, Kanis JA et al. The variable incidence of hip fracture in Southern Europe; the MEDOS Study. *Osteoporosis Int* 1994; **4**: 253–263.

6. Johnell O, Gullberg B, Allander E et al. The apparent incidence of hip fracture in Europe: a study of national register sources. MEDOS Study Group. *Osteoporosis Int* 1992; **2**: 298–302.

7. Lau EMC, Cooper C, Fung H et al. Hip fracture in Hong Kong over the last decade – a comparison with Britain. *J Public Health Med* 1999; **21**: 249–250.

8. Lau EMC, Lee JK, Suriwongpaisal P et al. The incidence of hip fracture in five Asian countries – the Asian Osteoporosis Study (AOS). *Osteoporosis Int* 2001; **12**: 239–243.

9. Cooper C, Campion G & Melton LJ III. Hip fractures in the elderly: a worldwide projection. *Osteoporosis Int* 1992; **2**: 285–289.

10. Gullberg B, Duppe H, Nilsson B et al. Incidence of hip fractures in Malmö, Sweden. *Bone* 1993; **14**: S23–S29.

11. Nungu S, Olerud C & Rehnberg L. The incidence of hip fracture in Uppsala Country. *Acta Orthop Scand* 1993; **64**: 75–78.

12. Jéquier V, Burnand B, Vader J-P et al. Hip fracture incidence in the Canton of Vaud, Switzerland, 1986–1991. *Osteoporosis Int* 1995; **5**: 191–195.

13. Agnusdei D, Camporeale A, Gerardi D et al. Trends in the incidence of hip fracture in Siena, Italy, from 1980 to 1991. *Bone* 1993; **14**: S31–S34.

14. Spector TD, Cooper C & Fenton Lewis A. Trends in admission for hip fracture in England and Wales, 1968–85. *BMJ* 1990; **300**: 1173–1174.

15. Evans JG, Seagroatt V & Goldacre MJ. Secular trends in proximal femur fracture, Oxford record linkage study area and England 1968–86. *J Epidemiol Community Health* 1997; **51**: 424–429.

16. Melton LJ III, Atkinson EJ & Madhok R. Downturn in hip fracture incidence. *Public Health Rep* 1996; **111**: 146–150.

17. Gullberg B, Johnell O & Kanis JA. Worldwide projections for hip fracture. *Osteoporosis Int* 1997; **7**: 407–413.

18. Ettinger B, Black DM, Nevitt MC et al. The Study of Osteoporotic Fractures Research Group. Contribution of vertebral deformities to chronic back pain and disability. *J Bone Miner Res* 1992; **7**: 449–456.

19. Melton LJ III, Lane AW, Cooper C et al. Prevalence and incidence of vertebral deformities. *Osteoporosis Int* 1993; **3**: 113–119.

20. Jones G, White C, Nguyen T et al. Prevalent vertebral deformities: relationship to bone mineral density and spinal osteophytosis in elderly men and women. *Osteoporosis Int* 1996; **6**: 233–239.

21. O'Neill TW, Felsenberg D, Varlow J et al. The prevalence of vertebral deformity in European men and women: the European Vertebral Osteoporosis Study. *J Bone Miner Res* 1996; **11**: 1010–1018.

22. Ross PD, Fujiwara S, Huang C et al. Vertebral fracture prevalence in women in Hiroshima compared to Caucasians or Japanese in the US. *Int J Epidemiol* 1995; **24**: 1171–1177.

23. Lau EMC, Chan HHL, Woo J et al. Normal ranges for vertebral height ratios and prevalence of vertebral fracture in Hong Kong Chinese: a comparison with American Caucasians. *J Bone Miner Res* 1996; **11**: 1364–1368.

24. Jacobsen SJ, Cooper C, Gottlieb MS et al. Hospitalization with vertebral fracture among the aged: a national population-based study, 1986–1989. *Epidemiology* 1992; **3**: 515–518.

25. Bauer RL & Deyo RA. Low risk of vertebral fracture in Mexican American women. *Arch Intern Med* 1987; **147**: 1437–1439.

26. Cooper C, Atkinson EJ, O'Fallon WM et al. The incidence of clinically diagnosed vertebral fracture: a population-based study in Rochester, Minnesota. *J Bone Miner Res* 1992; **7**: 221–227.

27. Bengnèr U, Johnell O & Redlund-Johnell I. Changes in the incidence and prevalence of vertebral fractures during 30 years. *Calcif Tissue Int* 1988; **42**: 293–296.

28. Cooper C, Atkinson EJ, Kotowicz M et al. Secular trends in the incidence of postmenopausal vertebral fractures. *Calcif Tissue Int* 1992; **51**: 100–104.

29. Cooper C & Melton LJ III. Epidemiology of osteoporosis. *Trends Endocrinol Metab* 1992; **314**: 224–229.

30. Hagino H, Yamamoto K, Teshima R et al. The incidence of fractures of the proximal femur and the distal radius in Tottori prefecture, Japan. *Arch Orthop Trauma Surg* 1989; **109**: 43–44.

31. Griffin MR, Ray WA, Fought RL et al. Black–white difference in fracture rates. *Am J Epidemiol* 1992; **136**: 1378–1385.

32. Sexson SB & Lehner JT. Factors affecting hip fracture mortality. *J Orthop Trauma* 1988; **1**: 298–305.

33. Magaziner J, Simonsick EM, Kashner TM et al. Survival experience of aged hip fracture patients. *Am J Public Health* 1989; **79**: 274–278.

34. Bonar SK, Tinetti ME, Speechley M et al. Factors associated with short- versus long-term skilled nursing facility placement among community-living hip fracture patients. *J Am Geriatr Soc* 1990; **38**: 1139–1144.

35. Ettinger B, Block JE, Smith R et al. An examination of the association among vertebral deformities, physical disabilities and psychosocial problems. *Maturitas* 1988; **10**: 283–296.

36. Ettinger B, Black DM, Nevitt MC et al. Contribution of vertebral deformity, chronic back pain and disability. *J Bone Miner Res* 1992; **7**: 449–456.

37. Lau EMC, Woo J, Chan H et al. The health consequences of vertebral deformity in elderly Chinese men and women. *Calcif Tissue Int* 1998; **63**: 1–4.

38. Ray NF, Chan JK, Thamer M et al. Medical expenditures for the treatment of osteoporotic fractures in the United States in 1995: Report from the National Osteoporosis Foundation. *J Bone Miner Res* 1997; **12**: 24–35.

39. Torgerson D & Cooper C. Osteoporosis as a candidate for disease management: Epidemiological and cost of illness considerations. *Dis Manage Health Outcomes* 1998; **3**: 207–214.

40. Randell A, Sambrook PN, Nguyen TV et al. Direct clinical and welfare costs of osteoporotic fractures in elderly men and women. *Osteoporosis Int* 1995; **5**: 427–432.

Chapter 3
Pathogenesis of osteoporosis

Clifford J. Rosen

INTRODUCTION

Osteoporosis is a disorder characterized by reduced bone mass and a propensity to fractures. For decades, this disease was considered to be a syndrome characterized by back pain, fractures and osteopoenia on plain X-ray films. In the past 10 years, however, significant progress has been made in both defining this disorder and understanding its complex pathogenesis. Most importantly, however, a consensus has emerged concerning the strength of the association between low bone mineral density (BMD) and fracture risk. Almost all population studies have confirmed that for every one standard deviation below mean in bone mineral density (at virtually any skeletal site) there is an early two-fold greater risk of a subsequent hip fracture.[1] Momentum increased dramatically after the World Health Organization published its recommendations in 1994, so that by the turn of this century, most clinicians and investigators confidently defined osteoporosis solely on a BMD of less than 2.5 standard deviations below the young normal reference ranges.[2] Although this 'bar' has been used to establish prevalence estimates and to define high-risk individuals who should be considered for treatment, it has also become evident that even the definition demands a better understanding of the pathophysiological processes that result in a low bone mass. In this paper, I will review the mechanisms responsible for altered bone density and strength that enhance the probability of fragility fractures. Irrespective of the aetiology and pathogenesis of osteoporosis, the end result is significant morbidity and mortality. Thus, understanding how this disorder develops and progresses has important socio-economic as well as medical consequences.

RISK FACTORS FOR LOW BONE MASS

Several risk factors predispose individuals to osteoporosis fractures. For a hip fracture, these include age greater than 65 years, a previous spine or hip fracture, a maternal history of a hip fracture, poor neuromuscular function, weight loss after the age of 50 and a low body mass index.[1,3] Falls are a major cause of fracture, and in all clinical situations, some degree of trauma can be linked to the injury.[4] Many osteoporotic patients, however, suffer fractures with very minimal trauma, and this is pathognomic of the skeletal fragility that accompanies a low BMD. It is for this reason that the most consistent risk factor for fractures of the spine, hip or wrist remains low BMD.[5] The continuous but inverse relationship between BMD and fracture is consistent at all points below the mean, suggesting that there is no threshold effect.[5,6] It is also applicable at virtually every skeletal site from the spine to finger to the calcaneus. Moreover, the advent of newer technology to measure bone mass has allowed widespread screening for risk as well as defining risk reduction with therapy.

A bone mass measurement is a relatively simple technique for defining mineral content per area of bone. In the laboratory, BMD as measured by dual-energy absorptiometry (DXA) is a very strong predictor of bone strength and accounts for about 80% of the variability in the breaking strength of a single femur. Thus, low BMD can be linked to increased skeletal fragility with a high degree of confidence. There are, however, other determinants of bone strength, including the rate of bone turnover, the extent of trabecular connectivity, cortical and periosteal bone size, and skeletal morphometry. Still, in vivo, BMD represents the most accurate, the most cost-effective and the easiest parameter for risk assessment.[5] In part, two-dimensional DXA measurements integrate actual bone mineral content in both the trabecular and cortical compartments with bone size. Because of the strong association between BMD and future fractures, this phenotype has become an excellent surrogate for defining both the genetic and the acquired components of the disease process.

Adult bone mass represents the sum of two processes, the acquisition of peak bone mass during adolescence and the maintenance of bone density during the middle and later years. Changes in bone mass result from physiological and pathophysiological processes in the bone remodelling cycle.[7] This can occur during the stage of accelerated linear growth in adolescence, or much later in life, usually after the menopause in women. The bone remodelling cycle is a tightly coupled process whereby bone is resorbed at approximately the same rate as new bone is formed. Basic multicellular units compose the remodelling unit of bone and include: osteoclasts, which resorb bone; osteoblasts, which are responsible for new bone formation; and osteocytes, older osteoblasts entombed by bone, present in a reduced state of activity, but likely important in signalling resting osteoblasts and transducing mechanical signs.[8] The activation of the remodelling cycle serves two functions in the adult skeleton:

1. To produce a supply, acutely as well as chronically, of calcium to the extracellular space.
2. To provide elasticity and strength to the skeleton.

When the remodelling process is uncoupled so that resorption exceeds formation, bone is lost. On the other hand, during peak bone acquisition, formation exceeds resorption, resulting in a net gain of bone. Remodelling is more pronounced in cancellous bone (e.g. the spine, calcaneus and proximal femur), which is the most metabolically active component of the skeleton, partly because of its proximity to the marrow space. Cancellous bone is, however, also extremely vulnerable to perturbations by local or systemic factors that can cause a significant imbalance in bone turnover.

BONE REMODELLING AND ITS RELATIONSHIP TO BONE MASS

The bone remodelling cycle begins with the activation of resting osteoblasts on the surface of bone and stromal cells in the marrow. This is followed by a cascade of signals to osteoclasts designed to stimulate the recruitment and differentiation of these multinucleated cells from haemopoietic stem cells.[7] After osteoclast-induced bone resorption, matrix components such as transforming growth factor-beta (TGF-β) and insulin-like growth factor-1 (IGF-1), as well as collagen, osteocalcin and other protein and mineral components, are released into the micro-environment. The growth factors released by resorption contribute to the recruitment of new osteoblasts to the bone surface, which begin the process of collagen synthesis and biomineralization. In healthy adults, as many as 2 million remodelling sites may be active at any given time, and it is estimated that nearly one-quarter of all cancellous bone is remodelled each year. In general, resorption takes only 10–13 days, while formation is a much slower process and can take upwards of 3 months.

In ideal circumstances the amount of bone resorbed by the end of the cycle equals the amount reformed. Osteoporosis has been classically defined as an uncoupling disorder in which resorption exceeds formation, leading to a net loss of bone; however, it is also apparent that some individuals have impaired peak bone acquisition. This scenario may be more common than previously appreciated and almost certainly represents inherited or acquired alterations in the rate of either bone formation or bone resorption during a critical period when several hormones (e.g. growth hormone, IGF-1, androgens and oestrogens) acting in synchrony orchestrate the increase in bone mass.

There are several key components of the remodelling cycle that are susceptible to systemic and local alterations and, when perturbed, can lead to a deleterious change in bone mass. In particular, the activation of remodelling and the recruitment of osteoclasts represent the two most vulnerable sites in the cycle. Increased activation of remodelling occurs following oestrogen deprivation or in response to endogenous parathyroid hormone

fluxes, cytokine stimulation, growth hormone surges, glucocorticoid excess or changes in serum calcium level. For the most part, oestrogen deprivation remains one of the most common and critical elements in shifting the resorption rate to a higher set point. Although bone formation can initially 'catch up', the length of time for each component of the remodelling cycle clearly favours resorption over formation as the process of laying down new bone requires the delicate and time-consuming interaction of several distinct processes.

It is, however, still unclear why a falling oestrogen level, a universal event during the menopausal years, can cause rapid bone loss in a relatively small percentage of women. Clearly, factors such as the peripheral conversion of testosterone to oestradiol, adrenal androgen production and other local signals may also be important. It is, in addition, still not clear whether there are heritable determinants that predispose some women to acute and rapid bone loss during the early phase of the menopause. Indeed, in inbred strains of mice, rates of bone loss after ovariectomy are considerably different, despite an absolute and consistent fall in oestradiol levels (Bouxsein, unpublished observation). In genetically susceptible individuals following oestrogen deprivation, uncoupling of the remodelling cycle can be dramatic, as a result of rapid bone resorption; this leads to significant bone loss and markedly increased skeletal fragility.

The second and most systematically examined component of the remodelling cycle is the osteoblast, with its inherent signalling to the osteoclast to ensure the activation of resorption (Figure 3.1). External signals (such as parathyroid hormone, growth hormone, interleukin-1 (IL-1) and oestrogen deprivation) to resting osteoblasts and stromal cells cause these cells to release a pot-pourri of cytokines (interleukins such as IL-1, -6 and -11, as well as macrophage colony-stimulating factor (m-CSF), tumour necrosis factor (TNF) and TGF-β) and most importantly, receptor activator of NF-κB ligand (RANKL), which enhance the recruitment and differentiative function of multinucleated giant cells destined to become bone resorbing cells.[7–9]

Elucidation of the RANK–RANKL–OPG pathway of osteoclast activation has prompted investigators to successfully delineate the osteoblast–osteoclast interaction scheme. Osteoprotegerin (OPG) is a soluble peptide originally described as a factor that markedly inhibited bone resorption and osteoclast differentiation in vitro.[10] This protein is a member of the TNF receptor superfamily, its role in bone remodelling being to act as a decoy receptor for the ligand now known as osteoprotegrin ligand (OPGL, TRANCE or RANKL).[11] RANKL is in fact a surface peptide that, when expressed on the osteoblast, can bind to the true OPG receptor (also called RANK receptor activator of the NF-κB ligand) on osteoclasts and initiate the cell–cell contact necessary for osteoclast activation and subsequent bone resorption.[11,12] The identification of OPG, OPGL and RANK has led investigators to synthesize both recombinant OPG and a systemic antibody to RANKL. The latter is currently being investigated in human trials as a potential therapeutic agent to slow

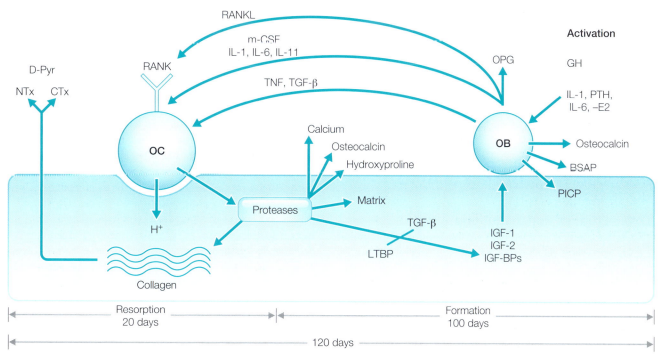

Figure 3.1. The bone remodelling cycle. The osteoblast (OB) orchestrates the orderly process of bone remodelling through activation signals from systemic factors, including growth hormone (GH), interleukins (IL-1, IL-6), parathyroid hormone (PTH) and the withdrawal of oestrogen (−E2). m-CSF and RANKL are the two major OB-mediated factors that regulate the recruitment and differentiation of the osteoclast (OC). Osteoprotogerin (OPG) is also synthesized by OBs and serves as a dummy receptor, binding avidly to RANKL. The inhibition or knock-out of these signals from OB–OC results in a reduction in bone resorption. The IGFs are released during bone resorption and serve as coupling factors to recruit new OBs to the surface. These peptides may also be important for osteoclast activity. BP, binding protein; BSAP, bone-specific alkaline phosphatase; CTx, C-telopeptide; D-Pyr, deoxypyridinoline; IGF, insulin-like growth factor; LTBP, latent transforming growth factor binding protein; NTx, N-telopeptide; PICP, procollagen I peptide; TGF-β, transforming growth factor-beta; TNF, tumour necrosis factor.

or inhibit bone resorption. Preliminary studies with this agent, administered once every 6 months, are very encouraging (McClung, personal observation).

The osteoblast functions not only to signal osteoclasts during remodelling, but also to lay down collagen and orchestrate the mineralization of previously resorbed lacunae in the skeletal matrix. This complex function is tied to the differentiation of mesenchymal stem cells that become osteoblasts and rest on the surface of the remodelling space.[7] The recruitment of stem cells to osteoblasts, rather than adipocytes, is a critical step in bone formation and requires a series of factors that enhance differentiation. One of the most important components of this process is Cbfa1, a transcription factor that is essential in the early differentiative pathway of stem cells to bone and away from adipocytes.[13] The regulation of Cbfa1 has become a major focus of work in the past 3 years as investigators have begun to consider novel ways of enhancing bone formation. Another recently described osteoblast pathway is through the Wnt/Lrp5/β-catenin signalling system. Wnt 10b, for example, is a very potent stimulator of osteoblast maturation.[14] On the other hand, the role of adipocyte differentiation factors, such as Pparg (peroxisome proliferator gamma), which can antagonize both Cbfa1 and Wnt ligands, has also received considerable attention

recently.[15] Exogenous activators of Pparg, such as rosiglitazone, have been shown to enhance marrow adipogenesis and reduce bone formation and bone mass in susceptible strains of mice. These preliminary studies are extremely important and will lead to new insights into the pathogenesis of osteoporosis.

With the activation of resting osteoblasts, osteoblastic cells begin to synthesize several types of collagen as well as elaborating a series of growth factors such as IGF-1, IGF-2, TGF-β and others, which are necessary for the further recruitment of bone-forming cells.[16] In addition, osteoblasts deposit these growth factors in the skeletal matrix, where they are stored in latent forms and released during subsequent remodelling cycles. After the deposition of new bone, some osteoblasts are encased by matrix. These cells, called osteocytes, are still viable, although less metabolically active, and can, through newly developed caniculi, provide signals to other bone cells. Indeed, there is some evidence that osteocytic signals are important in the so-called 'mechanostat', the gravity-sensing device that modulates bone formation.

In summary, the bone remodelling cycle is extremely complex and redundant. The two major players, osteoblasts and osteoclasts, arise from very different stem cells (mesenchymal and haemopoietic respectively) and are under the control of various factors that in harmony orchestrate an orderly remodelling sequence. Their birth and death (i.e. the cycle of recruitment, proliferation and programmed cell death), as well as the regulatory factors that control those events, are also complex yet vitally important for understanding the pathogenesis of osteoporosis. Alterations at any stage along the process of recruitment, activation, differentiation and cell death can lead to imbalances in remodelling that will eventually result in bone loss or reduced bone mass. Some of those perturbations are noted below.

SYSTEMIC ALTERATIONS IN THE BONE REMODELLING SEQUENCE LEAD TO BONE LOSS

Low oestradiol concentrations

The importance of oestrogen in maintaining calcium homeostasis in the post-menopausal woman was first established by Fuller Albright more than 60 years ago.[17] Since that time, more evidence has accumulated from randomized intervention trials demonstrating that hormone replacement (oestrogen with or without progesterone) reduces bone turnover and increases bone mass.[18]

These data, however, provide only indirect evidence that the oestrogen level is important as a pathogenic component of the osteoporosis syndrome. More recent studies provide stronger evidence of the association between low oestradiol concentration and low bone mass. Several investigators have demonstrated that the lowest oestradiol level in post-menopausal women (i.e. <5 pg/ml) is associated with the lowest BMD and the greatest likelihood of fracture.[19] In addition, at least one study has shown that males with osteoporosis have a lower serum level of oestradiol than do age-matched men who do not have a low bone mass.[20] Moreover, there are now two case reports describing mutations in either aromatase activity or the oestrogen receptor, which have produced a phenotype of severe osteoporosis in men.[21,22] In the former case, oestrogen replacement therapy for this young man resulted in a marked increase in spine and hip bone mineral density. In both situations, the lack of functional oestrogen, despite a normal-to-high level of testosterone, resulted in a severely low bone mineral density.[23]

Although a declining oestradiol level contributes to the osteoporosis syndrome, the precise molecular events or sequences that result from a change in the ambient hormonal concentration are not clear. In some animal models, oestrogen deprivation is associated with a marked increase in IL-6 and RANKL synthesis (and a decrease in OPG) from stromal cells. This is consistent with experimental findings demonstrating that oestrogen regulates the transcriptional activity of the IL-6 promoter.[24] Results from other studies are, however, conflicting. In other experimental paradigms, changes in TNF, IL-11 and IL-1 can all be associated with increased bone resorption.[25] It seems likely that several cytokines, working in concert, are active during oestrogen deprivation, and each can accelerate the process of bone resorption. Bone loss from oestrogen deprivation results when the bone formation rate cannot keep up with the rate of bone resorption in both men and women.[26]

Low androgen level

In contrast to the plethora of studies on bone loss and oestrogen, there are few good studies relating androgen deprivation to bone loss in women. Androgen receptors are present on osteoblasts. However, both in vitro and in vivo studies in men have yielded conflicting results. Like oestrogen, androgens can regulate the IL-6 promoter, and in experimental animals orchidectomy has been associated with increased IL-6 production and bone loss.[25] In men, a chronically low androgen level has been associated with a low bone mass, and testosterone replacement can enhance bone mineral density.[27] It is, however, unclear what role androgens play in the maintenance of bone mass in both men and women.

Secondary hyperparathyroidism and calcium deficiency syndromes

Although bone loss is sometimes accelerated immediately after the menopause, recent studies have demonstrated that markers of bone resorption are very high in later life. In particular, women in their eighties and nineties have been noted to lose bone at a rate of greater than 1% per year from the spine and hip.[28] Contrary to earlier studies, it is now evident that the older woman who is not as physically active, and is not taking oestrogen, is at an extremely high risk of bone loss and subsequent fracture.

The pathogenesis of this process is almost certainly multifactorial, although dietary calcium deficiency, leading to secondary hyperparathyroidism, certainly plays a central role. The average calcium intake of women in their eighth and ninth decades of life is between 500 and 600 mg per day.[29] If vitamin D intake is also suboptimal (the serum level of 25-hydroxyvitamin D being less than 25 ng/ml), secondary hyperparathyroidism is assured. Parathyroid hormone stimulates osteoblasts and provokes the remodelling sequence, including the elaboration of several cytokines that accelerate bone resorption. Unfortunately, in most of the elderly, bone formation is not enhanced, although the reason for this is not entirely clear, this resulting in further uncoupling in the bone remodelling cycle and significant bone loss.

Among older people with a low calcium intake who live in northern latitudes, seasonal changes in vitamin D can aggravate bone loss even further and may account for as much as 3% of bone loss during the winter months.[30,31] Whether increased bone loss is an independent risk factor for future fractures in the elderly remains somewhat controversial, necessitating further studies to define such a risk.

Vitamin D deficiency and osteoporosis

There is now abundant evidence that a declining serum level of vitamin D stimulates parathyroid hormone release, leading to an increase in bone turnover. As noted above, such a change is often not associated with a concomitant increase in bone formation, particularly in the elderly, thereby accelerating bone loss. Many older individuals already have established osteoporosis. Coincidental vitamin D deficiency resulting from poor intake, absent sunlight exposure or an impaired conversion of vitamin

D to its active metabolite can result in osteomalacia as well as aggravating pre-existent osteoporosis.[32] LeBoff et al.[33] reported that more than 50% of older people in Boston, MA, who presented with a hip fracture, were frankly vitamin D deficient. Other studies have confirmed these findings in other geographic areas outside of the north-east. Combining vitamin D deficiency with inadequate calcium intake enhances the likelihood of rapid bone loss in susceptible populations.

It is unclear how secondary hyperparathyroidism causes bone loss. A chronic elevation in parathyroid hormone secretion caused by primary or tertiary hyperparathyroidism has been associated with low BMD at several skeletal sites, particularly the radius. An elevated parathyroid hormone level in older women has been associated with bone loss in some studies but not others. In elderly individuals, it has been reported that the parathyroid hormone level is closely correlated with an increased synthesis of an IGF-binding protein (IGFBP-4), which suppresses the action of IGF on bone cells.[16,34] Since IGF-1 is an important growth factor for osteoblasts, it is conceivable that parathyroid hormone down-regulates IGF activity during states of relative calcium/and or vitamin D deficiency. This would shift the remodelling balance towards preserving the intravascular calcium concentration while inhibiting any new incorporation of calcium into the skeletal matrix. This response makes teleological sense, although further studies are needed to assess whether serum IGFBP-4 is a reliable marker of calcium deficiency in older individuals.[35] In sum, there is little doubt that calcium and vitamin D insufficiency are prominent causes of accelerated bone loss in the elderly. The scope of this 'epidemic' is not limited to the USA, but is certain to be one of the principal causes of age-related osteoporosis in most countries. Efforts to combat vitamin D deficiency are only now being launched and time will determine whether specific public health initiatives, such as greater vitamin D supplementation in food products, will impact the prevalence of low BMD and fractures in the elderly.

Glucocorticoid excess

A high circulating level of glucocorticoids has a significant impact on bone mass. In 1932, Harvey Cushing[36] recognized the syndrome of endogenous steroid excess that included marked osteopoenia, fractures and fat redistribution. A long-term exposure to glucocorticoids results in significant bone loss, and pharmacological treatment with prednisone or other glucocorticoids causes a dramatic uncoupling in the remodelling sequence by enhancing bone resorption and suppressing bone formation. Moreover, it is likely that adipocyte differentiation is preferably enhanced by glucocorticoids, leading to a shift in lineage allocation away from osteoblasts. In addition to having a direct effect on the osteoclast and osteoblast, glucocorticoids also induce secondary hypogonadism and hyperparathyroidism, impaired vitamin D metabolism, muscle atrophy and hypercalciuria, all of which contribute to a rapid and sustained loss of bone during the first few months of steroid therapy.[37]

The addition of other immunosuppressants such as cyclosporin has been shown to aggravate bone loss by further increasing bone resorption. As the number of organ transplants has increased exponentially over the past decade, the prevalence of post-transplantation osteoporosis has risen substantially. Steroid-induced osteoporosis is now considered to be the second most common cause of low bone mass in the general population.[38]

PATHOGENIC FACTORS THAT IMPAIR PEAK BONE MASS

Peak bone mass is acquired between the ages of 12 and 16 years. It is the high point of bone acquisition and represents the sum of several processes, including a marked increase in bone formation.[39] Boys tend to reach this peak 2 years later than girls, and their bone mineral density is higher than that of women at all skeletal sites. This partly relates to a greater cross-sectional bone area in males than females.[40] Peak bone mass results from a linear growth and consolidation of the cortical and trabecular components. Acquisition is most rapid during the latter stages of puberty and coincides with maximum growth hormone secretion, a high serum IGF-1 level, and rising concentrations of oestradiol and testosterone. In addition, calcium absorption is maximum and skeletal accretion optimal. All these processes combine over a relatively short period of time to produce a bone mass that subsequently plateaus and then falls during later life. It is estimated that more than 60% of adult bone mass can be related to peak acquisition. Hence, understanding the mechanisms responsible for a low bone mass must include perturbations in peak bone acquisition.

Hormonal status

There are several hormonal, environmental and heritable determinants of peak bone mass. These include oestrogen/testosterone, growth hormone/IGF-1, calcium/vitamin D and unknown genetic factors. If any is disturbed, a dramatic alteration in peak bone mass may occur, setting the stage for low bone density throughout life. Gonadal steroids are important not only to bone maintenance, but also to acquisition.

During puberty, oestrogen and testosterone levels rise and contribute to the consolidation of bone mass. Oestrogen is also necessary for epiphysial closure. Studies of a male with an oestrogen receptor mutation and men with an aromatase deficiency have established that oestradiol is critical for bone acquisition.[21–23] These young men share several phenotypic characteristics, including tall stature, unfused epiphyses and a very low bone mass. There must thus be a threshold effect for oestradiol in men, and this effect must be time dependent. Similar conclusions can be drawn from studies in women. Acquired deficiencies in oestrogen, such as anorexia nervosa or chemotherapy-induced ovarian dysfunction, result in a low peak bone mass and lead to a subsequent risk of osteoporosis.[41,42] Similar findings have been noted in patients with untreated Turner's syndrome and in men with Klinefelter's syndrome.

The timing of gonadal steroid surges is critical for bone acquisition since there is a relatively short window of time in which bone formation is favoured and matrix synthesis is markedly enhanced. That window is likely to be less than 3 years, and earlier in girls than boys. The study that has addressed this issue best is probably a retrospective analysis of men in their thirties who underwent late onset of puberty (at the age of 17 or 18) but were otherwise normal on full endocrine testing.[43] The semen had significantly lower bone mineral density than age-matched men who went through puberty at the normal time. These data suggest that the timing as well as the quantity of gonadal steroids is critical for bone acquisition.

Pubertal surges of oestrogen and androgens are also important for priming the growth hormone IGF-1 axis. A rising level of both contributes to growth hormone surges, which lead to an increase in the circulating level and tissue expression of IGF-1, an essential growth factor for chondrocyte hypertrophy and expansion. IGF-1 may also be critical in defining the cross-sectional size of bone, a potentially important determinant of bone strength.[44]

Once again, studies in growth hormone-deficient or growth hormone-resistant individuals have established that a low level of circulating IGF-1, especially during puberty, is associated with reduced bone mass.[45] In addition, rhGH replacement has been shown to restore linear growth and improve peak bone mass acquisition. Several studies in experimental animals, including inbred strains of mice, have established that IGF-1 is important for bone acquisition, the timing of IGF-1 peaks coinciding with the maximal rates of bone formation.[46,47] An impairment in the production of IGF-1 resulting from acquired disorders such as anorexia nervosa, malnutrition or diabetes mellitus can also impede peak bone acquisition.

Hormonal abnormalities may not only enhance bone resorption in older individuals, but also blunt the capacity of bone cells to maximize bone formation during adolescence. Clearly, hypogonadal boys and girls have impaired peak bone mass, resulting in a low adult bone mineral density. Even one form of contraception, Depo-Provera, reduces oestrogen concentrations enough in a teenage girl to reduce her capacity to acquire peak bone mass. This has recently prompted a black box warning for this contraceptive, noting the possibility of bone loss with continued use of Depo-Provera, and the likelihood that peak bone mass will be impaired. Similarly, it seems probable, although not proven, that smoking during the teenage years might impair osteoblast activity and flatten projected trajectories for peak bone acquisition. Finally, teenage pregnancies may put a greater burden on the maternal skeleton for calcium, than what is noted in adult mothers. This in turn could reduce peak bone mass and set the stage for osteoporosis later in life.

Calcium and dietary intake

In order to mineralize newly synthesized bone, calcium must become bioavailable to the skeletal matrix. In experimental studies in rodents and humans, it is clear that the several pools of available calcium are markedly enhanced during puberty. These include calcium efflux from the gastrointestinal tract and the calcium pool available for incorporation in the matrix. It is

no coincidence that growth hormone surges not only increase IGF-1 (thereby enhancing skeletal growth and matrix biosynthesis), but also result in an increase in the level of 1,25-dihydroxyvitamin D (possibly via the IGF-1 induction of 1α-hydroxylase activity), the active metabolite of vitamin D, which markedly enhances calcium absorption from the gut.[48]

Although there are no longitudinal studies in pubertal individuals with prolonged calcium deficiency, several randomized placebo-controlled trials in pubertal and pre-pubertal girls and boys have established that supplemental calcium can enhance BMD. In a twin study, in which one twin received 1200 mg of calcium supplementation and one received placebo, the radial bone mineral density increased by as much as 5% after 3 years when compared with placebo.[49] This study suggests that there is a significant gene–environment interaction and that even in those individuals with heritable determinants of low peak bone mass, calcium supplementation may provide an important and relatively simple means of protecting individuals from future osteoporotic fracture.

Probably the most important determinant of peak bone mass, but one that has lacked clear definition, is the genetic contribution. As noted above, low peak bone mass may be the most important pathogenic factor in the osteoporosis syndrome of later life, and it appears that at least 50% of peak bone mass is determined by genetic factors.[50–52] What are these determinants and how are they modified by environmental factors? Efforts to define the heritable determinants of peak bone mass have been plagued by a number of issues that are also common to other complex diseases. These include:[53]

1. A quantifiable phenotype.
2. Heterogeneity within a given population under study.
3. The polygenic nature of the disorder.
4. Epistasis (gene–gene interaction) pleitrophy, phenotypic differences with identical genotypes, and gene by environmental interactions (e.g. low bone density gene modified by high calcium diet).

Notwithstanding these barriers, it is now clear that BMD is an acceptable phenotype for defining heritable determinants. In addition, bone density is fully quantifiable and is therefore amenable to complex trait analysis. Moreover, bone density in the population is distributed in a gaussian manner, thereby allowing analyses at the extremes (outside ±2.0 SD) of the density distribution. Large homogeneous populations are, however, needed to ascertain various genetic determinants of bone density in humans.

Candidate loci identified by studying polymorphisms in genes, such as the vitamin D receptor, collagen 1A1, the oestrogen receptor, IL-1, IGF-1 and parathyroid hormone, have often produced conflicting results, depending on the population, the phenotype and the number of individuals studied. However, a polymorphism in the regulatory region of the collagen type 1α gene has been more consistently linked to low bone mass and osteoporotic fracture.[54] Twin studies examining discordant or concordant phenotypes can also be helpful, as are sib pair studies, although the results have been somewhat disappointing.[55] Very recently, Recker and colleagues[56] identified an extended family with high BMD and have fine-mapped this locus to a mutation in the Lrp5 gene, resulting in a single amino acid mutation in the external propeller of this receptor. Other groups have confirmed and extended those original observations; moreover, a loss of function mutation in the same gene results in a much rarer syndrome named osteoporosis pseudoglioma, characterized by severe osteoporosis and blindness in children.[57] Recently, several groups have also identified polymorphisms in the Lrp5 gene in men which are responsible for significant differences in adult BMD.[58] Ongoing genetic studies of inbred strains of mice may also shed light on the complex polygenic phenotype of bone mass acquisition. Klein et al.[59] identified one gene, *Alox12/15*, which is responsible for a major effect on peak acquisition in two inbred strains. Further genes are likely to be identified from these animal studies in the near future.

Intervention studies in adolescents have provided some fresh insight into the complex dilemma of gene–environmental interaction.[49] The famous twin study in Indiana revealed that as long as calcium supplementation continued during puberty, young boys could enhance their peak bone mass. In a Swiss study, younger pre-pubertal girls supplemented with a protein product had a significant increase in spine bone density, as did a cohort of pubertal girls receiving a milk powder in England.[60,61] Remarkably, in the latter cohort, the serum IGF-1 level also rose dramatically, providing further indirect evidence of a link between pubertal status, bone mass and the growth hormone/IGF-1 axis.

SUMMARY

The pathogenesis of osteoporosis is complex and multifactorial. Alterations in BMD almost certainly represent the final common pathway by which pathological factors affect the risk of future osteoporotic fracture. The interplay of various physiological processes that result in peak bone mass and the maintenance of adult bone mass are key to understanding the pathogenesis of this disease. Changes in hormonal status, particularly of oestradiol, are clearly important factors in both the formation and the resorption of bone in men and women. Perturbations in growth hormone activity, musculoskeletal function, the dietary intake of calcium and vitamin D, and genetic determinants are also important pathogenic factors.[62] Defining the role of genetic factors and their interaction with many of the environmental and hormonal determinants that have been established as potential aetiological agents responsible for low bone mass will certainly be the most difficult challenge facing basic and clinical researchers well into the next century. On the other hand, the strength of data from bench and clinical studies over the past decade now allows practitioners confidently to diagnose and treat osteoporosis.

PRACTICE POINTS

- There are multiple risk factors for osteoporosis, including bone density, age and history of previous fracture.

- Understanding the pathogenesis of bone loss in adults increases the chances of using the most effective therapy

RESEARCH AGENDA

- A better understanding of genetic factors that determine bone mass.

- Clarifying the role of local growth factors such as IGF-1 in the bone remodelling process.

REFERENCES

1. Cummings SR, Nevitt MC, Browner WS et al. Risk factors for hip fracture in white women. *N Engl J Med* 1995; **332**: 767–773.
2. Kanis JA, Melton LJ, Christiansen C et al. The diagnosis of osteoporosis. *J Bone Miner Res* 1994; **9**: 1137–1141.
3. Stewart A, Walker LG, Potter RW et al. Prediction of a second hip fracture: the potential role of DXA, ultrasound, and other risk factors for targeting of preventive therapy. *J Clin Densitom* 1999; **2**: 363–371.
4. Tinetti ME, Speechley M & Gunter SF. Risk factors for falls among elderly persons living in the community. *N Engl J Med* 1988; **319**: 1701–1707.
5. Miller PD. Guidelines for the clinical utilization of bone mass measurements in the adult population. *Calcif Tissue Int* 1995; **57**: 252–265.
6. Riggs BL, Wahner HW & Seeman E. Changes in bone mineral density of the proximal femur and spine with aging: differences between the postmenopausal and senile osteoporosis syndromes. *J Clin Invest* 1982; **70**: 716–723.
7. Lian JB & Stein GS. The cells of bone. In: Seibel MJ, Robbins S & Bilezikian JP, eds. *Principles of Bone and Cartilage Metabolism*. San Diego: Academic Press, 1999; 165–185.
8. Lorenzo JA & Raisz LG. Cytokines and prostaglandins. In: Seibel MJ, Robbins S & Bilezikian JP, eds. *Principles of Bone and Cartilage Metabolism*. San Diego: Academic Press, 1999; 97–109.
9. Udagawa N, Takahashi N, Jimi E et al. Osteoblasts/stromal cells stimulate osteoclast differentiation factor/RANKL but not macrophage colony stimulating factor. *Bone* 1999; **25**: 517–523.
10. Emery JG, McDonnell P, Burke MB et al. Osteoprotegrin is a receptor for the cytotoxic ligand TRAIL. *J Biol Chem* 1998; **273**: 14363–14367.
11. Suda T, Takahashi N & Martin TJ. Modulation of osteoclast differentiation. *Endocr Rev* 1992; **12**: 66–80.
12. Indridason OS, Franzson L & Sigurdsson G. Serum osteoprotegerin and its relationship with bone mineral density and markers of bone turnover. *Osteoporosis Int* 2005; **16**(4): 417–423.
13. Ducy P, Zhang RR, Geoffroy V et al. Osf2/Cbfal: a transcriptional activator of osteoblast differentiation. *Cell* 1997; **89**: 747–754.
14. Holmen SL, Zylstra CR, Mukherjee A et al. Essential role of beta-catenin in postnatal bone acquisition. *J Biol Chem* 2005; **280**: 21162–21168.
15. Rzonca SO, Suva LJ, Gaddy D et al. Bone is a target for the antidiabetic compound rosiglitazone. *Endocrinology* 2004; **145**(1): 401–406.

16. Rosen CJ. Growth hormone, IGF-I and the elderly: clues to potential therapeutic intervention. *Endocrine* 1997; **7**: 39–40.

17. Albright F. Postmenopausal osteoporosis. *JAMA* 1941; **116**: 2465–2474.

18. Chestnust C, Notelovitz M, Clark G et al. Use of the N-telopeptide of type I collagen to monitor the effect of therapy and predict changes in bone mineral density in postmenopausal women treated with hormone replacement therapy. *Am J Med* 1997; **102**: 29–37.

19. Ettinger B, Pressman A, Sklarin P et al. Associations between low levels of serum estradiol, bone density and fractures among elderly women: SOF. *J Clin Endocrinol Metab* 1998; **83**: 2239–2243.

20. Greendale GA, Edelstein S & Barrett-Connor E. Endogenous sex steroids and bone mineral density in older women and men. *J Bone Miner Res* 1997; **12**: 1833–1837.

21. Smith EP, Boyd J, Frank GR et al. Estrogen resistance caused by a mutation in the estrogen receptor gene in a man. *N Engl J Med* 1994; **331**: 1056–1061.

22. Morishima A, Grumbach MM, Simpson ER et al. Aromatase deficiency in male and female siblings caused by a novel mutation in the physiological role of estrogens. *J Clin Endocrinol Metab* 1995; **80**: 3689–3698.

23. Carani C, Quin K, Simoni M et al. Effect of testosterone and estradiol in a man with aromatase deficiency. *N Engl J Med* 1997; **337**: 91–95.

24. Jilka RG, Girsole GH, Passeri G et al. Increased osteoclast development after estrogen loss: mediation by IL-6. *Science* 1992; **257**: 88–91.

25. Pacifici R, Brown C & Puscheck E. The effect of surgical menopause and estrogen replacement on cytokine release from human blood monocytes. *Proc Natl Acad Sci USA* 1991; **88**: 5134–5138.

26. Manolagas SC & Jilka RL. Emerging insights into the pathophysiology of osteoporosis. *N Engl J Med* 1995; **332**: 305–311.

27. Snyder PJ, Peachey H, Hannoush P et al. Effect of testosterone treatment on body composition and muscle strength in men over 65. *J Clin Endocrinol Metab* 1999; **84**: 2647–2653.

28. Dresner-Pollak R, Parker RA, Poku M et al. Biochemical markers of bone turnover reflect femoral bone loss in elderly women. *Calcif Tissue Int* 1996; **59**: 328–333.

29. Food and Nutrition Board Institute of Medicine. *Dietary Reference Intakes for Calcium, Phosphorus, Magnesium, Vitamin D and Fluoride.* Washington, DC: National Academy Press, 1997.

30. Storm D, Smith-Porter E, Musgrave KO et al. Calcium supplementation prevents seasonal bone loss and changes in biochemical markers of bone turnover in elderly New England women: a randomized placebo-controlled trial. *J Clin Endocrinol Metab* 1998; **83**: 3817–3826.

31. Rosen CJ, Morrison A, Zhou H et al. Elderly women in northern New England exhibit seasonal changes in bone mineral density and calciotropic hormones. *Bone Miner* 1994; **25**: 83–92.

32. Holick MF. Vitamin D: new horizons for the 21st century. *J Nutr* 1996; **124**: 1159S–1164S.

33. LeBoff MS, Kohlmeier L, Hurwitz S et al. Occult vitamin D deficiency in postmenopausal US women with acute hip fracture. *JAMA* 1999; **282**: 1505–1511.

34. Rosen C, Donahue LR, Hunter S et al. The 24/25kD serum insulin-like growth factor binding protein is increased in elderly women with fractures. *J Clin Endocrinol Metab* 1992; **74**: 24–28.

35. Heaney RP, McCarron DA, Dawson Hughes B et al. Dietary changes favorably affect bone remodeling in older adults. *J Am Diuret Assoc* 1999; **99**: 1228–1233.

36. Cushing H. Basophile adenomas of the pituitary body and their clinical manifestations. *Bull Johns Hopkins Hosp* 1932; **50**: 137–145.

37. Rosen CJ & Adler RA. Glucorticoids and bone mass. *Clin Endocrinol Metab* 1994; **23**: 641–654.

38. Reid IR, Veale AG & France JT. Glucocorticoid osteoporosis. *J Asthma* 1994; **31**: 7–18.

39. Teegarden D, Proulx WR & Martin BR. Peak bone mass in young women. *J Bone Miner Res* 1995; **10**: 711–715.

40. Gilsanz V, Loro ML, Roe TF et al. Gender differences in vertebral size in adults: biomechanical implications. *J Clin Invest* 1995; **95**: 2332–2337.

41. Bachrach LK, Guido D, Katzman D et al. Decreased bone density in adolescent girls with anorexia nervosa. *Pediatrics* 1990; **86**: 440–447.

42. Prior JC, Vigna Y, Schechter MT et al. Spinal bone loss and ovulatory disturbances. *N Engl J Med* 1990; **323**: 1221–1227.

43. Finkelstein JS, Neer RM, Biller BMK et al. Osteopenia in men with a history of delayed puberty. *N Engl J Med* 1992; **326**: 600–604.

44. Mora S, Pitukcheewanont P, Nelson JC et al. Serum levels of IGF-I and the density volume and cross-sectional area of bone in children. *J Clin Endocrinol Metab* 1999; **84**: 2780–2783.

45. Bing-You RG, Denis MC & Rosen CJ. Low bone mineral density in adults with previous hypothalamic-pituitary tumors: correlation with growth hormone, responses to GHRH, IGF-I and IGFBP-3. *Calcif Tissue Int* 1993; **52**: 183–187.

46. Rosen CJ, Dimai HP, Vereault D et al. Circulating and skeletal IGF-I concentrations in two inbred strains of mice with different bone densities. *Bone* 1997; **21**(3): 217–223.

47. Beamer WG, Donahue LR, Rosen CJ et al. Genetic variability in adult bone density among inbred strains of mice. *Bone* 1996; **18**(5): 397–405.

48. Menaa C, Vrtovsnik F, Freidlander G et al. IGF-I, a unique calcium dependent stimulator of 1,25-vitamin D production. *J Biol Chem* 1995; **270**: 25461–25467.

49. Johnston CC, Miller JZ, Slemenda CW et al. Calcium supplementation and increases in bone mineral density in children. *N Engl J Med* 1992; **327**: 82–87.

50. McKay HA, Bailey DA, Wilkinson AA et al. Familial comparison of bone mineral density at the proximal femur and lumbar spine. *Bone Miner* 1994; **24**: 95–107.

51. Smith DM, Nance WE, Kang KW et al. Genetic factors in determining bone mass. *J Clin Invest* 1973; **52**: 2800–2808.

52. Seeman E. Genetic determinants of the population variance in bone mineral density. In: Rosen CJ, Glowacki J & Bilezikian JP, eds. *The Aging Skeleton.* San Diego: Academic Press, 1999; 77–84.

53. Rogers J, Mahaney MC, Beamer WG et al. Beyond one gene–one disease: alternative strategies for deciphering genetic determinants of osteoporosis. *Calcif Tissue Int* 1997; **60**: 225–228.

54. Ralston SH. The genetics of osteoporosis. *QJ Med* 1997; **90**: 247–251.

55. Utterlinden AG, Burger H, Huang Q et al. Relation of alleles of the collagen type I alpha 1 gene to bone density and the risk of osteoporotic fractures in postmenopausal women. *N Engl J Med* 1998; **338**: 1016–1021.

56. Johnson ML. The high bone mass family – the role of Wnt/Lrp5 signaling in the regulation of bone mass. *J Musculoskelet Neuronal Interact* 2004; **4**(2): 135–138.

57. Gong Y, Vikkula M, Boon L et al. Osteoporosis-pseudoglioma syndrome, a disorder affecting skeletal strength and vision, is assigned to chromosome region 11q12-13. *Am J Hum Genet* 1996; **59**(1): 146–151.

58. Ferrari SL, Deutsch S, Choudhury U et al. Polymorphisms in the low-density lipoprotein receptor-related protein 5 (LRP5) gene are associated with variation in vertebral bone mass, vertebral bone size, and stature in whites. *Am J Hum Genet* 2004; **74**(5): 866–875.

59. Klein RF, Allard J, Avnur Z et al. Regulation of bone mass in mice by the lipoxygenase gene Alox15. *Science* 2004; **303**(5655): 229–232.

60. Bonjour JP, Carrie AL & Ferrari S. Calcium enriched foods and bone mass growth in prepubertal girls: a randomized double blind placebo controlled trial. *J Clin Invest* 1997; **99**: 1287–1294.

61. Cadogan J, Blumsehn A, Barker M et al. A longitudinal study of bone gain in pubertal girls: anthropometric and biochemical correlates. *J Bone Miner Res* 1998; **13**: 1602–1612.

62. Weaver CM, Peacock M & Johnston CC. Adolescent nutrition in the prevention of postmenopausal osteoporosis. *J Clin Endocrinol Metab* 1999; **84**: 1839–1843.

Chapter 4

Prenatal and childhood influences on osteoporosis

M. Kassim Javaid and Cyrus Cooper

Osteoporosis is a skeletal disorder characterized by low bone mass and microarchitectural deterioration of bone tissue with a consequent increase in bone fragility and susceptibility to fracture.[1] It is a widespread condition, often unrecognized in clinical practice, which may have devastating health consequences through its association with fragility fractures. The term 'osteoporosis' was first used in the 19th century as a histological description for aged bone tissue, but its clinical consequences were not appreciated until Sir Astley Cooper recognized over 150 years ago that hip fractures might result from an age-related reduction in bone mass or quality. Because one disadvantage of a fracture-based definition is that diagnosis and treatment will be delayed when prevention is considered optimal treatment, an expert panel convened by the World Health Organization (WHO) has suggested that both low bone mineral density (BMD) and fracture be combined in a stratified definition of osteoporosis.[2]

Population-based data from the USA suggest that while the majority of white women aged under 50 years have normal bone density, osteoporosis becomes increasingly prevalent with advancing age.[3] However, prospective studies indicate that the risk of osteoporotic fracture increases continuously as BMD declines, with a 1.5- to 3-fold increase in the risk of fracture for each standard deviation fall in BMD.[4]

There does not appear to be a threshold value for BMD above which the fracture risk is stable, and the risk gradient for this relationship is as steep as that between blood pressure and stroke. The use of this density-based definition allows early diagnosis and therefore early initiation of preventive strategies.

Using the WHO criteria, it has been estimated that most American women under the age of 50 years have normal BMD and that osteoporosis is rare. With advancing age, an increasing number of women have osteoporosis, so that by the age of 80 years 27% are osteopoenic and 70% are osteoporotic at the hip, lumbar spine or forearm. Epidemiological studies from North America[3] have estimated the lifetime risk of common fragility fractures to be 17.5% for hip fracture, 15.6% for clinically diagnosed vertebral fracture and 16% for distal forearm fracture among white women aged 50 years. Corresponding risks among men are 6%, 5% and 2.5%. Estimates from Europe suggest that about 23% of women aged 50 years and over have osteoporosis according to the WHO definition. Fracture rates in Britain are somewhat lower than those in the USA: for women, lifetime fracture incidence rates are 14%, 11% and 13% at hip, spine and distal forearm respectively, while for men the corresponding figures are 3%, 2% and 2%[5] (Table 4.1). Osteoporosis-related fractures are estimated to cost about £1.7 billion annually, and the associated morbidity burden is considerable.

Table 4.1. Impact of osteoporotic fractures in British men and women.

	Hip	Vertebra	Wrist
Lifetime risk (%)			
Women 50 years	14	11	13
Men 50 years	3	2	2
Mean age (years)	79	67	65
Mortality (relative survival)	0.83	0.82	1.00
Functional impairment (%)	30	10	10

The bone mass of an individual in later adult life depends upon the peak obtained during skeletal growth and the subsequent rate of bone loss (Figure 4.1). Preventive strategies against osteoporosis may be aimed at either increasing the peak bone mass obtained or reducing the rates of bone loss. There is evidence to suggest that peak bone mass is inherited, but current genetic markers are able to explain only a small proportion of the variation in individual bone mass or fracture risk.[6] It is likely that environmental influences during early life interact with the genome in establishing the functional level of a variety of metabolic processes involved in skeletal growth. This chapter covers the normal patterns of skeletal growth during intrauterine life, childhood and adolescence; the environmental determinants of peak bone mass, including childhood nutrition and exercise; and the role played in establishing the risk of osteoporosis by influences during intrauterine or very early postnatal life. It also addresses the conceptual basis of the foetal origins hypothesis by considering epidemiological studies pointing to the foetal programming of later osteoporosis risk and animal evidence relating to the programming of skeletal growth and metabolism.

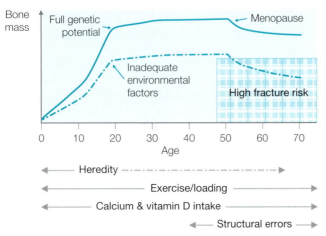

Figure 4.1. Schematic representation of determinants of peak bone mass. Reproduced with permission from: Heaney et al. *Osteoporosis Int* 2000; **11**: 985.

NORMAL SKELETAL GROWTH

Peak bone mass

At any age, the amount and quality of an individual's skeleton reflects everything that has happened from intrauterine life through the years of growth into young adulthood. The skeleton grows as the body grows, in length, breadth, mass and volumetric density. For men and women of normal body weight, total skeletal mass peaks a few years after fusion of the long bone epiphysis. The exact age at which bone mineral accumulation reaches a plateau varies with skeletal region and with how bone mass is measured. Areal density, the most commonly used measurement with dual-energy X-ray absorptiometry (DXA), peaks earliest (prior to age 20 years) at the proximal femur, while total skeletal mass peaks 6–10 years later.[7] However, total skeletal mass does not reflect the considerable heterogeneity in mineral accrual at other skeletal sites. Thus, the skull continues to increase in bone mass throughout life; certain regions, such as the femoral shaft and vertebral bodies, continue to increase in diameter in late adulthood.

The importance of peak bone mass for bone strength during later life was initially suggested by cross-sectional observations that the dispersion of bone mass does not widen with age.[8] This led to the proposition that bone mass tracks throughout life and that an individual at the high end of the population distribution at age 30 years is likely to remain at that end at age 70 years. Recent longitudinal studies have confirmed this tracking, at least across the pubertal growth spurt.[9] Using statistical modelling variation in peak bone mass accrual has been demonstrated to have a greater effect on delaying the onset of osteoporosis than either the timing of the menopause or rate of bone loss in later life.[10]

Bone growth in utero

The foetal skeleton develops in two distinct components, intramembranous (the skull and facial bones) and endochondral (the remainder of the skeleton) ossification. Intramembranous ossification begins with a layer or membrane of mesenchymal cells which becomes highly vascular; the mesenchymal cells then differentiate into isolated osteoblasts, which begin to secrete osteoid. The osteoid matrix is mineralized at the end of the embryonic period to form bony spicules, which are precursors of the lamellae of the Haversian systems. There is no cartilage model preceding ossification in this type of bone development.

Endochondral ossification is responsible for the formation of the bones that are the main sites of fragility fracture in later life. This form of ossification depends on a pre-existing cartilaginous model that undergoes invasion by osteoblasts and is only subsequently mineralized. The development of this cartilage model can be seen by 5 weeks gestation with the migration and condensation of mesenchymal cells in areas destined to form the bone.[11] These pre-cartilagenous anlagen reflect the shape, size, position and number of skeletal elements that will be present in the mature skeleton.

There is then an ordered differentiation of mesenchymal stem cells into chondrocyte precursors, proliferative chondrocytes, prehypertrophic chondrocytes and hypertrophic chondrocytes (Figure 4.2). During these stages of differentiation there is expansion of the bony template and production of an extracellular matrix rich in cytokines, which facilitate vascular invasion and mineralization. The major regulator of the proliferation of chondrocytes in PTHrP,[12] which is secreted by the perichondral cells; other proliferative stimuli include cytokines of the growth hormone (GH)/insulin-like growth factor (IGF) axis.[13] 1,25-Dihydroxyvitamin D_3[14] and tri-iodothyronine[15] are stimuli for the differentiation of the chondrocytes through different stages. Once the cartilage model has been formed, vascular growth factors embedded in the matrix are released by chondrocyte metalloproteinases. This stimulates angiogenesis and, under the influence of Cbfa1,[16] osteoblasts from the perichondrium invade and lay down matrix which is then mineralized.

During the period of a normal human pregnancy the foetus accumulates approximately 30 g of calcium; the majority of this is accrued during the third trimester.[17] To supply this demand, there is a requirement for: (i) an adequate maternal supply of calcium to the placenta; and (ii) increased placental calcium transfer to maintain a foetal serum calcium concentration higher than that in the mother.[18] This materno-foetal gradient emerges as early as 20 weeks of gestation.[19]

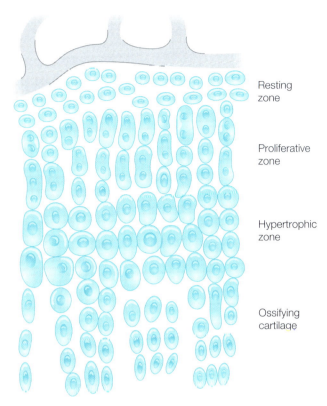

Resting zone

Proliferative zone

Hypertrophic zone

Ossifying cartilage

Figure 4.2. Diagram showing ordered differentiation of chondrocytes in the epiphyseal plate from a resting zone, through proliferative, hypertrophic and ossifactor stages. Reproduced with permission from Mosby. Source: Cormack DH, ed. *Human Histology*, 1997.

There is increased calcium absorption from the gut and also bone resorption to meet this demand. A rise in maternal serum PTHrP and 1,25-dihydroxyvitamin D_3[20] is thought to drive the maternal supply of calcium to the foetus. Net resorption of the maternal skeleton, liberating calcium, starts early in gestation,[21] at a time when the foetal demand is small, and this contributes to maternal calciuria during pregnancy.[22]

During the last trimester, maternal bone formation increases to balance bone resorption.[23] However, there is an overall decrease in the maternal bone mass of up to 10% during pregnancy.[22] Active calcium transfer across the placenta takes place in the cytotrophoblasts and involves specific calcium channels, intracellular calcium-binding proteins in the cytoplasm and calcium ATPases on the placental/foetal interface.[24] While in the mother 1,25-dihydroxyvitamin D_3 is the principle stimulus for calcium absorption, the mid portion of PTHrP is essential at the placenta for the maintenance of the materno-foetal gradient.[25] Secretion of PTHrP by the foetal parathyroid glands also enhances foetal renal calcium reabsorption. The rate of materno-foetal calcium transfer increases dramatically after 24 weeks, such that about two-thirds of total body calcium, phosphorus and magnesium are accumulated in a healthy term human foetus during this period. Factors that increase placental calcium

transport capacity as gestation proceeds are only partly genetically controlled, and are probably achieved through regulatory hormones, including 1,25 dihydroxyvitamin D_3, parathyroid hormone, PTH-related peptide and calcitonin. As the majority of foetal bone is gained during the last trimester, one of the major variables affecting bone mass at birth is gestational age.

Other factors known to influence neonatal bone mineral content (BMC) include environmental variables such as season of birth and maternal lifestyle. Newborn total body bone mineral content has been demonstrated to be lower among winter births than among infants born during the summer.[26] This observation is concordant with lower cord serum dihydroxyvitamin D concentrations observed during winter months, consequent upon maternal vitamin D deficiency. Other postulated contributors to impaired bone mineral acquisition during intrauterine life include maternal smoking, alcohol consumption, caffeine intake and diabetes mellitus.[27]

Bone mineral accrual in infancy and early childhood

During infancy, average whole body BMC increases by 389% and total body bone mineral density increases by 157%.[28] Weight and length are strong predictors of areal BMC and BMD during infancy.[29] However, because no studies of volumetric BMD have been done during the first year of life, it is not clear whether true volumetric density changes during this period. Gilsanz et al.[30] found no significant difference in true volumetric density of the lumbar spine, measured using computed tomography, between male and female, black or white children aged greater than 2 years.

Bone mineral accrual during childhood and adolescence

Cross-sectional and longitudinal studies of bone accretion during childhood have been reported in several Western populations.[31–37] As observed for infants, weight and height emerge as strong predictors of both areal BMC and BMD. Gender and ethnic differences have also been reported. Boys have higher BMC than girls, but these differences are not reflected in areal BMD or volumetric bone density.

Puberty is the period during which the characteristic difference in bone mass observed in adults becomes fully expressed. There is no evidence for a gender difference in bone mass of either the axial or the appendicular skeleton at birth. Similarly, the volumetric bone mineral density also appears similar between male and female neonates. This gender similarity is maintained until the onset of puberty. The most important difference to emerge during pubertal maturation is the greater increase in bone size, consequent upon an increase in the cortical shell in males as compared with females.[38] These gender differences in size contrast with similar values for volumetric bone mineral density between sexes. Studies based on histomorphometry and quantitative computed tomography indicate no difference in volumetric trabecular density at the end of the period of pubertal maturation.

Longitudinal studies using DXA indicate that, during pubertal maturation, areal BMC and BMD at the lumbar spine and proximal femur increase by four- to six-fold over a 3-year period (11–14 years in girls, 13–16 years in boys) (Figure 4.3). The increase in BMD during the corresponding pubertal period appears to be less marked in the diaphyses of long bones such as the radial or femoral shaft, where only two-fold increases are observed.[39]

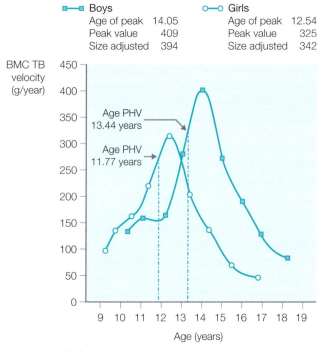

Figure 4.3. Whole body bone mineral content and peak height velocity (PHV). Reproduced with permission of the American Society for Bone and Mineral Research. Source: Bailey DA et al. *J Bone Miner Res* 1999; **14**: 1672–1679.[37]

There is also heterogeneity in linear skeletal growth. Growth of distal limb segments precedes that of proximal segments. Appendicular growth is more rapid than axial growth before puberty, but decelerates at puberty when axial growth accelerates.[35] The differing tempo in bone growth could have important pathophysiological consequences. Regions growing rapidly or relatively distant from their peak may be more affected by illness than those growing slowly or near completion of growth. Depending on age and pubertal maturation, deficits may occur in limb dimensions (pre-pubertal), spine dimensions (early puberty) or volumetric BMD through interference with the phenomenon of consolidation that follows the marked decline in longitudinal growth. In pre-pubertal children, there is a tight relationship between bone mass at the spine or hip, and statural height.[40] This close relationship vanishes during pubertal maturation, with the appearance of the pattern observed in adults, among whom BMD values are poorly correlated with height. Prospective studies have indicated that the period of maximal height gain and maximal accrual of bone mineral are dissociated by approximately 2 years.

DETERMINANTS OF BONE MINERAL ACQUISITION DURING CHILDHOOD AND ADOLESCENCE

Many factors influence the accumulation of bone mineral during growth. These include heredity, gender, diet, mechanical factors (physical activity, body weight), endocrine status (gonadal steroids, calcitriol, IGF-1), and exposure to other risk factors. Evidence from several sources suggests a genetic influence on peak bone mass. Family studies have shown an aggregation of low BMD among the relatives of osteoporotic parents and among the daughters of osteoporotic mothers. More recently, it has been demonstrated that the family history of an osteoporotic fracture predicts low bone mass among both men and women.[41] This relationship appears strongest for a maternal history of hip fracture. Twin studies allow more detailed study of genetic influences, by comparing monozygotic and dizygotic twins. These have consistently demonstrated that monozygotic twin pairs have greater concordance for axial and appendicular BMD than do dizygotic twin pairs, with corresponding estimates of heritability suggesting that as much as 70% of the variance in BMD might be genetic. There is no single genetic marker denoting an inherited susceptibility to osteoporosis. To date, the genes that regulate bone mass are incompletely defined. Potential candidates include the genes for the vitamin D receptor (VDR), the gene encoding type 1 collagen, and genes for the oestrogen receptor, interleukin-6 and transforming growth factor β.

Although it is widely proposed that increasing calcium intake during childhood and adolescence will be associated with greater accrual of bone mass, the evidence relating dietary calcium intake with bone mass among children and young adults has been inconsistent.[42] These studies are difficult to interpret due to the potential confounding by other determinants of bone growth, and have been complemented in recent years by intervention studies. Overall, these studies indicate greater bone mineral accrual among children and adolescents receiving calcium supplementation over periods varying from 12 to 36 months.[43-48] The benefit of supplemental calcium appears greater in the appendicular than in the axial skeleton. Thus, in pre-pubertal children, calcium supplementation is more effective on cortical appendicular bone than on axial trabecular bone.

The skeleton also appears more responsive to calcium supplementation before the onset of pubertal maturation. Finally, the method of administration of calcium is also important, with more pronounced gains observed during administration of milk or calcium phosphate salts from milk extract (Figure 4.4) than from administration of calcium carbonate or calcium citrate salts alone. It remains uncertain whether the gains resulting from such interventions are lost after discontinuation of calcium supplementation. In addition, there is a growing body of evidence to suggest that a proportion of the long-term benefit in areal BMD is due to an earlier onset of puberty in those supplemented with calcium.

Several reports in children and adolescents involved in competitive sport or ballet indicate that intense exercise is associated

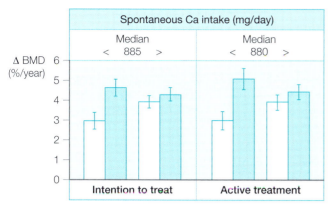

Figure 4.4. Gain in BMD at six skeletal sites among 149 prepubertal girls randomized to receive calcium phosphate supplementation from milk extract (shaded bars), compared with placebo (open bars). (In each analysis, results are divided into those subjects with low and high spontaneous calcium intake.) Reproduced with permission from: Bonjour et al. *J Clin Invest* 1997; **99**: 1287–1294.

with an increase in bone mineral accrual at weight-bearing skeletal sites.[49–51] In some of these investigations, intense exercise seems to be associated with a greater gain in bone size than in volumetric bone mineral density. However, the more relevant issue for public health programmes is the effect of moderate exercise on bone mass acquisition. Some prospective studies have indicated that exercise programmes undertaken in schools may serve to increase the acquisition of bone mass.[52,53] It remains uncertain to what extent the greater gains in areal BMD observed in such studies translate into an increase in bone strength and a reduction in later fracture risk.

Other factors that influence peak bone mass include cigarette smoking, alcohol consumption and the presence of anorexia nervosa or exercise-induced amenorrhoea. The potential beneficial influence of using oral contraceptives remains uncertain.

INTRAUTERINE PROGRAMMING OF OSTEOPOROSIS AND FRACTURE

Epidemiological studies of coronary heart disease performed over a decade ago demonstrated strong geographical associations between death rate from the disorder in 1968–1978 and infant mortality in 1901–1910.[54] Subsequent research, based on individuals whose birth records had been preserved for seven decades, revealed that men and women who were undernourished during intrauterine life, and therefore had low birth weight or were thin at birth, had an increased risk for coronary heart disease, hypertension, non-insulin-dependent diabetes and hypercholesterolaemia.[55] These associations are explained by a phenomenon known as programming or the developmental origins of adult disease;[56] this term describes persisting changes in structure and function caused by environmental stimuli acting at critical periods during early development. During embryonic life, the basic form of the human baby is laid down in miniature. However, the body does not increase greatly in size until the foetal period, when a rapid growth phase

commences, which continues until after birth.[57] The main feature of foetal growth is cell division. Different tissues of the body grow during periods of rapid cell division, so-called 'critical' periods.[58] The timing differs for different tissues; for example, the kidney has a critical period during the weeks immediately before birth, while the long bones accelerate their rate of growth during the second trimester of gestation. The main adaptive response to a lack of nutrients and oxygen during this period of growth is to slow the rate of cell division, especially in tissues that are undergoing critical periods at the time. This reduction in cell division is either direct, or mediated through altered concentrations of growth factors or hormones (in particular insulin, growth hormone and cortisol).

It is not in question that the human skeleton can be programmed by undernutrition. Rickets has served as a long-standing example of undernutrition at a critical stage of early life, leading to persisting changes in structure. What is new is the realization that some of the body's 'memories' of early undernutrition become translated into pathology and thereby determine disease in later life. Evidence has now accumulated that such intrauterine programming contributes to the risk of osteoporosis in later life.

Evidence that the risk of osteoporosis might be modified by environmental influences during early life stems from four groups of studies: (a) bone mineral measurements undertaken in cohorts of adults whose detailed birth and/or childhood records have been preserved; (b) detailed physiological studies exploring the relationship between candidate endocrine systems which might be programmed (GH/IGF-1; hypothalamic–pituitary–adrenal, gonadal steroid) and age-related bone loss; (c) studies characterizing the nutrition, body build and lifestyle of pregnant women and relating these to the bone mass of their newborn offspring; and (d) studies relating childhood growth rates to the later risk of hip fracture.

Epidemiological studies

The first epidemiological evidence that the risk of osteoporosis might be programmed came from a study of 153 women born in Bath during 1968–1969 who were traced and studied at 21 years of age.[59] Data on childhood growth were obtained from linked birth and school health records. There were statistically significant (P < 0.05) associations between weight at 1 year and BMC, but not density, at the lumbar spine and femoral neck; these relationships were independent of adult weight and body mass index. The data suggested a discordance between the processes that govern skeletal growth and those that influence mineralization. They also provide direct evidence that the trajectory of bone growth might be programmed, an assertion previously supported only by inference from measurements of body height. The association between weight in infancy and adult bone mass was replicated in a second cohort study of 238 men and 201 women, aged 60–75 years, who were born and still lived in Hertfordshire.[60] In this study, there were highly significant relationships between weight at 1 year and adult bone area at the spine and hip (P < 0.005); the relationships with BMC at these two sites were

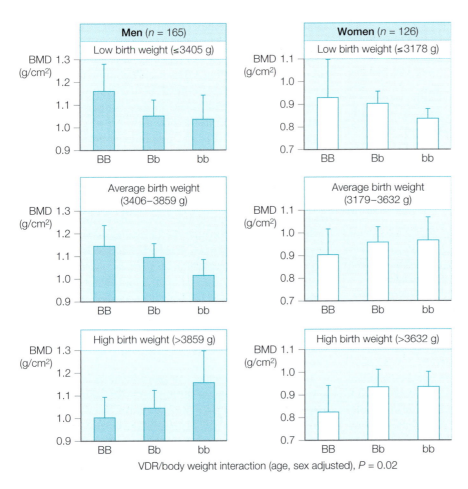

Figure 4.5. Relation between VDR genotype (BB, Bb, bb), birth weight and lumbar spine BMD among 165 men and 126 women resident in Hertfordshire. Reproduced with permission from Blackwell Science Ltd. Source: Dennison EM et al. *Paediatr Perinatal Epidemiol* 2001; **15**: 211–219.[62]

weaker but remained statistically significant ($P < 0.02$). They also remained after adjustment for known genetic markers of osteoporosis risk, such as polymorphisms in the gene for the vitamin D receptor[61] and for collagen IAI, and after adjustment for lifestyle characteristics in adulthood that might have influenced bone mass (physical activity, dietary calcium intake, cigarette smoking and alcohol consumption). More detailed analyses of the interactions between polymorphism in the gene for the vitamin D receptor, birth weight and bone mineral density have recently been published from the same cohort study. In the cohort as a whole, there were no significant associations between either birth weight or VDR genotype and bone mineral density. However, the relationship between lumbar spine BMD and vitamin D receptor (VDR) genotype varied according to birth weight. Among individuals in the lowest third of birth weight, spine BMD was higher ($P = 0.01$) among individuals of genotype 'BB' after adjustment for age, sex and weight at baseline. In contrast, spine BMD was reduced ($P = 0.04$) in individuals of the same genotype who were in the highest third of the birth weight distribution. A statistically significant ($P = 0.02$) interaction was also found between VDR genotype and birth weight as determinants of BMD. These results suggest that genetic influences on adult bone size and mineral density may be modified by undernutrition in utero[62] (Figure 4.5). Subsequent studies from the USA, Australia and Scandinavia

Table 4.2. Growth in infancy and adult bone mass.*

Site		Birth weight	Weight at 1 year
BMC	L/S†	0.15 (0.10–0.20)	0.25 (0.19–0.32)
	F/N	0.12 (0.07–0.18)	0.20 (0.14–0.27)
	W/B	0.19 (0.10–0.28)	0.44 (0.35–0.52)
BMD	L/S	0.12 (0.07–0.16)	0.11 (0.04–0.18)
	F/N	0.12 (0.07–0.16)	0.05 (−0.02–0.12)
	W/B	0.24 (0.17–0.30)	0.25 (0.15–0.35)

*Figures are correlation coeffcients with 95% CI. Data are derived from published studies ($n = 10$) relating weight in infancy and adult bone mass.
†L/S, lumbar spine; F/N, femoral neck; W/B, whole body.

have replicated these relationships between weight in infancy and adult bone mass (Table 4.2).

Physiological studies

To explore further the potential role of hypothalamic/pituitary function and its relevance to the pathogenesis of osteoporosis, profiles of circulating GH and cortisol were compared with bone density among groups of men and women whose birth records had been preserved. These studies revealed that birth weight and weight in infancy were predictors of basal levels of GH and cortisol during later adult life.[63–65] The levels of these two skeletally active hormones were also found to be determinants of prospectively determined bone loss rate. The data are compatible with the hypothesis that environmental stressors during intrauterine or early postnatal life alter the sensitivity of the growth plate to GH and cortisol. The consequence of such endocrine programming would be to reduce peak skeletal size, perhaps also to reduce mineralization, and to predispose to an accelerated rate of bone loss during later life.[63–65]

Maternal nutrition, lifestyle and neonatal bone mineral

The third piece of epidemiological evidence that osteoporosis might be programmed stems from investigation of a series of mothers through pregnancy; anthropometric and lifestyle maternal characteristics were related to the bone mineral of their newborn offspring.[66,67] After adjusting for sex and gestational age, neonatal bone mass was strongly positively associated with birth weight, birth length and placental weight. Other determinants included maternal and paternal birth weight, and maternal triceps skinfold thickness at 28 weeks (Figure 4.6). Maternal smoking and maternal energy intake at 18 weeks gestation were negatively associated with neonatal BMC at both the spine and whole body (Figure 4.7). The independent effects of maternal and paternal birth weight on foetal skeletal development support the notion that paternal influences – for example, through the imprinting of growth promoting genes such as IGF-2 – contribute strongly to the establishment of the early skeletal growth trajectory, while maternal nutrition and body

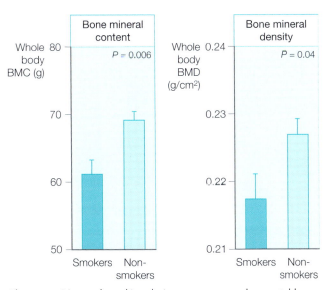

Figure 4.7. Maternal smoking during pregnancy and neonatal bone mineral among 144 term neonates. Values are mean ± SE P-values adjusted for sex and gestation. Reproduced with permission of the American Society for Bone and Mineral Research. Source: Godfrey K et al. *J Bone Miner Res* 2001; **16**: 1694–1703.[67]

build modify foetal nutrient supply and subsequent bone accretion, predominantly through influences on placentation.

Childhood growth and hip fracture

Most evidence relating the intrauterine environment to later osteoporosis stems from studies utilizing non-invasive assessment of bone mineral. The clinically important consequence of reduced bone mass is fracture, and data are now available that directly link growth rates in childhood with the risk of later hip fracture.[68] Studies of a unique Finnish cohort, in whom birth and childhood growth data were linked to later hospital discharge records for hip fracture, have permitted follow-up of about 7000 men and women who were born in Helsinki University Central Hospital during the period 1924–1933. Body size at birth was recorded and an average of 10 measurements were obtained of height and weight throughout childhood. The incidence of hip fracture was assessed in this cohort using the Finnish hospital discharge registration system. After adjustment for age and sex, there were two major determinants of hip fracture risk: tall maternal height ($P < 0.001$), and low rate of childhood growth (height, $P = 0.006$; weight, $P = 0.01$) (Figure 4.8). The effects of maternal height and childhood growth rate were statistically independent of each other, and remained after adjusting for socio-economic status. More important, hip fracture risk was also elevated ($P = 0.05$) among babies born short. These data are compatible with endocrine programming influencing the risk of hip fracture. In addition, the observation that fracture subjects were shorter at birth, but of average height by age 7 years, suggests that the risk of hip fracture might be particularly elevated among children in whom growth of the skeletal envelope is forced ahead of the capacity to mineralize, a phenomenon that is accelerated during pubertal growth.

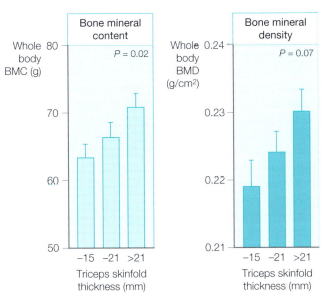

Figure 4.6. Maternal triceps skinfold thickness in early pregnancy and neonatal bone mineral among 144 term neonates. Values are mean ± SE P-values adjusted for sex and gestation. Reproduced with permission of the American Society for Bone and Mineral Research. Source: Godfrey K et al. *J Bone Miner Res* 2001; **16**: 1694–1703.[67]

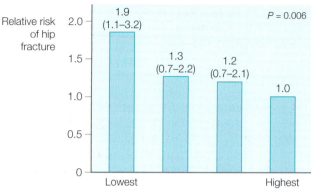

Figure 4.8. Rate of childhood height gain between age 7 and 15 years, and later risk of hip fracture among 3639 men and 3447 women born in Helsinki University Central Hospital between 1924 and 1933. Reproduced with permission from: Cooper C et al. *Osteoporosis Int* 2001; **12**: 623–629.[68]

Mechanisms of programming

Numerous animal experiments have shown that hormones, undernutrition and other influences that affect development during sensitive periods of early life permanently programme the structure and physiology of the body's tissues and systems. A remarkable example is the effect of temperature on the sex of reptiles.[69] If the eggs of an American alligator are incubated at 30°C, all the offspring are female. If incubated at 33°C, all the off-spring are male. At temperatures between 30 and 33°C, there are varying proportions of females and males. It is believed that the fundamental sex is female, and a transcription factor is required to divert growth along a male pathway. Instead of the transcription factor being controlled genetically by a sex chromosome, it depends on the environment, specifically temperature.

Organ systems in the body are most susceptible to programming during periods when they are growing rapidly. During the first 2 months of life, the embryonic period, there is extensive differentiation of progenitor cells, without rapid cell replication. Thereafter, in the foetal period, the highest growth rates are observed. Growth slows in late gestation and continues to slow in childhood. The high growth rates of the foetus compared with the child are mostly the result of cell replication; the proportion of cells that are dividing becomes progressively less as the foetus becomes older. Slowing of growth is a major adaptation to undernutrition. Experiments on rats, mice, sheep and pigs have demonstrated that protein or calorie restriction of the mother during pregnancy and lactation is associated with smaller offspring.[69–72] In general, the earlier in life that undernutrition occurs, the more likely it is to have permanent effects on body size.[73] Early in embryonic life, growth is regulated by the supply of nutrients and oxygen. At some point shortly after birth, growth begins to track. In humans, tracking is demonstrated by the way in which infants grow along centile curves. Once tracking is established it is no longer possible to make animals grow faster by offering them unlimited food. The rate of growth has become set, homeostatically controlled by feedback systems. After a period of undernutrition, they will regain their expected size. This contrasts with the effects of undernutrition during intrauterine life, in which skeletal development is slowed and the peak skeletal proportions attained following the completion of linear growth are reduced.

There are three cellular mechanisms for the induction of programming. First, the nutrient environment may permanently alter gene expression; one example of this is permanent change in the activity of metabolic enzymes such as HMG-CoA reductase.[74] Second, early nutrition may permanently reduce cell numbers. The small but normally proportioned rat produced by undernutrition before weaning has been shown to have fewer cells in its organs and tissues.[75] Growth-retarded human babies have reduced numbers of cells in their pancreas, which may limit insulin secretion,[76] and reduced size of their airways, which may limit respiratory function.[77] Third, certain clones of cells may be altered by environmental adversity during development; for example, an altered balance of the TH-1 and TH-2 lymphocyte subtypes might predispose to atopic disease in later life.[78] Evidence from the human studies outlined above suggests that skeletal development might be programmed as a consequence of the first two of these mechanisms.

In the most recent work, data from mother offspring cohorts has demonstrated that maternal vitamin D status during late pregnancy and neonatal calcium status at birth may have persisting effects on the bone mass of her offspring which are evident in the pre-pubertal age group.[79]

Summary

Undernutrition and other adverse influences arising in foetal life or immediately after birth have a permanent effect on body structure, physiology and metabolism. The specific effects of undernutrition depend on the time and development at which it occurs; rapidly growing foetuses and neonates are more vulnerable. Its effects include altered gene expression, reduced cell numbers, imbalance between cell types, altered organ structure, and changes in the pattern of hormonal release and tissue sensitivity to these hormones. Evidence is now accumulating from human studies that programming of bone growth might be an important contributor to the later risk of osteoporotic fracture. Body weight in infancy is a determinant of adult bone mineral content, as well as of the basal levels of activity of the GH/IGF-1 and HPA axes. Epidemiological studies have suggested that maternal smoking and nutrition during pregnancy and vitamin D status influence intrauterine skeletal mineralization. Finally, childhood growth rates have been directly linked to the risk of hip fracture many decades later. Further studies of this phenomenon are required in order that effective preventive strategies against osteoporosis throughout the life course may be delineated and more effectively applied.

CONCLUSIONS

Several modifiable factors influence the growing skeleton and permit it to achieve its full genetic potential. These may act during intrauterine or early postnatal life, childhood, or adolescence. While many important research questions need to be addressed in this area, concerted action in health policy should be directed at: (1) optimizing maternal nutrition and intrauterine growth; (2) improving the calcium intake and general nutritional levels of all children; (3) increasing the general exercise level of pre-pubertal and pubertal children; (4) ensuring adequate vitamin D status, not just during infancy but throughout the period of growth and during pregnancy. Further research into the interaction between the genome and early environmental risk factors for osteoporotic fracture is urgently required in order that environmental modification can be targeted to those at the greatest risk. Finally, intervention studies exploring the role of maternal lifestyle and nutrition on bone mineral accrual among the offspring of these mothers will provide much needed evidence on this approach to the reduction in fracture risk of future generations.

ACKNOWLEDGEMENTS

We are grateful to the Medical Research Council, the Wellcome Trust, the Arthritis Research Campaign and the National Osteoporosis Society for support of our research programme into the foetal origins of osteoporotic fracture. Dr Kassim Javaid was in receipt of an ARC Clinical Research Fellowship. The manuscript was prepared by Gill Strange.

PRACTICE POINTS

- Environmental influences during intrauterine and early postnatal life lead to persisting alterations in bone mineral accrual during childhood and adolescence, which modify fracture risk in later decades.

- Maternal lifestyle (smoking, undernutrition and physical activity), as well as maternal vitamin D insufficiency, independently modify placental calcium transport and thereby reduce the rate of intrauterine and postnatal bone mineral accrual. Maintenance of adequate vitamin D status among mothers during pregnancy will reduce the risks of osteoporosis in their offspring.

RESEARCH AGENDA

- Further studies to elucidate the underlying molecular mechanisms of skeletal programming. This would assist the early identification of those at higher risk of fragility fracture in later adulthood.

- The identification of critical periods during early life, during which safe interventions can be instituted leading to long-term augmentation of peak bone mass.

- Randomized controlled trials of dietary interventions in the mother and child to improve the child's peak bone mass.

REFERENCES

1. Consensus Development Conference. Prophylaxis and treatment of osteoporosis. *Osteoporosis Int* 1991; **1**: 114–117.

2. World Health Organization. Assessment of fracture risk and its application to screening for post-menopausal osteoporosis. *WHO Technical Report Series.* Geneva: WHO, 1994.

3. Melton LJ III. How many women have osteoporosis now? *J Bone Miner Res* 1995; **10**: 175–177.

4. Cummings SR, Black DM, Nevitt MC et al. Bone density at various sites for prediction of hip fractures. *Lancet* 1993; **341**: 72–75.

5. Dennison E & Cooper C. The epidemiology of osteoporosis. *Br J Clin Pract* 1996; **50**: 33–36.

6. Ralston SH. Do genetic markers aid in risk assessment? *Osteoporosis Int* 1998; **8**: S37–S42.

7. Matkovic V, Jelic T, Wardlaw GM et al. Timing of peak bone mass in Caucasian females and its implication for the prevention of osteoporosis. *J Clin Invest* 1994; **93**: 799–808.

8. Newton John HF & Morgan BD. The loss of bone with age: osteoporosis and fractures. *Clin Orthop* 1970; **71**: 229–232.

9. Ferrari S, Rizzoli R, Slosman D et al. Familial resemblance for bone mineral mass is expressed before puberty. *J Clin Endocrinol Metab* 1998; **83**: 358–361.

10. Hernandez CJ, Beaupre GS & Carter DR. A theoretical analysis of the relative influences of peak BMD, age-related bone loss and menopause on the development of osteoporosis. *Osteoporosis Int* 2003; **14**: 843–847.

11. DeLise AM, Fischer L & Tuan RS. Cellular interactions and signaling in cartilage development. *Osteoarth Cartil* 2000; **8**: 309–334.

12. Karaplis AC, Luz A, Glowacki J et al. Lethal skeletal dysplasia from targeted disruption of the parathyroid hormone-related peptide gene. *Genes Dev* 1994; **8**: 277–289.

13. Bhaumick B & Bala RM. Differential effects of insulin-like growth factors I and II on growth, differentiation and glucoregulation in differentiating chondrocyte cells in culture. *Acta Endocrinol (Copenh)* 1991; **125**: 201–211.

14. Sylvia VL, Del Toro F, Hardin RR et al. Characterization of PGE(2) receptors (EP) and their role as mediators of 1alpha,25-(OH)(2)D(3) effects on growth zone chondrocytes. *J Steroid Biochem Molec Biol* 2001; **78**: 261–274.

15. Quarto R, Campanile G, Cancedda R et al. Modulation of commitment, proliferation, and differentiation of chondrogenic cells in defined culture medium. *Endocrinology* 1997; **138**: 4966–4976.

16. Ducy P. Cbfa1: a molecular switch in osteoblast biology. *Devl Biol* 2000; **219**: 461–471.

17. Widdowson EM, Southgate DAT & Hey E. Fetal growth and body composition. *Perinatal Nutr* 1988; **4**: 14.

18. Schauberger CW & Pitkin RM. Maternal–perinatal calcium relationships. *Obstet Gynecol* 1979; **53**: 74–76.

19. Forester F, Daffos F, Rainaut M et al. Blood chemistry of normal human fetuses at mid-trimester of pregnancy. *Paediatr Res* 1987; **21**: 579.

20. Ardawi MS, Nasrat HA & BA'Aqueel HS. Calcium-regulating hormones and parathyroid hormone-related peptide in normal human pregnancy and postpartum: a longitudinal study. *Eur J Endocrinol* 1997; **137**: 402–409.

21. Purdie DW, Aaron JE & Selby PL. Bone histology and mineral homeostasis in human pregnancy. *Br J Obstet Gynaecol* 1988; **95**: 849–854.

22. Gambacciani M, Spinetti A, Gallo R et al. Ultrasonographic bone characteristics during normal pregnancy: longitudinal and cross-sectional evaluation. *Am J Obstet Gynecol* 1995; **173**: 890–893.

23. Black AJ, Topping J, Durham B et al. A detailed assessment of alterations in bone turnover, calcium homeostasis, and bone density in normal pregnancy. *J Bone Miner Res* 2000; **15**: 557–563.

24. Hosking DJ. Calcium homeostasis in pregnancy. *Clin Endocrinol (Oxford)* 1996; **45**: 1–6.

25. Kovacs CS, Lanske B, Hunzelman JL et al. Parathyroid hormone-related peptide (PTHrP) regulates fetal–placental calcium transport through a receptor distinct from the PTH/PTHrP receptor. *Proc Natl Acad Sci USA* 1996; **93**: 15233–15238.

26. Namgung R, Tsang RC, Li C et al. Low total body bone mineral content and high bone resorption in Korean winter-born versus summer-born newborn infants. *J Paediatr* 1998; **132**: 285–288.

27. Specker BL, Namgung R & Tsang RC. Bone mineral acquisition in utero, during infancy, and throughout childhood. In: Marcus R, Feldman D & Kelsey J, eds. *Osteoporosis*, 2nd edn, Vol. 1. New York: Academic Press, 2001; 599–620.

28. Koo WWK, Bush AJ, Walters J et al. Postnatal development of bone mineral status during infancy. *J Am Coll Nutr* 1998; **17**: 65–70.

29. Li JY, Specker BL, Ho ML et al. Bone mineral content in black and white children 1–6 years of age. *Am J Dis Child* 1989; **143**: 1346–1349.

30. Gilsanz V, Roe TF, Mora S et al. Changes in vertebral bone density in black girls and white girls during childhood and puberty. *N Engl J Med* 1991; **325**: 1597–1600.

31. Ellis KJ, Shypailo RJ, Hergenroeder A et al. Total body calcium and bone mineral content: comparison of dual energy X-ray absorptiometry with neutron activation analysis. *J Bone Miner Res* 1996; **11**: 843–848.

32. Moro M, Vandermeulen MCH, Kiratli BJ et al. Body mass is the primary determinant of mid-femoral bone acquisition during adolescent growth. *Bone* 1996; **19**: 519–526.

33. Molgaard C, Thomsen BL & Michaelsen KF. Whole body bone mineral accretion in healthy children and adolescents. *Arch Dis Child* 1999; **81**: 10–15.

34. Nelson DA, Simpson PM, Johnson CC et al. The accumulation of whole body skeletal mass in third and fourth grade children: effects of age, gender, ethnicity and body composition. *Bone* 1997; **20**: 73–78.

35. Bass S, Delmas PD, Pearce G et al. The differing tempo of growth in bone size, mass and density in girls is region-specific. *J Clin Invest* 1999; **104**: 795–804.

36. Gilsanz V, Gibbens D, Roe T et al. Vertebral bone density in children: effect of puberty. *Radiology* 1988; **166**: 847–850.

37. Bailey DA, McKay HA, Mirwald RL et al. A six year longitudinal study of the relationship of physical activity to bone mineral accrual in growing children. The University of Saskatchewan bone mineral accrual study. *J Bone Miner Res* 1999; **14**: 1672–1679.

38. Seeman E. From density to structure: growing up and growing old on the surfaces of bone. *J Bone Miner Res* 1997; **12**: 509–521.

39. Theintz G, Buchs B, Rizzoli R et al. Longitudinal monitoring of bone mass accumulation in healthy adolescents: evidence for a marked reduction after 18 years of age at the levels of the lumbar spine and femoral neck in female subjects. *J Clin Endocrinol Metab* 1992; **75**: 1060–1065.

40. Bonjour JP, Theintz G, Buchs B et al. Critical years and stages of puberty for spinal and femoral bone mass accumulation during adolescence. *J Clin Endocrinol Metab* 1991; **73**: 555–563.

41. Walker-Bone K, Dennison E & Cooper C. Osteoporosis. In: Silman AJ & Hochberg MC, eds. *Epidemiology of the Rheumatic Diseases*, 2nd edn. Oxford: Oxford University Press, 2001; 259–292.

42. Rizzoli R, Bonjour JP & Ferrari SL. Osteoporosis, genetics and hormones. *J Molec Endocrinol* 2001; **26**: 79–94.

43. Matkovic V, Fontana D, Tominac C et al. Factors that influence peak bone mass formation: a study of calcium balance and the inheritance of bone mass in adolescent females. *Am J Clin Nutr* 1990; **52**: 878–888.

44. Johnston CC, Millar JZ, Slemenda CW et al. Calcium supplementation and increases in bone mineral density in children. *N Engl J Med* 1992; **327**: 82–87.

45. Lloyd T, Andon MB, Rollings N et al. Calcium supplementation and bone mineral density in adolescent girls. *JAMA* 1993; **270**: 841–844.

46. Lee WTK, Leung SFF, Wang SH et al. Double-blind controlled calcium supplementation and bone mineral accretion in children accustomed to a low calcium diet. *Am J Clin Nutr* 1994; **60**: 744–750.

47. Nowson CA, Green RM, Hopper JL et al. A co-twin study of the effect of calcium supplementation on bone density during adolescence. *Osteoporosis Int* 1997; **7**: 219–225.

48. Zamora SA, Rizzoli R, Belli DC et al. Vitamin D supplementation during infancy is associated with higher bone mineral mass in prepubertal girls. *J Clin Endocrinol Metab* 1999; **84**: 4541–4544.

49. Karlsson MK, Johnell O & Obrandt KJ. Is bone mineral density advantage maintained long-term in previous weight lifters? *Calcif Tissue Int* 1995; **57**: 325–328.

50. Bass S, Pearce G, Bradney M et al. Exercise before puberty may confer residual benefits in bone density in adulthood: studies in active, prepubertal and retired female gymnasts. *J Bone Miner Res* 1998; **13**: 500–507.

51. Kannus P, Haapasalo H, Sankelo M et al. Effect of starting age of physical activity on bone mass in the dominant arm of tennis and squash players. *Ann Intern Med* 1995; **123**: 27–31.

52. Morris FL, Naughton GA, Gibbs JL et al. Prospective 10-month exercise intervention in pre-menarcheal girls: positive effects on bone and lean mass. *J Bone Miner Res* 1997; **12**: 1453–1462.

53. Bradney M, Pearce G, Naughton G et al. Moderate exercise during growth in prepubertal boys: changes in bone mass size, volumetric density and bone strength. A controlled prospective study. *J Bone Miner Res* 1998; **13**: 1814–1821.

54. Barker DJP. Fetal origins of coronary heart disease. *BMJ* 1995; **311**: 171–174.

55. Barker DJP. The fetal origins of adult disease. *Proc R Soc Lond, Ser B* 1995; **262**: 37–43.

56. Lucas A. Programming by early nutrition in man. In: Bock GR & Whelan J, eds. *The Childhood Environment and Adult Disease*. New York: John Wiley, 1991; 38–55.

57. Wolpert L. *The Triumph of the Embryo*. Oxford: Oxford University Press, 1991.

58. Widdowson EM & McCance RA. The determinants of growth and form. *Proc R Soc Lond, Ser B* 1974; **185**: 1–17.

59. Cooper C, Cawley MID, Bhalla A et al. Childhood growth, physical activity and peak bone mass in women. *J Bone Miner Res* 1995; **10**: 940–947.

60. Cooper C, Fall C, Egger P et al. Growth in infancy and bone mass in later life. *Ann Rheum Dis* 1997; **56**: 17–21.

61. Keen R, Egger P, Fall C et al. Polymorphisms of the vitamin D receptor, infant growth and adult bone mass. *Calcif Tissue Int* 1997; **60**: 233–235.

62. Dennison EM, Arden NK, Keen RW et al. Birthweight, vitamin D receptor genotype and the programming of osteoporosis. *Paediatr Perinatal Epidemiol* 2001; **15**: 211–219.

63. Fall C, Hindmarsh P, Dennison E et al. Programming of growth hormone secretion and bone mineral density in elderly men; an hypothesis. *J Clin Endocrinol Metab* 1998; **83**: 135–139.

64. Dennison E, Hindmarsh P, Fall C et al. Profiles of endogenous circulating cortisol and bone mineral density in healthy elderly men. *J Clin Endocrinol Metab* 1999; **84**: 3058–3063.

65. Phillips DIW, Barker DJP, Fall CHD et al. Elevated plasma cortisol concentrations: a link between low birthweight and the insulin resistance syndrome? *J Clin Endocrinol Metab* 1998; **83**: 757–760.

66. Dennison E, Godfrey K, Wheeler T et al. Determinants of neonatal bone mass. *Bone* 1997; **20**: 26S (abstract).

67. Godfrey K, Walker-Bone K, Robinson S et al. Neonatal bone mass: influence of parental birthweight, maternal smoking, body composition, and activity during pregnancy. *J Bone Miner Res* 2001; **16**: 1694–1703.

68. Cooper C, Eriksson JG, Forsén T et al. Maternal height, childhood growth and risk of hip fracture in later life: a longitudinal study. *Osteoporosis Int* 2001; **12**: 623–629.

69. Barker DJP. Programming the baby. In: Barker DJP, ed. *Mothers, Babies and Health in Later Life*. London: Churchill Livingstone, 1998; 13–41.

70. McCance RA & Widdowson EM. The determinants of growth and form. *Proc R Soc Lond, Ser B* 1974; **185**: 1–17.

71. Smart JL, Massey RF, Nash SC et al. Effects of early life undernutrition in artificially reared rats: subsequent body and organ growth. *Br J Nutr* 1987; **58**: 245–255.

72. Chow BF & Lee CJ. Effect of dietary restriction of pregnant rats on body weight gain of the offspring. *J Nutr* 1964; **82**: 10–18.

73. McCance RA & Widdowson EM. Nutrition and growth. *Proc R Soc Lond, Ser B* 1962; **156**: 326–337.

74. Brown SA, Rogers LK, Dunn JK et al. Development of cholesterol homeostatic memory in the rat is influenced by maternal diets. *Metabolism* 1990; **39**: 468–473.

75. McLeod KI, Goldrick RB & Whyte HM. The effect of maternal malnutrition on the progeny in the rat: studies on growth, body composition and organ cellularity in first and second generation progeny. *Aust J Exp Biol Med Sci* 1972; **50**: 435–446.

76. Snoeck A, Remacle C, Reusens B et al. Effect of a low protein diet during pregnancy on the fetal rat endocrine pancreas. *Biol Neonate* 1990; **57**: 107–118.

77. Matsui R, Thurlbeck WM, Fujita Y et al. Connective tissue, mechanical, and morphometric changes in the lungs of weanling rats fed a low protein diet. *Pediatr Pulmonol* 1989; **7**: 159–166.

78. Godfrey KM, Barker DJP & Osmond C. Disproportionate fetal growth and raised IGE concentration in adult life. *Clin Exp Allergy* 1994; **24**: 641–648.

79. Javaid MK, Crozier SR, Harvey NC et al. Maternal vitamin D status during pregnancy and childhood bone mass at age 9 years: a longitudinal study. *Lancet* 2006; **367**: 36–43.

Chapter 5
Glucocorticoid-induced osteoporosis

Ian R. Reid

INTRODUCTION

It is now more than 50 years since the introduction of gluco-corticoids into clinical practice, and their continued widespread use attests to their unrivalled efficacy in a number of major illnesses, including obstructive respiratory disease, inflammatory conditions such as rheumatoid arthritis, temporal arteritis and inflammatory bowel disease. They also continue to have a major role in the management of organ transplantation. Their substantial therapeutic efficacy is counterbalanced by a number of major side-effects, which sometimes produce morbidity comparable to that of the original illness. One of these is the development of osteoporosis. An emphasis on this particular problem is most appropriate at this time, since developments in both diagnostics and therapeutics have made it possible to predict those who will have fractures, and to effectively intervene to prevent this eventuality. Thus, the assessment of fracture risk and the appropriate use of interventions have moved from only being on the research agenda to now being a major responsibility incumbent on any doctor prescribing glucocorticoid drugs.

PATHOGENESIS

Because of the widespread distribution of the glucocorticoid receptor, these agents are able to impact on bone and calcium metabolism at many levels.

Osteoblasts

The most consistently demonstrated effects of glucocorticoids on bone are in the osteoblast. In general, glucocorticoids can be characterized as increasing osteoblast differentiation and decreasing the proliferation of these cells,[1,2] though these findings are dependent on the experimental conditions used.[3] Increased differentiation may be partly attributable to increased production of bone morphogenic protein-6,[4] and the reduced proliferation to reduced expression of cyclin-dependent kinases and cyclin-D3, together with enhanced transcription of inhibitors of cyclin-dependent kinases.[5] There is also evidence for glucocorticoid regulation of a number of important osteoblast genes, including those for type I collagen, osteocalcin, osteopontin, fibronectin, β-1 integrin, bone sialoprotein, alkaline phosphatase, collagenase, and the nuclear proto-oncogenes c-myc, c-fos, c-jun and dickkopf-1.[6] The induction of dickkopf-1 provides an antagonist to Wnt signalling, which is a crucial regulator for bone formation, so is likely to contribute to the reduced osteoblast anabolism of glucocorticoid excess. The effects on type I collagen mRNA are reflected in reduced intracellular immunoreactivity for type I procollagen in osteoblasts treated with dexamethasone, as well as reduced levels of procollagen propeptides in the culture medium.[7]

Osteoblasts produce factors which act in an autocrine manner to regulate their own activity. Insulin-like growth factors (IGFs)-1 and -2 act in this way, and their local synthesis is inhibited by glucocorticoids. Their local activity is modulated by the interplay of specific binding proteins and there is now evidence for a reduction in the levels of the stimulatory binding proteins, IGFBP-3 and IGFBP-5, and for increased production of IGFBP-6, an inhibitor of IGF-2 activity. However, blocking the effects of endogenous IGFs does not abrogate the effect of glucocorticoids on osteoblast proliferation and collagen synthesis. Transforming growth factor-β is a further important autocrine factor modulated by glucocorticoids.

Osteoblast factors play important paracrine roles in regulating the differentiation and activity of osteoclasts, through the production of osteoprotegerin and receptor activator of NF-κB ligand (RANKL). Hofbauer et al.[8] have shown that glucocorticoids promote osteoclastogenesis by inhibiting osteoprotegerin production and by stimulating RANKL production in a variety of osteoblastic cell models. These effects on osteoprotegerin have been confirmed by others.[2] Von Tirpitz et al.[9] have found the same pattern of changes in circulating levels of these two proteins in patients with Crohn's disease treated with glucocorticoids, and Sasaki et al.[10,11] also found that steroid treatment reduced circulating osteoprotegerin, though this protein appears to be increased in patients with Cushing's syndrome.[12] Following heart transplantation, serum osteoprotegerin falls by almost 50%, accounting for 67% of the variance in bone loss over the first 6 months, and is related to fracture risk.[13]

A major contributor to the negative effects of glucocorticoids on osteoblasts is their promotion of apoptosis, both in these cells and in osteocytes.[14] The latter may be a key contributor to the loss of skeletal strength caused by glucocorticoids, since transgenic mouse models of steroid treatment in which there is bone loss but not osteoblast/osteocyte apoptosis do not show a loss of vertebral compressive strength.[15] Assessments of biochemical markers of bone formation consistently show evidence of reduced bone formation (Table 5.1).

Osteoclasts

The direct effects of glucocorticoids on osteoclasts are contradictory. There is evidence that glucocorticoids increase rodent osteoclast formation from precursor cells in bone marrow,[16,17] but also that they lead to apoptosis of mature rodent osteoclasts.[18,19] In human cell cultures, glucocorticoids stimulate the proliferation and differentiation of osteoclast precursors but inhibit the bone-resorbing activity of mature osteoclasts.[20] These opposing effects may account for the findings that glucocorticoids can either increase or decrease bone resorption in organ culture, depending on the culture conditions.[21–23] In organ culture, glucocorticoid effects may also be contributed to

by their effects on osteoprotegerin and RANKL, as discussed above, and by inhibition of local production of cytokines such as interleukin-1 and the tumour necrosis factors, which are important regulators of bone resorption.

Animal and human studies are also difficult to interpret, showing an increase in the eroded bone surface but a decrease in the number of osteoclasts. These findings could be accounted for by a reduced rate of recruitment of osteoblasts to the sites at which bone has been resorbed, leaving eroded surfaces unfilled for a greater time than normal. Thus, there is probably not an increased rate of bone resorption, and most of the human studies of biochemical markers of bone resorption would be consistent with this conclusion (Table 5.1).

Intestinal and renal handling of calcium and phosphate

Clinical studies have consistently demonstrated an inhibition of calcium absorption associated with glucocorticoid treatment. This is not mediated by changes in vitamin D metabolites and is therefore likely to represent a direct effect on the small intestine.

Within weeks of glucocorticoid treatment there is a substantial rise in urine calcium excretion,[24] which is not accounted for

Table 5.1. Prospective studies of the effects of glucocorticoids on biochemical markers of bone turnover.

	Study reference												
	122	123	26	124	40	125	126	127	128	129	130	9	11
Duration	12W	4W	5W	8d	5d	3d	1W	1W	4m	1W	2y	3m	6m
Formation markers													
Osteocalcin	↓	→	↓↓	↓	↓		↓		↓	↓	↓	↓	↓
Total ALP	↓	↓		→	↓		↓						
Bone ALP	↓				→				↓				↓
PICP				↓		↓	↓	↓					
PINP										↓			
Resorption markers													
ICTP				↓		↓	↓	→*					
Pyridinoline			→	↓			→	↓					
Deoxypyridinoline				↓	→	→		↓				→	
Hydroxyproline	→	↑	→	→			↓				→		
TRAP			↑		→								↑
sCTX										→			
uCTX											→		
Urine calcium	↑	↑		→			↑				↑		

ALP, alkaline phosphatase; ICTP, type I collagen C-telopeptide; PICP, procollagen type I carboxy-propeptide; PINP, procollagen type I amino-propeptide; sCTX, serum C-telopeptide of type I collagen; TRAP, tartrate-resistant acid phosphatase; uCTX, urine C-telopeptide of type I collagen.
*Changes inversely related to age – mean change, nil.
Copyright © Reid IR, used with permission.

by changes in the serum ionized calcium or the glomerular filtration rate. This suggests that glucocorticoids directly regulate tubular resorption of calcium.[25] There is also evidence for malabsorption of phosphate in both the gut and renal tubule associated with glucocorticoid use.[26]

Vitamin D

There is little evidence to support the contention that changes in vitamin D metabolism contribute significantly to the development of steroid osteoporosis. Prospective studies of patients or normal subjects beginning steroid therapy have shown no changes in 25-hydroxyvitamin D or 24,25-dihydroxyvitamin D, but significant increases in 1,25-dihydroxyvitamin D 2–15 days after initiation of therapy.[26] These are likely to be secondary to changes in parathyroid hormone and/or serum phosphate concentrations. There is no evidence for glucocorticoid effects on concentrations of vitamin D binding protein.[27]

Parathyroid hormone

Hyperparathyroidism has been inconsistently demonstrated in human and animal studies spanning durations of steroid use from minutes to years. Some cross-sectional studies of patients receiving chronic glucocorticoid therapy show elevations of parathyroid hormone levels 50–100% above those of control subjects, though others show no effect. Glucocorticoids appear to directly stimulate parathyroid hormone secretion though, in vivo, calcium malabsorption in both the gut and the renal tubule probably also contribute.

Sex hormones

Sex hormones are important regulators of bone metabolism, and hypogonadism in either sex is associated with the development of osteoporosis. Glucocorticoids acutely depress plasma levels of testosterone in men[28] and their chronic use is associated with a dose-dependent reduction in free testosterone concentrations of approximately 50%.[29] These changes appear to result from inhibition of gonadotropin secretion and a reduction in numbers of gonadotropin-binding sites in the testis. Circulating oestradiol and adrenal androgen concentrations are also reduced in men on glucocorticoids.[30] High-dose steroid therapy is associated with oligomenorrhoea in women, suggesting a similar effect on the pituitary–gonadal axis.

EFFECTS ON BONE DENSITY

Within hours of steroid administration there is a fall in circulating levels of osteocalcin, a bone matrix protein produced by osteoblasts. This change in osteoblast activity is followed by a fall in bone mass, which is maximal over the first few months of therapy. The losses may be considerable and depend to some extent on the method of their estimation. In a study assessing bone loss using biopsies, trabecular bone volume decreased by almost 30%, most of this loss occurring over the first 6 months.[31] Patients in this study were treated with 10–25 mg/day of prednisone. Laan et al.[32] demonstrated an average loss of 8%

of trabecular bone density and 2% of cortical bone density in the lumbar spine over a 20-week period in response to treatment with a mean dose of prednisone of 7.5 mg/day.

Increased rates of bone loss persist, even in patients who have already been taking steroids for some years. Saito et al.[33] demonstrated rates of loss two to three times higher than that of control subjects in older men and women who had already been using steroids for a mean period of 2 years. Continuing bone loss is particularly likely in subjects requiring more than 10 mg/day of prednisone.[34] As a result, bone density in steroid-treated subjects studied cross-sectionally is related both to the duration of their steroid treatment and to the average dose of these drugs,[34–36] as well as to factors that influence pretreatment bone density, such as body weight and age.[37]

Cross-sectional assessments of bone density in steroid-treated patients show values extending from the middle of the age-appropriate normal range to substantially below it. The fact that a number of steroid-treated patients thus have normal bone density is sometimes interpreted as indicating that some individuals are resistant to the osteopoenic effects of glucocorticoids. This is theoretically possible, since there are polymorphisms of the glucocorticoid receptor that might result in differences between subjects in sensitivity to these hormones.[38] However, there is little clinical evidence that this is of practical importance, and the limited prospective data that are available indicate that virtually all subjects lose bone.[32,39] Biochemical studies have also failed to identify a subgroup of steroid-treated patients who do not show suppression of markers of osteoblast activity.[40] Therefore, the fact that some steroid-treated patients still have bone densities within the normal range is probably a reflection of the fact that the mean value has been displaced downwards by an amount which is less than the width of the normal range. For example, in antero-posterior dual energy X-ray absorptiometry (DXA) scans of the lumbar spine, the normal range is 80–120% of the mean normal value. An average bone loss of 20% in patients receiving steroids results in a range in these subjects of 60–100% of the mean normal value.[41] The fact that bone density in steroid-treated patients remains normally distributed with a standard deviation the same as that in normal subjects indicates that a uniform reduction in bone density must have occurred, and rules out the existence of a significant number of subjects who do not undergo any bone loss when taking these drugs long term.

Cross-sectional studies of patients treated for periods of 5 years show that integral bone density of the lumbar spine and proximal femur is about 20% below control values.[41] However, the more rapid loss of trabecular bone results in decrements approaching 40% when lumbar spine density is assessed by quantitative computed tomography[34] or by DXA in the lateral projection.[42] The more rapid loss of trabecular bone is a reflection of the greater surface-to-volume ratio of trabecular bone. Since bone remodelling takes place only at bone surfaces, trabecular bone responds more rapidly to either positive or negative changes in bone balance.

The bone loss induced by glucocorticoids is substantially reversible following the withdrawal of these drugs. Two prospective studies have demonstrated a reaccumulation of bone density over approximately the same time span as its loss occurred.[32,39] Substantial increases in bone density have been reported after cure of Cushing's syndrome and we have demonstrated that bone density is normal in subjects cured of Cushing's syndrome for a mean period of 9 years.[43] Alternate day administration of the glucocorticoids, however, does not diminish bone loss.[44,45]

EFFECTS ON FRACTURE INCIDENCE

Because glucocorticoids have their greatest effect on trabecular bone, fractures are most common in regions of the skeleton that are predominantly trabecular, such as the vertebral bodies and ribs. Hip and forearm fractures are also more common.[46,47] The increase in fracture risk is seen within a few months of the initiation of glucocorticoid therapy (Figure 5.1) and has been confirmed in at least one randomized controlled trial.[48] It is related to the dose, duration of use, age, body weight (inversely) and to female sex.[46,49] A recent prospective study found current dose and bone density to be the principal determinants of fracture risk[50] (Figure 5.2), though prior facture is also important[51] and risk is increased above what BMD alone would predict.[50,51] Approximately 20% of older men and post-menopausal women had vertebral fractures in the first year of steroid treatment in the placebo arms of two clinical trials of therapies for the prevention of steroid osteoporosis.[52,53] Approximately one-third of patients have evidence of vertebral fractures after 5–10 years of glucocorticoid treatment,[54] though this can be very much higher in older patients.[55]

LOCALLY ADMINISTERED STEROIDS

In some conditions it is possible to administer steroids locally, thereby reducing systemic side-effects. However, there is usually some systemic absorption of locally administered steroids, evidenced by growth retardation in children receiving inhaled steroids[56,57] and the development of cataracts in adults.[58] Both beclomethasone and budesonide can affect osteoblast markers in doses as low as 800 μg/day, though fluticasone appears to have lesser effects on bone when given in doses with the same anti-asthmatic effect.[59] Some cross-sectional studies have indicated that bone density is reduced in those using inhaled glucocorticoids (reviewed in reference 57), but this has not been the finding of the small number of prospective studies available,[60,61] suggesting that the cross-sectional studies are confounded by the effects of past oral steroid use or the underlying disease. The large epidemiological study of Van Staa et al.[62,63] supports this contention, by showing that fractures are more common in users of inhaled steroids when compared with normal subjects, but not when compared with users of inhaled bronchodilators. Randomized controlled trials of fluticasone in doses up to 500 μg twice daily show no effect on bone loss over

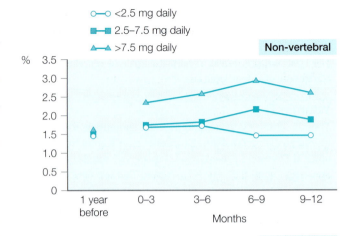

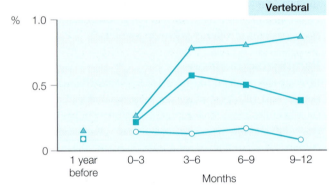

Figure 5.1. Risk of non-vertebral and vertebral fractures before and during the first year of glucocorticoid therapy, stratified by dose. Reproduced with permission of Springer-Verlag. Copyright © 2002 Springer-Verlag. Source: Van Staa TP, Leufkens HGM & Cooper C. *Osteoporosis Int* 2002; **13**: 777–787.[46]

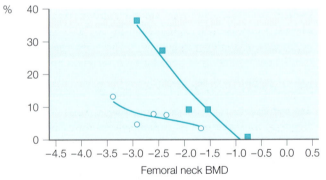

Figure 5.2. Annual incidence of vertebral fracture in patients receiving glucocorticoids (squares) compared with non-users of glucocorticoids (circles), by baseline femoral neck bone mineral density (BMD) quintile. The solid lines have been fitted to these individual point estimates. Reprinted with permission of Wiley-Liss, Inc., a subsidiary of John Wiley & Sons, Inc. Copyright © 2003 Wiley-Liss, Inc. Source: Van Staa TP et al. *Arthritis Rheum* 2003; **48**: 3224–3229.[50]

a 2-year period.[64,65]. However, a recent trial of 412 patients with chronic obstructive pulmonary disease randomized to inhaled triamcinolone (600 μg), or placebo, twice daily, found greater bone loss at 3 years in the treated group (1.8% between-group difference at the femoral neck and 1.3% at the spine).[66] However, while there is usually some systemic absorption of locally administered steroids, they are to be preferred to systemic therapy because their ratio of therapeutic benefit to bone loss is substantially greater.

ASSESSMENT OF FRACTURE RISK

Most individuals using glucocorticoid drugs in doses greater than 5 mg prednisone per day, or its equivalent, will experience bone loss and may be at increased risk of fractures. In addition to dose, the other key risk factor is bone density, which is usually measured in the lumbar spine and proximal femur by DXA. Ultrasound of the heel has also been investigated as a method of assessing bone loss in steroid-treated patients.[67,68] While the data are promising, ultrasound is not used routinely in clinical practice for fracture risk assessment at present. Bone turnover markers have not been consistently shown to be helpful in predicting bone loss or fracture risk in steroid-treated patients.[34,69–73]

A determination of when intervention is appropriate is arbitrary and depends to some extent on the cost and potential side-effects of the available interventions. Figure 5.2 shows that, in post-menopausal women, bone density T-scores below –1.5 are associated with a steeply rising fracture risk, above levels observed in post-menopausal osteoporosis. This suggests that this is a sensible threshold for the introduction of anti-osteoporotic therapies. In an individual beginning steroid therapy, it can be predicted that bone density will drop a further one standard deviation in the first year of treatment, and this should be factored into the decision-making process. A past history of fracture after minimal trauma is also a major reason for weighting the balance in favour of intervention, since it implies that the individual's skeleton is already of marginal adequacy to withstand the trauma of daily living.

INTERVENTIONS TO INCREASE BONE MASS

Most of the therapies used in post-menopausal osteoporosis have also been assessed in steroid osteoporosis. However, efficacy in the former context is not necessarily generalizable, since the pathogeneses are different. Furthermore, the size and number of studies carried out in steroid osteoporosis are both considerably smaller than in post-menopausal osteoporosis, so the evidence for the anti-fracture efficacy of some agents is absent. Some studies distinguish between the use of anti-osteoporotic therapies at the time of introduction of steroids versus the treatment of established osteoporosis in those already having had long-term steroid treatment. In general, this distinction is not important, since efficacy of most agents is similar in both situations.

The general measures that should be considered in all osteoporotic patients (e.g. mobilization, attention to nutrition, cessation of smoking, moderation of alcohol intake) are appropriate in those receiving steroids, whatever their bone density. In those with a higher risk of fracture, pharmacological intervention is usually also necessary. The therapeutic options are as follows.

Calcium and vitamin D

Calcium and vitamin D have been used for several decades as an empirical therapy for osteoporosis of various aetiologies. Their use in combination in trials obscures their relative contributions to any beneficial effects. There is extensive observational data on the effect of calcium supplementation on steroid-induced bone loss, in that the 'control' groups in trials of most other agents have been given calcium. These data indicate that considerable bone loss still occurs despite calcium supplementation. However, calcium does reduce biochemical indices of bone resorption in steroid-treated patients[74] and hydroxyapatite tablets have been shown to slow forearm bone loss in one study.[75]

Two studies of calcium and vitamin D combinations have been reported. Buckley et al.[76] studied patients with rheumatoid arthritis receiving low-dose prednisone who were randomized to receive placebo or calcium (500 mg/day) plus vitamin D (500 IU/day). Those receiving calcium and vitamin D showed 2% more positive changes in bone density than those receiving placebo. The vitamin D status of the study subjects was not assessed. In contrast, Adachi et al.[77] failed to show any benefit on lumbar spine density from the use of calciferol (50,000 u/week) plus calcium (1000 mg/day) in a randomized controlled trial over 3 years.

At present, it seems reasonable to provide calcium supplementation to those whose dietary intake is less than 1–1.5 g/day (i.e. four to six servings of dairy products) and in whom there are not contraindications (e.g. renal calculi). There is increasing evidence that vitamin D deficiency has deleterious effects on the skeleton in the frail elderly population, and this is likely to be relevant to frail steroid-treated patients who are seldom outdoors. Therefore, assessment of vitamin D status (by a measurement of serum 25-hydroxyvitamin D) and, where necessary, supplementation with vitamin D itself (e.g. calciferol, 500–1000 u/day or 20,000–50,000 u/month) is appropriate for steroid-treated patients at risk.

Vitamin D metabolites

The case for using vitamin D metabolites to treat osteoporosis is mixed, since these agents increase both intestinal calcium absorption and bone resorption, thus potentially accelerating bone loss as well as placing the patient at risk of hypercalcaemia. This balance of the potential benefits and risks may be different for different agents and doses.

Trials in this area have recently been reviewed[78] and suggest a small beneficial effect of these agents on bone density. Calcitriol has been assessed in several randomized controlled trials. Dykman et al.[79] found no difference between calcitriol (0.4 μg/day) and placebo in their effects on forearm bone density. Sambrook et al.[80] have reported a large, 1-year study in which patients beginning glucocorticoid therapy were randomly assigned to receive calcium, calcium plus calcitriol (mean dose 0.6 μg/day) or these two agents combined with calcitonin. Bone losses from the lumbar spine were 4.3%, 1.3% and 0.2% in the respective groups. There was a similar, non-significant trend in distal radial bone loss, but no evidence of reduced bone loss in the proximal femur (3% in all groups). The same group studied heart transplant patients over 2 years, and found protection in the femur but not in the spine.[81] Another larger trial over 3 years in cardiac transplant patients showed no effect on lumbar spine density from calcitriol (0.25 μg/day).[82] A trial comparing the use of calcitriol (0.5 μg/day) with hormone replacement therapy in hypogonadal young women with systemic lupus erythematosus showed progressive bone loss in those taking the vitamin D analogue in comparison with increases in density observed in those receiving hormones (between-group difference at the spine of 3.7% at 2 years).[83] There was also a significant difference between groups at the distal radius. A similar study in eugonadal premenopausal women with lupus suggested that calcitriol use resulted in spine density changes that were about 1.5% more positive than in placebo, though these differences were not significant.[84] Henderson et al.[85] have shown comparable protection after heart transplantation with either calcitriol or etidronate over 6 months.

Following cardiac transplantation, alfacalcidol has been shown to slow but not completely prevent femoral neck and lumbar spine bone loss.[86] A similar attenuation of lumbar spine bone loss has been reported in a predominantly non-transplant population with the use of alfacalcidol (1 μg/day), though femoral bone density was not measured in this study.[87] In a population of patients with established steroid osteoporosis, Ringe et al.[88] have shown a beneficial effect at the lumbar spine (2.5% between groups at 3 years) of alfacalcidol (1 μg/day) in comparison with calciferol plus calcium supplements. There was no significant effect in the proximal femur. Thus, there is some consistency in the results with this particular agent.

The variability of outcomes with the various agents in this class make it difficult to generalize with respect to the use of vitamin D metabolites in the management of steroid osteoporosis. The most consistent data are with alfacalcidol, though its effects are generally less than those of the bisphosphonates. Their best use may be as adjunctive therapy to bisphosphonates in patients with severe steroid osteoporosis, or as a second-line therapy in patients for whom these other agents are not acceptable.

Bisphosphonates

Bisphosphonates are currently the treatment of choice in steroid osteoporosis. The bisphosphonate nucleus consists of two phosphate groups joined through a central carbon atom, the individual members of the group differing only in the side-groups attached to that carbon atom. The clinically relevant differences between individual bisphosphonates are their route of administration, their side-effects and their anti-resorptive potency, though most of the newer agents appear to achieve a comparable maximal inhibition of bone resorption. All bisphosphonates are very insoluble and therefore have a low oral bioavailability. To achieve benefit from oral dosing, they must be taken fasting with water at least 30 minutes before food, and separated by some hours from the ingestion of mineral supplements (such as calcium or iron) or antacids. Occasionally, oral aminobisphosphonates cause upper gastrointestinal irritation, sometimes being associated with oesophageal erosions in those with disordered oesophageal motility. Bisphosphonates were originally used in steroid osteoporosis because their inhibition of bone resorption offered the potential to directly redress the imbalance between bone formation and resorption. Recently it has been demonstrated, in vitro, that they reverse the increase in osteocyte and osteoblast apoptosis caused by glucocorticoids, so they may have a more specific role in this condition.[89]

Oral pamidronate was the first bisphosphonate demonstrated to be effective in steroid osteoporosis,[90] but its use intravenously (either a 90 mg infusion annually or 3-monthly administration of 30–60 mg) appears to be comparably effective.[91,92] Similar regimens are reported to be effective in children.[93] The more potent intravenous bisphosphonate, ibandroante, has also been assessed in steroid osteoporosis. Injections at 3-month intervals have been shown to prevent bone loss and vertebral deformities in renal transplant patients[94] and in other steroid-treated subjects.[95]

There are a number of studies showing that cyclic etidronate is an effective therapy in steroid-treated subjects, and this treatment has high patient acceptability since medication is only taken for 2 weeks every 3 months. A large randomized controlled trial of etidronate has been reported,[52] and demonstrated prevention of bone loss in both the lumbar spine and proximal femur in patients recently started on steroid treatment. The beneficial effects of etidronate persisted beyond the 12-month administration period.[96] Furthermore, the study suggested that etidronate reduced fracture rates by 50% and that height loss was also diminished. Another study over 5 years in patients receiving glucocorticoids for asthma showed that etidronate significantly increased bone density at the lumbar spine but not at the hip and had little protective effect against fractures, except possibly in post-menopausal women.[97] Combination of etidronate with calcium treatment had no advantage, but increased unwanted effects. A meta-analysis of some of these studies indicates that etidronate use does decrease fractures, and that it has beneficial effects on bone density at both the spine and hip.[98]

A major trial of alendronate has been reported.[99] This study included patients already established on steroid treatment as well as those just commencing. Beneficial effects on bone density throughout the skeleton were found with both 5 and 10 mg/day of alendronate, though the higher dose tended to be more effective. Gains in bone mass occurred irrespective of the duration of previous steroid use. At 2 years, there were four morphometric vertebral fractures in 59 subjects on placebo, compared with one in 143 subjects taking alendronate (P =

0.026). All fractures occurred in women. Further studies have demonstrated the effectiveness of alendronate in steroid treated children,[100] in Chinese women receiving inhaled steroids and in patients with sarcoidosis or Cushing's syndrome.

Risedronate has been evaluated in both the prevention and treatment of steroid osteoporosis.[53,101] The changes in bone density (with respect to placebo) were comparable to those seen with etidronate and alendronate, and data from pooling the two studies[102] indicated a more than 50% reduction in fractures in the first year of treatment (16% of placebo patients had fractures at 1 year, 7% of those assigned to risedronate, 2.5 mg/day, and 5% of those on risedronate, 5 mg/day, $n = 509$, $P = 0.01$). Efficacy of risedronate in prevention of bone loss has also been shown in patients with rheumatoid arthritis treated with glucocorticoids.[103]

Of the various agents investigated to date, the bisphosphonates have produced the most consistently positive results on bone density in steroid-treated subjects, and the only evidence of reduced fracture rates. They can be used in virtually all steroid-treated patients, including the young and sex hormone replete.

Sex hormones

Oestrogen and testosterone have been used for a number of years in steroid-treated hypogonadal patients, as a treatment for coexisting sex hormone deficiency. The increases in bone density they produce in steroid-treated patients are comparable to those seen in patients not taking steroids.[104–108] Because sex steroids have actions on many tissues, their use involves consideration of a number of potential beneficial and harmful effects.[109]

Anabolic steroids, which are androgens modified to reduce their virilizing effects, have also been used for treating steroid-induced osteoporosis. They would seem to have little place in the management of men, in whom they are likely to further reduce testosterone levels and in whom testosterone itself can be used if a deficiency is demonstrable. Their use in women is associated with beneficial effects on bone mass, but also with virilizing side-effects in almost one-half of treated patients. Of these adverse effects, deepening of the voice is of particular concern since it is often irreversible.

Fluoride

Fluoride ion is a potent osteoblast mitogen capable of producing sustained gains in lumbar spine bone density when used long term. This unique beneficial effect is counterbalanced by its interference with the normal mineralization of bone when present in bone crystal at high concentrations. These opposing effects have made it difficult to translate fluoride's beneficial effects on bone mass into reduced fracture incidence.

There is now clear evidence that fluoride increases spinal bone density[110–113] and trabecular bone volume of the iliac crest[114] in steroid-treated subjects. However, its anti-fracture efficacy in this context remains to be established and it should not be used as a first-line agent in steroid osteoporosis.

Calcitonin

Calcitonin acts via specific receptors on osteoclasts, reducing bone resorption. It has been used in some countries for the management of post-menopausal osteoporosis, though its effectiveness is generally less than that of hormone replacement therapy or the bisphosphonates. In steroid-treated subjects some,[115,116] but not all,[117] studies suggest that calcitonin injections slow bone loss. Similar results using intranasal calcitonin have been reported.[118,119] Adachi et al.[119] studied 31 patients starting steroids for polymyalgia rheumatica, who were randomized to intranasal calcitonin (200 iu daily) or placebo over a 12-month period. Mean spinal bone density changed from 1.11 to 1.08 g/cm² in the placebo group and from 1.06 to 1.04 g/cm² in those on calcitonin. These results are statistically different, but the clinical significance of such a small difference must be marginal. In the proximal femur, the between-group trends were of similar magnitude but in the opposite direction, and in the total body scans the two groups responded identically. Thus, the clinical utility of intranasal calcitonin must remain in doubt.

Parathyroid hormone

Parathyroid hormone is the focus of much attention in post-menopausal osteoporosis because of the substantial increases in axial bone density it has been shown to produce. This effect has now been demonstrated in post-menopausal women receiving steroid therapy and sex hormone replacement in a randomized controlled trial carried out over 12 months, in which 11% increases in spine density were found.[120] Further positive changes in density were seen in the year after parathyroid hormone was discontinued.[121] However, parathyroid hormone is expensive, requires daily injections and some concerns regarding its safety remain to be resolved.

TREATMENT DECISIONS

Figure 5.3 sets out an approach to both the evaluation of a steroid-treated patient and the making of therapeutic decisions, and these are summarized as 'Practice Points'. Optimization of dietary and lifestyle variables is applicable to all subjects receiving steroids. In those with a history of minimal trauma fracture, treatment will usually be offered, but bone densitometry is still useful since it further defines the fracture risk and provides a baseline against which to assess subsequent change. In individuals whose bone density is at the lower end of the young normal range, intervention with a single agent is appropriate, usually a bisphosphonate, though sex hormone replacement is an option in those with demonstrable deficiency. In a patient with more marked bone loss, these agents can be combined with each other, and/or with other interventions such as alfacalcidol, though the anti-fracture efficacy of such combination regimens is unknown.

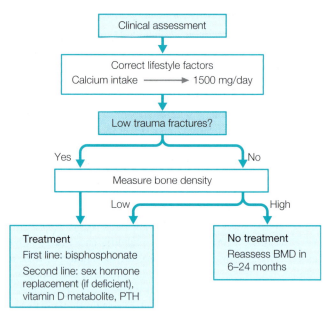

Figure 5.3. Flow chart for the evaluation and treatment of osteoporosis in patients receiving glucocorticoid therapy. Copyright © Reid IR, used with permission.

CONCLUSION

The availability of effective interventions in this condition places a responsibility of any prescriber of glucocorticoids to assess fracture risk in patients and to provide prophylaxis against bone loss when appopriate. The widespread adoption of this strategy will result in many fewer patients receiving glucocorticoids having to accept the morbidity of multiple fractures on top of that of their other medical conditions.

REFERENCES

1. Walsh S, Jordan GR, Jefferiss C et al. High concentrations of dexamethasone suppress the proliferation but not the differentiation or further maturation of human osteoblast precursors in vitro: relevance to glucocorticoid-induced osteoporosis. *Rheumatology* 2001; **40**: 74–83.
2. Atkins GJ, Kostakis P, Pan BQ et al. RANKL expression is related to the differentiation state of human osteoblasts. *J Bone Miner Res* 2003; **18**: 1088–1098.
3. Pereira RMR, Delany AM & Canalis E. Cortisol inhibits the differentiation and apoptosis of osteoblasts in culture. *Bone* 2001; **28**: 484–490.
4. Boden SD, Hair G, Titus L et al. Glucocorticoid-induced differentiation of fetal rat calvarial osteoblasts is mediated by bone morphogenetic protein-6. *Endocrinology* 1997; **138**: 2820–2828.
5. Rogatsky I, Trowbridge JM & Garabedian MJ. Glucocorticoid receptor-mediated cell cycle arrest is achieved through distinct cell-specific transcriptional regulatory mechanisms. *Molec Cell Biol* 1997; **17**: 3181–3193.
6. Ohnaka K, Taniguchi H, Kawate H et al. Glucocorticoid enhances the expression of dickkopf-1 in human osteoblasts : novel mechanism of glucocorticoid-induced osteoporosis. *Biochem Biophys Res Commun* 2004; **318**: 259–264.
7. Hernandez MV, Guanabens N, Alvarez L et al. Immunocytochemical evidence on the effects of glucocorticoids on type I collagen synthesis in human osteoblastic cells. *Calcif Tissue Int* 2004; **74**: 284–293.
8. Hofbauer LC, Gori F, Riggs BL et al. Stimulation of osteoprotegerin ligand and inhibition of osteoprotegerin production by glucocorticoids in human osteoblastic lineage cells: potential paracrine mechanisms of glucocorticoid-induced osteoporosis. *Endocrinology* 1999; **140**: 4382–4389.
9. Von Tirpitz C, Epp S, Klaus J et al. Effect of systemic glucocorticoid therapy on bone metabolism and the osteoprotegerin system in patients with active Crohn's disease. *Eur J Gastroenterol Hepatol* 2003; **15**: 1165–1170.
10. Sasaki N, Kusano E, Ando Y et al. Glucocorticoid decreases circulating osteoprotegerin (OPG): possible mechanism for glucocorticoid induced osteoporosis. *Nephrol, Dial, Transplant* 2001; **16**: 479–482.
11. Sasaki N, Kusano E, Ando Y et al. Changes in osteoprotegerin and markers of bone metabolism during glucocorticoid treatment in patients with chronic glomerulonephritis. *Bone* 2002; **30**: 853–858.
12. Ueland T, Bollerslev J, Godang K et al. Increased serum osteoprotegerin in disorders characterized by persistent immune activation or glucocorticoid excess – possible role in bone homeostasis. *Eur J Endocrinol* 2001; **145**: 685–690.

13. Fahrleitner A, Prenner G, Leb G et al. Serum osteoprotegerin is a major determinant of bone density development and prevalent vertebral fracture status following cardiac transplantation. *Bone* 2003; **32**: 96–106.

14. Weinstein RS, Jilka RL, Parfitt AM et al. Inhibition of osteoblastogenesis and promotion of apoptosis of osteoblasts and osteocytes by glucocorticoids – potential mechanisms of their deleterious effects on bone. *J Clin Invest* 1998; **102**: 274–282.

15. O'Brien CA, Jia D, Plotkin LI et al. Glucocorticoids act directly on osteoblasts and osteocytes to induce their apoptosis and reduce bone formation and strength. *Endocrinology* 2004; **145**: 1835–1841.

16. Shuto T, Kukita T, Hirata M et al. Dexamethasone stimulates osteoclast-like cell formation by inhibiting granulocyte-macrophage colony-stimulating factor production in mouse bone marrow cultures. *Endocrinology* 1994; **134**: 1121–1126.

17. Kaji H, Sugimoto T, Kanatani M et al. Dexamethasone stimulates osteoclast-like cell formation by directly acting on hemopoietic blast cells and enhances osteoclast-like cell formation stimulated by parathyroid hormone and prostaglandin E-2. *J Bone Miner Res* 1997; **12**: 734–741.

18. Tobias J & Chambers TJ. Glucocorticoids impair bone resorptive activity and viability of osteoclasts disaggregated from neonatal rat long bones. *Endocrinology* 1989; **125**: 1290–1295.

19. Dempster DW, Moonga BS, Stein LS et al. Glucocorticoids inhibit bone resorption by isolated rat osteoclasts by enhancing apoptosis. *J Endocrinol* 1997; **154**: 397–406.

20. Hirayama T, Sabokbar A & Athanasou NA. Effect of corticosteroids on human osteoclast formation and activity. *J Endocrinol* 2002; **175**: 155–163.

21. Caputo CB, Meadows D & Raisz LG. Failure of estrogens and androgens to inhibit bone resorption in tissue culture. *Endocrinology* 1976; **98**: 1065–1068.

22. Lowe C, Gray DH & Reid IR. Serum blocks the osteolytic effect of cortisol in neonatal mouse calvaria. *Calcif Tissue Int* 1992; **50**: 189–192.

23. Gronowicz G, McCarthy MB & Raisz LG. Glucocorticoids stimulate resorption in fetal rat parietal bones in vitro. *J Bone Miner Res* 1990; **5**: 1223–1230.

24. Gray RE, Doherty SM, Galloway J et al. A double-blind study of deflazacort and prednisone in patients with chronic inflammatory disorders. *Arthritis Rheum* 1991; **34**: 287–295.

25. Reid IR & Ibbertson HK. Evidence for decreased tubular reabsorption of calcium in glucocorticoid-treated asthmatics. *Horm Res* 1987; **27**: 200–204.

26. Cosman F, Nieves J, Herbert J et al. High-dose glucocorticoids in multiple sclerosis patients exert direct effects on the kidney and skeleton. *J Bone Miner Res* 1994; **9**: 1097–1105.

27. Braun JJ, Juttman JR, Visser TJ et al. Short-term effect of prednisone on serum 1,25-hydroxy-vitamin D in normal individuals an in hyper- and hypoparathyroidism. *Clin Endocrinol* 1982; **17**: 21–28.

28. Doerr P & Pirke KM. Cortisol-induced suppression of plasma testosterone in normal adult males. *J Clin Endocrinol Metab* 1976; **43**: 622–629.

29. Reid IR, France JT, Pybus J et al. Low plasma testosterone levels in glucocorticoid-treated male asthmatics. *BMJ* 1985; **291**: 574.

30. Hampson G, Bhargava N, Cheung J et al. Low circulating estradiol and adrenal androgens concentrations in men on glucocorticoids: a potential contributory factor in steroid-induced osteoporosis. *Metab Clin Exp* 2002; **51**: 1458–1462.

31. LoCascio V, Bonucci E, Imbimbo B et al. Bone loss in response to long-term glucocorticoid therapy. *Bone Miner* 1990; **8**: 39–51.

32. Laan RFJM, Vanriel PLCM, Vandeputte LBA et al. Low-dose prednisone induces rapid reversible axial bone loss in patients with rheumatoid arthritis – a randomized, controlled study. *Ann Intern Med* 1993; **119**: 963–968.

33. Saito JK, Davis JW, Wasnich RD et al. Users of low-dose glucocorticoids have increased bone loss rates: a longitudinal study. *Calcif Tissue Int* 1995; **57**: 115–119.

34. Reid IR & Heap SW. Determinants of vertebral mineral density in patients receiving chronic glucocorticoid therapy. *Arch Intern Med* 1990; **150**: 2545–2548.

35. Hall GM, Spector TD, Griffin AJ et al. The effect of rheumatoid arthritis and steroid therapy on bone density in postmenopausal women. *Arthritis Rheum* 1993; **36**: 1510–1516.

36. Mateo L, Nolla JM, Rozadilla A et al. Bone mineral density in patients with temporal arteritis and polymyalgia rheumatica. *J Rheumatol* 1993; **20**: 1369–1373.

37. Thompson JM, Modin GW, Arnaud CD et al. Not all postmenopausal women on chronic steroid and estrogen treatment are osteoporotic – predictors of bone mineral density. *Calcif Tissue Int* 1997; **61**: 377–381.

38. Huizenga NATM, Koper JW, Delange P et al. A polymorphism in the glucocorticoid receptor gene may be associated with an increased sensitivity to glucocorticoids in vivo. *J Clin Endocrinol Metab* 1998; **83**: 144–151.

39. Rizzato G & Montemurro L. Reversibility of exogenous corticosteroid-induced bone loss. *Eur Respir J* 1993; **6**: 116–119.

40. Lane SJ, Vaja S, Swaminathan R et al. Effects of prednisolone on bone turnover in patients with corticosteroid resistant asthma. *Clin Exp Allergy* 1996; **26**: 1197–1201.

41. Reid IR, Evans MC, Wattie DJ et al. Bone mineral density of the proximal femur and lumbar spine in glucocorticoid-treated asthmatic patients. *Osteoporosis Int* 1992; **2**: 103–105.

42. Reid IR, Evans MC & Stapleton J. Lateral spine densitometry is a more sensitive indicator of glucocorticoid-induced bone loss. *J Bone Miner Res* 1992; **7**: 1221–1225.

43. Manning PJ, Evans MC & Reid IR. Normal bone mineral density following cure of Cushing's syndrome. *Clin Endocrinol* 1992; **36**: 229–234.

44. Gluck OS, Murphy WA, Hahn TJ et al. Bone loss in adults receiving alternate day glucocorticoid therapy. *Arthritis Rheum* 1981; **24**: 892–898.

45. Ruegsegger P, Medici TC & Anliker M. Corticosteroid-induced bone loss. A longitudinal study of alternate day therapy in patients with bronchial asthma using quantitative computed tomography. *Eur J Clin Pharmacol* 1983; **25**: 615–620.

46. Van Staa TP, Leufkens HGM & Cooper C. The epidemiology of corticosteroid-induced osteoporosis: a meta-analysis. *Osteoporosis Int* 2002; **13**: 777–787.

47. Baltzan MA, Suissa S, Bauer DC et al. Hip fractures attributable to corticosteroid use. Study of Osteoporotic Fractures Group [letter]. *Lancet* 1999; **353**: 1327.

48. Van Everdingen AA, Jacobs JWG, van Reesema DRS et al. Low-dose prednisone therapy for patients with early active rheumatoid arthritis: clinical efficacy, disease-modifying properties, and side effects – A randomized, double-blind, placebo-controlled clinical trial. *Ann Intern Med* 2002; **136**: 1–12.

49. Michel BA, Bloch DA, Wolfe F et al. Fractures in rheumatoid arthritis – an evaluation of associated risk factors. *J Rheumatol* 1993; **20**: 1666–1669.

50. Van Staa TP, Laan RF, Barton IP et al. Bone density threshold and other predictors of vertebral fracture in patients receiving oral glucocorticoid therapy. *Arthritis Rheum* 2003; **48**: 3224–3229.

51. Kanis JA, Johansson H, Oden A et al. A meta-analysis of prior corticosteroid use and fracture risk. *J Bone Miner Res* 2004; **19**: 893–899.

52. Adachi JD, Bensen WG, Brown J et al. Intermittent etidronate therapy to prevent corticosteroid-induced osteoporosis. *N Engl J Med* 1997; **337**: 382–387.

53. Cohen S, Levy RM, Keller M et al. Risedronate therapy prevents corticosteroid-induced bone loss – A twelve-month, multicenter, randomized, double-blind, placebo-controlled, parallel-group study. *Arthritis Rheum* 1999; **42**: 2309–2318.

54. Walsh LJ, Wong CA, Oborne J et al. Adverse effects of oral corticosteroids in relation to dose in patients with lung disease. *Thorax* 2001; **56**: 279–284.

55. Walsh LJ, Lewis SA, Wong CA et al. The impact of oral corticosteroid use on bone mineral density and vertebral fracture. *Am J Respir Crit Care Med* 2002; **166**: 691–695.

56. Doull I, Freezer N & Holgate S. Osteocalcin, growth, and inhaled corticosteroids – a prospective study. *Arch Dis Child* 1996; **74**: 497–501.

57. Lipworth BJ. Systemic adverse effects of inhaled corticosteroid therapy – a systematic review and meta-analysis. *Arch Intern Med* 1999; **159**: 941–955.

58. Cumming RG, Mitchell P & Leeder SR. Use of inhaled corticosteroids and the risk of cataracts. *N Engl J Med* 1997; **337**: 8–14.

59. Pauwels RA, Yernault JC, Demedts MG et al. Safety and efficacy of fluticasone and beclomethasone in moderate to severe asthma. *Am J Respir Crit Care Med* 1998; **157**: 827–832.

60. Halpern MT, Schmier JK, Van Kerkhove MD et al. Impact of long-term inhaled corticosteroid therapy on bone mineral density: results of a meta-analysis. *Ann Allergy Asthma Immunol* 2004; **92**: 201–207.

61. Sorkness CA. Establishing a therapeutic index for the inhaled corticosteroids – part II. Comparisons of systemic activity and safety among different inhaled corticosteroids. *J Allergy Clin Immunol* 1998; **102**: S52–S64.

62. Van Staa TP, Leufkens HGM & Cooper C. Use of inhaled corticosteroids and risk of fractures. *J Bone Miner Res* 2001; **16**: 581–588.

63. Van Staa TP, Bishop N, Leufkens HGM et al. Are inhaled corticosteroids associated with an increased risk of fracture in children? *Osteoporosis Int* 2004; **15**: 785–791.

64. Li JTC, Ford LB, Chervinsky P et al. Fluticasone propionate powder and lack of clinically significant effects on hypothalamic–pituitary–adrenal axis and bone mineral density over 2 years in adults with mild asthma. *J Allergy Clin Immunol* 1999; **103**: 1062–1068.

65. Kemp JP, Osur S, Shrewsbury SB et al. Potential effects of fluticasone propionate on bone mineral density in patients with asthma: a 2-year randomized, double-blind, placebo-controlled trial. *Mayo Clin Proc* 2004; **79**: 458–466.

66. Scanlon PD, Connett JE, Wise RA et al. Loss of bone density with inhaled triamcinolone in Lung Health Study II. *Am J Respir Crit Care Med* 2004; **170**: 1302–1309.

67. Blanckaert F, Cortet B, Coquerelle P et al. Contribution of calcaneal ultrasonic assessment to the evaluation of postmenopausal and glucocorticoid-induced osteoporosis. *Rev Rhumat* 1997; **64**: 305–313.

68. Daens S, Peretz A, de Maertelaer V et al. Efficiency of quantitative ultrasound measurements as compared with dual-energy X-ray absorptiometry in the assessment of corticosteroid-induced bone impairment. *Osteoporosis Int* 1999; **10**: 278–283.

69. Hall GM, Spector TD & Delmas PD. Markers of bone metabolism in postmenopausal women with rheumatoid arthritis – Effects of corticosteroids and hormone replacement therapy. *Arthritis Rheum* 1995; **38**: 902–906.

70. Boulet LP, Milot J, Gagnon L et al. Long-term influence of inhaled corticosteroids on bone metabolism and density – Are biological markers predictors of bone loss? *Am J Respir Crit Care Med* 1999; **159**: 838–844.

71. Toogood JH, Hodsman AB, Fraher LJ et al. Serum osteocalcin and procollagen as markers for the risk of osteoporotic fracture in corticosteroid-treated asthmatic adults. *J Allergy Clin Immunol* 1999; **104**: 769–774.

72. Reeve J, Loftus J, Hesp R et al. Biochemical prediction of changes in spinal bone mass in juvenile chronic (or rheumatoid) arthritis treated with glucocorticoids. *J Rheumatol* 1993; **20**: 1189–1195.

73. Stepan JJ, Havrdova E, Tyblova M et al. Markers of bone remodeling predict rate of bone loss in multiple sclerosis patients treated with low dose glucocorticoids. *Clin Chim Acta* 2004; **348**: 147–154.

74. Reid IR & Ibbertson HK. Calcium supplements in the prevention of steroid-induced osteoporosis. *Am J Clin Nutr* 1986; **44**: 287–290.

75. Nilsen KH, Jayson MIV & Dixon AS. Microcrystalline calcium hydroxyapatite compound in corticosteroid-treated rheumatoid patients: a controlled study. *BMJ* 1978; **ii**: 1124.

76. Buckley LM, Leib ES, Cartularo KS et al. Calcium and vitamin D-3 supplementation prevents bone loss in the spine secondary to low-dose corticosteroids in patients with rheumatoid arthritis – a randomized, double-blind, placebo-controlled trial. *Ann Intern Med* 1996; **125**: 961–968.

77. Adachi JD, Bensen WG, Bianchi F et al. Vitamin D and calcium in the prevention of corticosteroid induced osteoporosis – a 3 year followup. *J Rheumatol* 1996; **23**: 995–1000.

78. Richy F, Ethgen O, Bruyere O et al. Efficacy of alphacalcidol and calcitriol in primary and corticosteroid-induced osteoporosis: a meta-analysis of their effects on bone mineral density and fracture rate. *Osteoporosis Int* 2004; **15**: 301–310.

79. Dykman TR, Haralson KM, Gluck OS et al. Effect of oral 1,25-dihydroxy-vitamin D and calcium on glucocorticoid-induced osteopenia in patients with rheumatic diseases. *Arthritis Rheum* 1984; **27**: 1336–1343.

80. Sambrook P, Birmingham J, Kelly P et al. Prevention of corticosteroid osteoporosis – a comparison of calcium, calcitriol, and calcitonin. *N Engl J Med* 1993; **328**: 1747–1752.

81. Sambrook P, Henderson NK, Keogh A et al. Effect of calcitriol on bone loss after cardiac or lung transplantation. *J Bone Miner Res* 2000; **15**: 1818–1824.

82. Stempfle HU, Werner C, Echtler S et al. Prevention of osteoporosis after cardiac transplantation – A prospective, longitudinal, randomized, double-blind trial with calcitriol. *Transplantation* 1999; **68**: 523–530.

83. Kung AWC, Chan TM, Lau CS et al. Osteopenia in young hypogonadal women with systemic lupus erythematosus receiving chronic steroid therapy: a randomized controlled trial comparing calcitriol and hormonal replacement therapy. *Rheumatology* 1999; **38**: 1239–1244.

84. Lambrinoudaki I, Chan DTM, Lau CS et al. Effect of calcitriol on bone mineral density in premenopausal Chinese women taking chronic steroid therapy. A randomized, double blind, placebo controlled study. *J Rheumatol* 2000; **27**: 1759–1765.

85. Henderson K, Eisman J, Keogh A et al. Protective effect of short-term calcitriol or cyclical etidronate on bone loss after cardiac or lung transplantation. *J Bone Miner Res* 2001; **16**: 565–571.

86. Van Cleemput J, Daenen W, Geusens P et al. Prevention of bone loss in cardiac transplant recipients – a comparison of biphosphonates and vitamin D. *Transplantation* 1996; **61**: 1495–1499.

87. Reginster JY, Kuntz D, Verdickt W et al. Prophylactic use of alfacalcidol in corticosteroid-induced osteoporosis. *Osteoporosis Int* 1999; **9**: 75–81.

88. Ringe JD, Coster A, Meng T et al. Treatment of glucocorticoid-induced osteoporosis with alfacalcidol/calcium versus vitamin D/calcium. *Calcif Tissue Int* 1999; **65**: 337–340.

89. Plotkin LI, Weinstein RS, Parfitt AM et al. Prevention of osteocyte and osteoblast apoptosis by bisphosphonates and calcitonin. *J Clin Invest* 1999; **104**: 1363–1374.

90. Reid IR, King AR, Alexander CJ et al. Prevention of steroid-induced osteoporosis with (3-amino-1-hydroxypropylidene)-1,1-bisphosphonate (APD). *Lancet* 1988; **i**: 143–146.

91. Boutsen Y, Jamart J, Esselinckx W et al. Primary prevention of glucocorticoid-induced osteoporosis with intravenous pamidronate and calcium: a prospective controlled 1-year study comparing a single infusion, an infusion given once every 3 months, and calcium alone. *J Bone Miner Res* 2001; **16**: 104–112.

92. Krieg MA, Seydoux C, Sandini L et al. Intravenous pamidronate as treatment for osteoporosis after heart transplantation: a prospective study. *Osteoporosis Int* 2001; **12**: 112–116.

93. Shaw NJ, Boivin CM & Crabtree NJ. Intravenous pamidronate in juvenile osteoporosis. *Arch Dis Child* 2000; **83**: 143–145.

94. Grotz W, Nagel C, Poeschel D et al. Effect of ibandronate on bone loss and renal function after kidney transplantation. *J Am Soc Nephrol* 2001; **12**: 1530–1537.

95. Ringe JD, Dorst A, Faber H et al. Intermittent intravenous ibandronate injections reduce vertebral fracture risk in corticosteroid-induced osteoporosis: results from a long-term comparative study. *Osteoporosis Int* 2003; **14**: 801–807.

96. Brown JP, Olszynski WP, Hodsman A et al. Positive effect of etidronate therapy is maintained after drug is terminated in patients using corticosteroids. *J Clin Densitom* 2001; **4**: 363–371.

97. Campbell IA, Douglas JG, Francis RM et al. Res Comm British Thoracic S. Five year study of etidronate and/or calcium as prevention and treatment for osteoporosis and fractures in patients with asthma receiving long term oral and/or inhaled glucocorticoids. *Thorax* 2004; **59**: 761–768.

98. Adachi JD, Roux C, Pitt PI et al. A pooled data analysis on the use of intermittent cyclical etidronate therapy for the prevention and treatment of corticosteroid induced bone loss. *J Rheumatol* 2000; **27**: 2424–2431.

99. Adachi JD, Saag KG, Delmas PD et al. Two-year effects of alendronate on bone mineral density and vertebral fracture in patients receiving glucocorticoids – A randomized, double-blind, placebo-controlled extension trial. *Arthritis Rheum* 2001; **44**: 202–211.

100. Rudge S, Hailwood S, Horne A et al. Effects of once-weekly oral alendronate on bone in children on glucocorticoid treatment. *Rheumatology* 2005; **44**: 813–818.

101. Reid DM, Hughes RA, Laan RFJM et al. Efficacy and safety of daily risedronate in the treatment of corticosteroid-induced osteoporosis in men and women: a randomized trial. *J Bone Miner Res* 2000; **15**: 1006–1013.

102. Wallach S, Cohen S, Reid DM et al. Effects of risedronate treatment on bone density and vertebral fracture in patients on corticosteroid therapy. *Calcif Tissue Int* 2000; **67**: 277–285.

103. Eastell R, Devogelaer JP, Peel NFA et al. Prevention of bone loss with risedronate in glucocorticoid-treated rheumatoid arthritis patients. *Osteoporosis Int* 2000; **11**: 331–337.

104. Grey AB, Cundy TF & Reid IR. Continuous combined oestrogen/progestin therapy is well tolerated and increases bone density at the hip and spine in post-menopausal osteoporosis. *Clin Endocrinol* 1994; **40**: 671–677.

105. MacDonald AG, Murphy EA, Capell HA et al. Effects of hormone replacement therapy in rheumatoid arthritis – a double blind placebo-controlled study. *Ann Rheum Dis* 1994; **53**: 54–57.

106. Reid IR, Wattie DJ, Evans MC et al. Testosterone therapy in glucocorticoid-treated men. *Arch Intern Med* 1996; **156**: 1173–1177.

107. Isoniemi H, Appelberg J, Nilsson CG et al. Transdermal oestrogen therapy protects postmenopausal liver transplant women from osteoporosis. A 2-year follow-up study. *J Hepatol* 2001; **34**: 299–305.

108. Hall GM, Daniels M, Doyle DV et al. Effect of hormone replacement therapy on bone mass in rheumatoid arthritis patients treated with and without steroids. *Arthritis Rheum* 1994; **37**: 1499–1505.

109. Rossouw JE, Anderson GL, Prentice RL et al. Risks and benefits of estrogen plus progestin in healthy postmenopausal women – Principal results from the Women's Health Initiative randomized controlled trial. *JAMA* 2002; **288**: 321–333.

110. Rizzoli R, Chevalley T, Slosman DO et al. Sodium monofluorophosphate increases vertebral bone mineral density in patients with corticosteroid-induced osteoporosis. *Osteoporosis Int* 1995; **5**: 39–46.

111. Guaydier-Souquieres G, Kotzki PO, Sabatier JP et al. In corticosteroid-treated respiratory diseases, monofluorophosphate increases lumbar bone density – a double-masked randomized study. *Osteoporosis Int* 1996; **6**: 171–177.

112. Lems WF, Jacobs WG, Bijlsma JWJ et al. Effect of sodium fluoride on the prevention of corticosteroid-induced osteoporosis. *Osteoporosis Int* 1997; **7**: 575–582.

113. Lems WF, Jacobs JWG, Bijlsma JWJ et al. Is addition of sodium fluoride to cyclical etidronate beneficial in the treatment of corticosteroid induced osteoporosis. *Ann Rheum Dis* 1997; **56**: 357–363.

114. Meunier PJ, Briancon D, Chavassieux P et al. Treatment with fluoride: bone histomorphometric findings. In: Christiansen C, Johansen JS & Riis BJ, eds. *Osteoporosis 1987*. Copenhagen: Osteopress; 1987: 824–828.

115. Rizzato G, Tosi G, Schiraldi G et al. Bone protection with salmon calcitonin (sCT) in the long-term steroid therapy of chronic sarcoidosis. *Sarcoidosis* 1988; **5**: 99–103.

116. Luengo M, Picado C, Del Rio L et al. Treatment of steroid-induced osteopenia with calcitonin in corticosteroid-dependent asthma. A one-year follow-up study. *Am Rev Respir Dis* 1990; **142**: 104–107.

117. Hay JE, Malinchoc M & Dickson ER. A controlled trial of calcitonin therapy for the prevention of post-liver transplantation atraumatic fractures in patients with primary biliary cirrhosis and primary sclerosing cholangitis. *J Hepatol* 2001; **34**: 292–298.

118. Montemurro L, Schiraldi G, Fraioli P et al. Prevention of corticosteroid-induced osteoporosis with salmon calcitonin in sarcoid patients. *Calcif Tissue Int* 1991; **49**: 71–76.

119. Adachi JD, Bensen WG, Bell MJ et al. Salmon calcitonin nasal spray in the prevention of corticosteroid-induced osteoporosis. *Br J Rheumatol* 1997; **36**: 255–259.

120. Lane NE, Sanchez S, Modlin GW et al. Parathyroid hormone treatment can reverse corticosteroid-induced osteoporosis – results of a randomized controlled clinical trial. *J Clin Invest* 1998; **102**: 1627–1633.

121. Lane NE, Sanchez S, Modin GW et al. Bone mass continues to increase at the hip after parathyroid hormone treatment is discontinued in glucocorticoid-induced osteoporosis: Results of a randomized controlled clinical trial. *J Bone Miner Res* 2000; **15**: 944–951.

122. Prummel MF, Wiersinga WM & Lips P. The couse of biochemical parameters of bone turnover during treatment with corticosteroids. *J Clin Endocrinol Metab* 1991; **72**: 382–386.

123. Morrison D, All NJ, Routledge PA et al. Bone turnover during short course prednisolone treatment in patients with chronic obstructive airways disease. *Thorax* 1992; **47**: 418–420.

124. Lems WF, Gerrits MI, Jacobs JWG et al. Changes in (markers of) bone metabolism during high dose corticosteroid pulse treatment in patients with rheumatoid arthritis. *Ann Rheum Dis* 1996; **55**: 288–293.

125. Wolthers OD, Heuck C, Hansen M et al. Serum and urinary markers of types I and III collagen turnover during short-term prednisolone treatment in healthy adults. *Scand J Clin Lab Invest* 1997; **57**: 133–139.

126. Lems WF, Vanveen GJM, Gerrits MI et al. Effect of low-dose prednisone (with calcium and calcitriol supplementation) on calcium and bone metabolism in healthy volunteers. *Br J Rheumatol* 1998; **37**: 27–33.

127. Bornefalk E, Dahlen I, Michaelsson K et al. Age-dependent effect of oral glucocorticoids on markers of bone resorption in patients with acute asthma. *Calcif Tissue Int* 1998; **63**: 9–13.

128. Pearce G, Tabensky DA, Delmas PD et al. Corticosteroid-induced bone loss in men. *J Clin Endocrinol Metab* 1998; **83**: 801–806.

129. Cooper MS, Blumsohn A, Goddard PE et al. 11-Beta-hydroxysteroid dehydrogenase type 1 activity predicts the effects of glucocorticoids on bone. *J Clin Endocrinol Metab* 2003; **88**: 3874–3877.

130. Van Everdingen AA, van Reesema DRS, Jacobs JWG et al. Low-dose glucocorticoids in early rheumatoid arthritis: discordant effects on bone mineral density and fractures? *Clin Exp Rheumatol* 2003; **21**: 155–160.

Chapter 6
Lower peak bone mass and its decline

MaryFran Sowers

INTRODUCTION

Low peak bone mineral density (BMD) is an important risk factor for osteoporosis and related fractures.[1] The achievement of optimal peak BMD, characterized as the amount of bone tissue present at the end of skeletal maturation,[2] involves an ongoing remodelling process of bone resorption and formation. It is thought that the achievement of optimal peak BMD occurs in the early third decade, followed by relatively stable BMD until the menopause transition.[3] However, while the levels of peak bone mass may be high relative to levels in old age, stochastic models developed by Horsman and Burkinshaw[4] have suggested that two-thirds of the risk for fracture can be predicted based on pre-menopausal BMD.

Lower BMD can be observed well before menopause[5] and bone loss may begin before menopause.[6] For example, serum follicle-stimulating hormone (FSH) levels rise prior to menopause[7–9] and bone turnover marker activity appears to correspond with this rise in FSH.[10] The longer that peak BMD is sustained in the pre- and peri-menopausal periods, the shorter the time interval the woman should be at risk for fracture.

What contributes to lower peak bone mass?

The World Health Organization (WHO) definition of osteoporosis references the mean peak bone mass observed in women, aged 20–45.[11] It is widely accepted that BMD of 95% of those with fracture will meet this WHO definition based on the reference to peak bone mass levels (–2.5 SD). However, in using this cut-off point, there will be 2.5% of healthy young adult women who can be classified as osteoporotic. Furthermore, this does not include those additional pre- or peri-menopausal women for whom osteopoenia or osteoporosis is secondary to disease states or the use of medications to treat disease. Finally, this definition does not encompass those women who may be losing bone prior to the menopausal transition.

In pre-menopausal women, the primary goal is to optimize or maintain BMD. With accumulating recommendations for environmental interventions, including diet and exercise, and the expanding portfolio of therapeutic interventions, there is a need to more clearly consider the following:

1. Who is at high risk for suboptimal peak bone mass?
2. What are disease-related conditions, or the treatments, associated with lower BMD?
3. When does measurable bone loss commence relative to the menopause?
4. Who is at high risk for greater bone loss around the menopause transition?

The subsequent disease frequency of osteoporosis in older women may be modifiable with implementation of intervention strategies during the period of peak bone mass and the peri-menopausal transition. This argues for early identification of high-risk groups based on risk factor identification or selective clinical diseases or treatment practices.

DEVELOPING PEAK BONE MASS

Relating life course stages to risk

The continuum of change in bone mass and architecture over the life span can be characterized by division into life course stages. Three stages, shown in Table 6.1, are related to the achievement of optimal bone mass, maintaining that level, and initiating the uncoupling of bone remodelling that will ultimately result in a decline of bone mass.

Three general classes of factors (shown in Table 6.2) can influence peak or pre-menopausal bone mass. This includes alterations in hormone concentrations, alternations in bone loading and alterations in nutritionally related or lifestyle factors. These factors may contribute singly, in multiples and cumulatively in their contribution to bone remodelling, leading to changes in BMD within the life course stages in each of the life course stages.

Table 6.1. Life course stages and bone mineralization.

- **Birth to age 20.** There is formation and mineralization of bone during growth and development. During adolescence, matrix formation may exceed mineralization, leading to an osteopoenia of adolescent growth

- **Ages 20—39.** Peak bone mass is achieved and maintained

- **Ages 39—59.** With the onset of the menopausal transition, there is a shift in ovarian hormone concentration production, leading to the eventual diminution of oestradiol concentrations, as well as the eventual predominance of bone resorption relative to formation

- **Ages 60—75.** Increasing numbers of women and, to a lesser degree, of men are at risk for osteoporosis primarily due to bone resorption

- **>75 years.** There is a high prevalence of osteoporosis with bone mineral loss and matrix deterioration (microfracture), accompanied by increasing frailty and the presence of co-morbid conditions

Table 6.2. Factors associated with suboptimal peak bone mass or bone loss.

- Alteration in reproductive, calciotrophic and other hormone concentrations

- Alterations in weight, strength, mobility or bone-loading

- Alterations in nutritional status and lifestyle presence of co-morbid conditions

ALTERATIONS IN PEAK BONE MASS

Alteration in reproductive hormone status

There appear to be at least four identifiable factors that are related to accessing reproductive hormone concentrations that could be associated with lower peak BMD but which are associated with Stage 1 of adolescence. These include late age at menarche, early age at first pregnancy, a failure to establish regular menstrual cycles, and amenorrhoea associated with low body fat, anorexia nervosa and/or intense physical activity.

Alterations in reproductive hormone status during adolescence

There is some evidence that in pregnancy at an early age, when the skeleton of both foetus and mother are simultaneously being mineralized, a competitive demand for calcium may result in lower peak bone density. Sowers et al.[12,13] observed that a first pregnancy during adolescence was associated with

significantly lower age-adjusted baseline radial BMD, lower follow-up radial BMD and greater 5-year radial BMD loss, an observation confirmed by Fox et al.[14] in a cross-sectional study of 1800 elderly women.

Numerous studies suggest that later age at menarche is associated with lower BMD and more rapid pre-menopausal bone loss.[13–15] Girls with late age at menarche (>14 years) are likely to be taller, have lower body fat and to have lower bone density.[15] Osteopoenia and osteoporosis are established complications of anorexia nervosa and other eating disorders where food consumption is curtailed in the face of the opportunity for a well-balanced, energy-sufficient diet.[16–19] Proposed mechanisms for osteopoenia include oestrogen deficiency, glucocorticoid excess, generalized malnutrition and calcium intake deficiency, with the potential for more than one mechanism to be operating simultaneously. Some investigators have reported that compulsive exercise that is frequently concurrent with anorexia nervosa was protective for bone loss,[19] whereas others have failed to observe this protective relation.[19,20] This discrepancy may be related to the degree and intensity of exercise practised by affected adolescents and women.

Because women with anorexia nervosa are frequently both underweight and amenorrhoeic, both factors need to be considered in treatment.[21] Bachrach et al.[19] found body size, age at onset and duration of anorexia nervosa, but not dietary calcium intake, physical activity level or duration of amenorrhea, to be correlated with BMD in adolescent girls, suggesting that the primary factors are the underlying hormonally mediated metabolic events. Dietary calcium supplementation has not sustained bone mineral; however, the difference may be associated with patient compliance with the therapy and the short duration of therapy programmes. With rare exceptions, the studies have failed to differentiate whether the subjects were women who had failed to acquire bone or women who had lost bone.

Reproductive hormone concentration in peak bone mass

Factors related to reproductive hormone concentrations that could be associated with lower peak BMD include the amenorrhoea of chronic endurance activity, nulliparity, use of medoxyprogesterone injectible contraceptive, oophorectomy and early ovarian failure. Adolescent and adult athletes frequently have lower body fat, leaner body mass and greater BMD than non-athletes. However, it has long been appreciated that chronic endurance exercise accompanied by menstrual dysfunction may be catabolic for bone rather than anabolic.[22–25] Reported menstrual cycle changes in women who exercise strenuously may include delay in menarche, shortened luteal phase of the menstrual cycle, menstrual irregularities, oligomenorrhoea and amenorrhoea.[26]

Some investigators have suggested that the hypothalamic–pituitary–ovarian–adrenal axis is suppressed by rigorous physical activity; subsequently, bone mass is lower because of lower concentrations of oestradiol and progesterone and higher concentrations of cortisol.[23,27–29] An alternative hypothesis is that lower BMD in female athletes is the consequence of repeated episodes of hyperprolactinaemia, although increased basal prolactin values have not been consistently identified in amenorrhoeic athletes.[21,30–33] Studies have shown that progesterone, prolactin and testosterone concentrations all increase with strenuous physical activity.[32,33] Prior et al.[34] concluded that decreases in spinal bone density among eumenorrhoeic women athletes correlated with asymptomatic disturbances of the ovulatory cycle and not with degree of physical activity.

Nulliparous women include those who lack reproductive competence, those who have not had the opportunity to conceive and those who choose not to conceive. The lack of reproductive competence may be related to lower bone mass. Sowers et al.,[13] in a longitudinal study of pre-menopausal women, found that nulliparity was highly predictive of reduced radial BMD, but not rate of change. Fox et al.[14] also identified that nulliparous women had significantly lower bone density of the distal radius in the post-menopausal women enrolled in the Study of Osteoporotic Fractures, suggesting that their risk may be associated with inability to conceive or maintain a pregnancy. Clomiphene citrate used for ovulation induction is stimulatory for the gonadotropins and highly stimulatory for oestrogens, but its effect on prolactin, testosterone, inhibins, activins and follistatin remains to be evaluated.[35]

In 2004, the United States Food and Drug administration mandated use of a warning label on medroxyprogesterone injectable contraceptive (Depo-Provera) about significant bone loss with use. The warning acknowledges that it is yet to be determined how much BMD recovery might occur with discontinuation (or the duration of time required for that recovery). A 2-year study of 178 first-time users had mean hip and spine BMD losses of 5.7%, while 145 controls had less than 0.9 % loss over the same period after a 24-month period. Increasing body mass index among DMPA users offered protection against DMPA-related BMD loss; however, calcium intake, physical activity and smoking did not influence BMD change in either group.[36] Two other studies of new DMPA users with a smaller number of users reported hip and spine BMD losses ranging from 1.5% to 3.3%.[37,38] Three longitudinal studies of predominantly long-term DMPA users reported minimal or no BMD loss,[39–41] but these data do not indicate the status of BMD prior to DMPA initiation.

Oophorectomy is a common example of iatrogenically induced hypo-oestrogenism with an impact on measures of calcium metabolism,[42] fracture[43] and bone mineral content in both white and Japanese women.[42–47] Aitken et al.[42] reported that bone density, as measured by standard aluminium equivalents, was lowest in women who had undergone oophorectomy at earlier ages.

Several studies have attempted to define the rate of bone loss following oophorectomy. Stepan et al.[46] suggested a mean loss of 2.8% of metacarpal cortical area and 8% of the lumbar spine (by dual photon densitometry) in the first year following oophorectomy. Based on statistical modelling, Reeves[47] projected that there was a doubling of bone resorption following oophorectomy. Genant et al.[48] estimated that annual bone mineral loss was approximately 8% in the vertebral spongiosum and 2% in the peripheral cortex when evaluated by quantitative computed tomography.

While oophorectomy provides a model for the evaluation of ovarian hormone deprivation and BMD, that relationship may be confounded by those events that gave rise to the oophorectomy. Oophorectomy and/or hysterectomy are performed for the treatment of malignancy, pelvic inflammatory disease, endometriosis, uterine fibroids and other conditions that may influence BMD independently of the surgical procedure and the hormone sequelae.

The impact of oestrogen replacement following oophorectomy is surprisingly poorly documented. Aitken et al.[42] estimated that women lost approximately 8% of metacarpal bone mass in the first 2 years following oophorectomy in comparison to no measurable loss in women treated with mestranol. While the women who were 3 years post-oophorectomy maintained bone density, women who were 6 years post-surgery were unresponsive to mestranol and continued to lose bone, suggesting an optimal therapeutic window following oophorectomy, when bone is more responsive to hormone replacement.

A number of alternative treatments for the bone loss associated with oophorectomy, apart from hormone replacement, have been evaluated.[49] Gambacciani et al.[50] reported no effect of synthetic flavonoid administration in women with oophorectomy/hysterectomy. The prophylactic administration of salmon calcitonin in women with oophorectomy apparently inhibited skeletal resorption as measured by radial bone mineral content and the behaviour of Gla protein and hydroxyproline concentrations.[51]

Women who experience early ovarian failure with chemotherapy for breast cancer are poorly described. Age is a major determinant of the likelihood of ovarian failure. It occurs in approximately 50% of women less than 40 years, as compared to 90% in older women. Observational studies have indicated that tamoxifen had modest positive effects on bone mass.[52,53] Several clinical trials have confirmed that tamoxifen reduced bone turnover[54] and has an effect on the bone remodelling rate similar to those of oestrogen.[55]

Several studies have suggested that marginal hormone status is important in establishing variation in pre-menopausal BMD, although there is little work that defines what constitutes 'marginal' and this state is unlikely to be defined with physical examination. Sowers et al.[56] described lower oestradiol and testosterone concentrations and higher luteinizing hormone (LH) values in a low BMD group compared to a control group. Women with lower peak BMD had different daily urinary hormone excretion patterns with lower LH peaks and a muted progesterone response.[5]

Sustaining peak bone mass and reproductive hormone concentrations

Pregnancy and lactation are characterized by significant alterations in the maternal hormone environment, notably oestrogen and prolactin concentrations, but apparently only transitory bone loss. Studies of bone mass published between 1960 and 1990 were highly inconsistent with respect to the impact of lactation. However, more recent longitudinal studies and clinical trials have consistently shown significant early losses of BMD at the spine and hip in amounts of 5–7%,[57,58] findings also reported in animal studies.[59] Importantly, BMD is largely restored in the 6- to 12-month period following weaning, as menses is re-established and appears to continue recovery during a subsequent pregnancy.[60] Lower BMD was not found among women who practised long-term lactation with 10–18 pregnancies.[61]

The acute changes in calcium homeostasis during reproduction appear to be independent of lifestyle, including dietary calcium intake and exercise. Bone loss and recovery experiences have been reported to occur in Gambian women with low calcium intakes, as well as groups of white women with greater calcium intakes.[62] Additionally, Little and Clapp[63] report that regular, self-selected, recreational exercise has no impact on early postpartum lactation-induced BMD loss.

A number of studies have reported an increase in bone mass with parity as measured with different measurement technologies at different bone sites with different parity classifications,[64,65] although this is not a consistent association in studies of pre-menopausal or post-menopausal women.[66,67]

Although bone loss accelerates when menses cease,[68] the timing and amount of pre-menopausal or peri-menopausal bone loss is just being elucidated. Some cross-sectional studies suggest that bone mass of the spine or proximal femur decreases prior to the menopause, though it is difficult to distinguish pre- from peri-menopausal loss in these studies.[69–72] Furthermore, historical differences in peak bone mass (a cohort effect) might explain these data. Three longitudinal studies of pre- or early peri-menopausal women failed to detect significant decreases in spine, radius or total body bone mass, although these studies had relatively small sample size and limited duration.[73–75] In contrast, other longitudinal studies have reported significant pre-menopausal or late peri-menopausal bone loss from the radius and spine.[13,76,77] A 4-year longitudinal study of women, aged 24–44 years at baseline, reported that bone loss in the pre-menopausal period was limited to the femoral neck and the rate of change was not clinically significant. However, women who had begun the transition, irrespective of chronological age, were more likely to be losing bone.[6] Information from the SWAN Study indicates that lumbar spine BMD values were lower in women with increasing FSH even among women whose menstrual bleeding pattern indicated they were pre- or early perimenopausal.[78]

In summary, there are a number of reproductive and hormone-level-related factors that influence the level of peak BMD attained, as well as the amount of bone loss. Thus, interventions that may be appropriate for the time period must consider whether the underlying defect is a failure to achieve higher levels of peak bone mass or greater rates of change. There are studies underway to consider the efficacy of hormone treatment to treat bone loss in the peri-menopause.

Where the lower BMD is secondary to disease process, as in cancers or anorexia, the focus should be placed on effective therapy for the primary condition, with plans to monitor bone status and consider appropriate intervention based on the findings from that monitoring. The findings of substantial bone loss with Depo-Provera use must be considered against the competing benefit of an effective contraceptive methodology.

Calciotrophic hormone factors and bone throughout the life course

The calciotrophic hormones include parathyroid hormone (PTH), PTHrP, 25-hydroxyvitamin D, 1,25-dixydroxyvitamin D and calcitonin. Modifications related to calciotrophic hormone concentrations, like the reproductive hormones, can impact the achievement of peak bone mass, the risk for bone loss and the rate of bone loss, and are potentially eligible for primary prevention strategies.

Measurable PTHrP concentrations in lactation and breast cancer are related to acute changes in bone status in pre-menopausal women. In lactation, changes in 1,25-dihydroxyvitamin D and 25-hydroxyvitamin D were not associated with either the bone loss or its subsequent recovery.[79] However, PTHrP, oestradiol and prolactin concentrations, or lactation status, were highly associated with the bone loss and recovery.[80] Lactation studies suggest that much, if not all, of bone mineral is recovered and there is no indication for 'treating' this rapid turnover state.

Elevated PTHrP concentrations occur in more than 50% of cases of malignancy-associated hypercalcaemia.[80] Among pre-menopausal women, this is particularly notable for breast cancer. Currently, therapy can include treatment with bisphosphonates to reduce osteolytic lesions.

Corticosteroid medications are the treatment of choice for inflammatory conditions that disproportionately affect pre-menopausal adult women, including rheumatoid arthritis, asthma and systemic lupus erythematosus. However, the use of oral corticosteroids is one of the most common causes of iatrogenically induced osteoporosis, depending upon the dose and duration of therapy. Skeletal problems have not been observed in asthmatic patients treated with inhaled corticosteroid therapy.[81] Of increasing concern is the appearance of fractures at greater levels of BMD than typically expected. Peel et al.[82] indicated a six-fold increase in risk of fracture with a 1 SD decrease of BMD.

Corticosteroids stimulate osteoclast action and bone resorption while inhibiting bone formation by osteoblasts.[83] Corticosteroids decrease calcium and phosphate absorption from the gut and increases urinary calcium excretion, potentially independent of vitamin D. These actions stimulate PTH, which in turn increases osteoblast activity as a mechanism to maintain intracellular and extracellular calcium concentrations. Corticosteroid use also impacts oestrogen metabolism.[84]

Treatment guidelines have been published for glucocorticoids.[85] The specific course of action is framed within the reference of the individual's lifestyle, menstrual history and family history, complete physical examination, recommended laboratory parameters and measurement of BMD.[85]

In summary, the major disruption in the vitamin D axis during peak bone maintenance is associated with corticosteroid hormone use. Currently, recommendations are to treat the underlying conditions that generated the need for treatment, to initiate monitoring to determine if significant bone loss occurs, and to treat the bone loss.

Alterations in other hormone concentrations

The actions of thyroid, insulin and growth hormone concentrations with bone cells are essential. Thyroid disease has been associated with poor bone health in women, potentially affecting more than 10% of the population. However, disease may impact the capacity of thyroxine and tri-iodothyronine to stimulate osteoclast activity.[86] A related problem is the ongoing use of thyroid medication inappropriately or in doses inconsistent with physiological requirements.[87] A meta-analysis of studies in which BMD was assessed in women receiving thyroid-stimulating hormone (TSH)-suppressive doses of thyroxine concluded that this treatment led to a 1% increase in annual bone loss among post-menopausal women.[88] However, thyroid hormone replacement therapy in the absence of TSH suppression did not appear to be associated with this substantial bone loss. There are no comparable studies in pre-menopausal women, though thyroid medication is widely used in this group.

In summary, the major actions with respect to thyroid disease among pre-menopausal women include appropriate diagnosis of hyper- or hypothyroidism and then monitoring of TSH concentrations among treated women. A bone density assessment at time of therapy may be appropriate, particularly if other risk factors for lower bone mass or its change are present.

ALTERATIONS IN WEIGHT, STRENGTH, MOBILITY OR BONE-LOADING

Frost[89] speculated that bone loss of ageing is secondary to decreases in muscle mass, strength and loading. The influence of weight, strength, mobility and bone-loading probably begins early in life. It is consistently observed that heavier pre- and peri-menopausal women have greater BMD that their less heavy peers. Greater BMD may be achieved because greater weight may result in greater bone-loading, thereby increasing BMD; greater weight may provide the opportunity for slightly greater oestrogen levels through aromatization in the adipocytes; and excess weight also includes an accumulation of greater lean mass. Adjusting for weight led to a reinterpretation of the relative levels of peak bone mass among women of different race/ethnic origins. Based on information from more than 2100 women, SWAN investigators reported that lumbar spine BMD was similar in African-American, Chinese and Japanese women, all of whom had higher BMDs than Caucasians, when comparisons are made among women of comparable weight. Femoral neck BMD is highest in African-Americans and similar in Chinese, Japanese and Caucasians. These findings may explain why African-Americans and Asians have lower fracture rates than Caucasians.[90]

Minimalization of weight-bearing activity due to paralysis, immobilization or limitation in physical functioning is associated with decrease in bone mass. It has been recognized that decline in bone mass can occur rapidly. For example, much of the decrease in bone mass following paralysis occurs within the first year.[91]

While there is an extensive literature about athletes and BMD, there is relatively less information about usual physical activity among women, especially pre-menopausal women. In young adults, bone tends to be better maintained in the physically active, although exercise during young adulthood that has a modest effect in pre-menopausal women may have no effect on bone in post-menopausal women.[92] Two studies have recently reported greater BMD in treated pre-menopausal women, but the difference between the treated and controls was not statistically significant.[93,94]

There is increasing belief that higher BMD observed in some physically active adults is a residual of the positive effect of exercise and activity during growth and development.[95] Two studies have indicated that participation in organized sports during adolescence is associated with greater maintenance of peak BMD,[96] while physical inactivity was associated with low bone mass.[97] There is a direct effect of physical activity on bone hypertrophy in growing children, but there is little bone increase due to moderate activity in young adults and the aged.[98] In a study of the spine, femur and total body BMD in Icelandic women aged 16–20 years, the highest levels of routine physical activity were associated with a 4–5% higher BMD in adolescents, but by age 20 the effect was halved.

Even though the observed effect of physical activity on bone mineral density in adults may account for a limited amount of explained variation, there could be other important effects.[95] Potentially, an additional advantage of physical activity to bone-related functioning is its contribution to muscle strength and neuromuscular coordination, both of which can contribute to fall prevention.[99] However, the importance of lean mass, muscle strength and physical activity is reinforced by newly acquired evidence indicating that bone loss occurs when there is suppression of reproductive hormone (by Depo-Provera) and weight gain is comprised of increased fat mass but not lean mass.[36]

NUTRITIONAL AND LIFESTYLE FACTORS AND BONE

Calcium is required for the growing skeleton, and supplementation may be needed during periods of peak growth if dietary intakes are inadequate. Because calcium is the major mineral in bone and important during adolescent growth, the Institute of Medicine recommendations for dietary calcium intake were increased for children and adolescents living in the USA.[100] However, there is a continuing debate about daily calcium intake recommendations for late adolescence and young adulthood, in part because of the absence of data, particularly data that address interactions with other nutrients, lifestyle practices and normal calcium metabolism.[101] For example, studies have identified that calcium supplementation in growing children with normal nutrition produces a transient 2% acceleration of growth but does not lead to increased peak bone mass. Moreover, the small temporary increase was lost after supplementation stopped. Additionally, greater dietary intake is typically associated with greater calcium excretion, primarily in the faeces.[102–104]

In normal young adults with reasonable access to an abundant variety of foods, there is limited correlation between dietary calcium intake and BMD. Several cross-sectional and prospective studies have not shown statistically significant associations between BMD and calcium intake.[96,105] Much nutrition research has considered dietary calcium intake alone without considering the context of other dietary factors that influence the excretion of calcium from the gut via faecal material or excretion of calcium by the kidneys via urine. Furthermore, many of the studies in pre-menopausal women have included relatively small numbers. Given that the demonstrable influence is likely to be of the magnitude of about 1% increase per year or less, studies of dietary calcium intake in healthy pre-menopausal women will have to include large enrolments, followed for extended periods, to provide convincing evidence of efficacy. In women at risk for lower peak bone mass or for rapid bone turnover, it is important that dietary calcium intake not be marginalized, but it is equally important to maintain an appropriate perspective on the limited impact that dietary calcium intake makes in the bone-compromised pre-menopausal woman.[101]

There is still important information to be developed about the role of dietary sodium, dietary protein, caffeine and plant sterols with weak oestrogenic activity in pre-menopausal women. The effects of dietary protein are paradoxical. A number of studies have reported that a high-protein diet is associated with increased urinary calcium excretion, with a projected loss of 1 mg of calcium from the urine for every 1 gram rise in dietary protein. The most frequently cited mechanism is that sulphur-containing amino acids result in a greater acid load, which is buffered by mineral from the skeleton. However, consumption of alkali-rich foods, including fruits and vegetables, can moderate this action, indicating the importance of considering total dietary intake.[106] Further, the relative role of dietary protein intake in peak bone mass is poorly studied.[106]

There is substantial interest in the potential for oestrogen mimics such as the soy-based isoflavone to modify peak bone mass, but study results have been inconsistent. For example, higher dietary genistein intake was associated with higher BMD in Japanese women, but not Chinese, Caucasian or African-American women.[107] Some intervention studies have suggested that, above some threshold dose, the isoflavones genistein and diadzein have a positive effect on BMD, but the effect may be dependent on both the dose and the enzymatic capacity to degrade the chemical configuration of the isoflavones.[108,109]

A review of the limited number of studies suggests that obese persons on very-low-calorie diets or histories of weight cycling have the potential for bone loss or lower BMD.[105]

Smoking, as originally hypothesized by Daniell,[110] increases the ageing loss of bone density and increases the fracture rate. Smoking appears to decrease calcium absorption and may increase PTH.[111,112] More pre-menopausal women are smoking and there is increasing risk of bone compromise. A meta-analysis by Law and Hackshaw[111] demonstrated the collective effect of smoking in post-menopausal women, but not in pre-menopausal women. Essentially, body weight and fat was lower in smokers and there is interference with oestrogen metabolism. Smoking has been universally linked with an earlier onset of menopause.[110]

Moderate alcohol intake has not been associated with lower peak bone mass. For example, consuming a drink per day or less was actually protective for maintaining peak bone mass in a 6-year longitudinal study.[96]

In contrast, it is likely that BMD has been impacted in approximately 8% of US women, aged 18–40 years, who misuse alcohol.[113,114] Although alcohol misuse is a widely cited risk factor for generalized osteoporosis, the studies are most frequently in men, and there are remarkably few studies of alcoholism and bone status in women. A recent study indicates that alcohol abuse and dependence was associated with lower femoral neck and lumbar spine peak BMD. Additionally, pre-menopausal women with histories of alcohol dependence had a higher lifetime prevalence of fractures and often reported that the onset of fractures occurred prior to the onset of problem drinking (often during adolescence), suggesting that factors other than acute intoxication could have contributed to the greater fracture prevalence.[115]

Several direct and indirect mechanisms may contribute to bone loss with excess alcohol use, including reduced bone formation and impaired mineralization[116] and vitamin D deficiency in alcoholism.[116] Alcohol misuse may be accompanied by factors associated with lower BMD, including nutritional deficiencies, greater frequency of smoking, earlier age of first pregnancy and more episodes of non-pregnancy-related amenorrhoea.[114]

PREVENTIVE MEASURES

In considering preventive measures, a primary consideration is whether pre- and peri-menopausal women should be screened for low BMD and rapid bone turnover. Screening women in the pre-menopausal, peri-menopausal and early post-menopausal years for high fracture risk by measuring their bone mass has achieved some popularity in recent years. However, there are many questions about the usefulness of such screening. These include who should be screened, whether multiple measurements over time are needed, what other risk assessment is needed apart from a measure of bone mass and what therapy should be used in those with various degrees of low bone mass. When considering the use of bone turnover markers, the requisite information includes understanding how the marker reflects short-term compared with long-term turnover and how that marker relates to the stage of bone (formation, maintenance, transition-based loss, ageing-related loss). In addition to understanding these measurement tools, other requirements for screening are important. This includes the cost of the screening and the availability of an effective therapy. At present, however, there is no consensus that any screening method should be used universally for healthy women in the general population.

Special groups would appear to be candidates for monitoring. These groups might include persons treated with therapies that disrupt the hypothalamic–pituitary–ovarian axis or with glucocorticosteroids. Women with amenorrhoea should be monitored for BMD and treatment considered. Evidence of vitamin D deficiency or alcoholism also qualify for monitoring and access to treatment. Certainly appropriate exercise, appropriate sunlight exposure and appropriate nutritional quality are important and could be considered a part of a general preventive health counselling programme.

PRACTICE POINTS

- Alterations in reproductive hormone levels that can affect attainment and maintenance of peak BMD may occur in adolescence and may include early age of pregnancy before age 17 and amenorrhoea from anorexia nervosa or exercise.

- Alterations in reproductive hormone levels during the reproductive years can affect BMD (i.e. oophorectomy, early ovarian failure and use of Depo-Provera).

- BMD may be affected by alterations in calciotrophic hormone concentrations associated with corticosteroid therapy use or breast cancer treatment.

- Lifestyle risk factors that may influence BMD include the misuse of alcohol and possibly smoking, physical inactivity or imbalance in dietary intake.

RESEARCH AGENDA

- Further studies of peak BMD and bone loss are needed to delineate the important risk factors in prediction of fracture and bone mineral density.

- Further studies are needed to delineate invention strategies appropriate to the pre-menopause and peri-menopause.

- Further epidemiological studies in non-white populations are needed.

REFERENCES

1. Consensus Development Conference. Prophylaxis and treatment of osteoporosis. JAMA 1991; 90: 107–110.
2. Bonjour JP, Theintz G, Law F et al. Peak bone mass: facts and uncertainties. Arch Pediatr 1995; 2: 460–468.
3. Riggs L. Overview of osteoporosis. West J Med 1991; 154: 63–77.
4. Horsman A & Burkinshaw L. Stochastic models of femoral bone loss and hip fracture risk. In: Kleerkoper MJ & Krane SM, eds. Clinical Disorders of Bone and Mineral Metabolism. New York: MA Liebert, 1989; 253–263.
5. Sowers MF, Crutchfield M, Shapiro B et al. Urinary ovarian and gonadotrophin hormone levels in premenopausal women with low bone mass. J Bone Miner Res 1998; 13: 1191–1202.
6. Sowers MF, Crutchfield M, Bandekar R et al. Bone mineral density and its change in pre- and perimenopausal white women: the Michigan Bone Health Study. J Bone Miner Res 1998; 13: 1134–1140.
7. Sherman BM & Korenman SG. Hormonal characteristics of the human menstrual cycle throughout reproductive life. J Clin Invest 1975; 55: 699–706.
8. Metcalf MG, Donald RA & Livesey JH. Pituitary–ovarian function in normal women during the menopausal transition. Clin Endocrinol 1981; 14: 245–255.
9. Lenton EA, Sexton L, Lee S et al. Progressive changes in LH and FSH and LH:FSH ratio in women throughout reproductive life. Maturitas 1988; 10: 35–43.
10. Garton M, Martin J, New S et al. Bone mass and metabolism in women aged 45–55. Clin Endocrinol 1996; 44: 563–570.
11. World Health Organization. Assessment of fracture risk and its application to screening for postmenopausal osteoporosis: Report of a WHO Study Group. Technical Report Series 843. Geneva: WHO, 1994.
12. Sowers MF, Wallace RB & Lemke JH. Correlates of mid-radius bone density among premenopausal women: a community study. Prev Med 1985; 14: 585–596.
13. Sowers MF, Clark MK, Hollis B et al. Radial bone mineral density in pre- and perimenopausal women: a prospective study of rates and risk factors for loss. J Bone Miner Res 1992; 7: 647–657.
14. Fox KM, Magaziner J, Sherwin R et al. Reproductive correlates of bone mass in elderly women. J Bone Miner Res 1993; 8: 901–908.
15. Galuska DA & Sowers MF. Menstrual history and bone density in young women. J Women's Health 1999; 8: 647–656.
16. Ayers JW, Gidwani GP, Schmidt IM et al. Osteopenia in hypoestrogenic young women with anorexia nervosa. Fertil Steril 1984; 41: 224–228.
17. Biller BM, Saxe V, Herzog DB et al. Mechanisms of osteoporosis in adult and adolescent women with anorexia nervosa. J Clin Endocrinol Metab 1989; 68: 548–554.
18. Rigotti NA, Nussbaum SR, Herzog DB et al. Osteoporosis in women with anorexia nervosa. N Engl J Med 1984; 311: 1601–1606.
19. Bachrach LK, Guido D, Katzman D et al. Decreased bone density in adolescent girls with anorexia nervosa. Pediatrics 1990; 86: 440–447.
20. Myerson M, Gutin R, Warren MP et al. Total body bone density in amenorrheic runners. Obstet Gynecol 1992; 79: 973–978.
21. Klibanski A & Greenspan SL. Increase in bone mass after treatment of hyperprolactinemic amenorrhea. N Engl J Med 1986; 315: 542–546.
22. Baker E & Demers L. Menstrual status in female athletes: correlation with reproductive hormones and bone density. Obstet Gynecol 1988; 72: 683–687.
23. Drinkwater BL, Nilson K, Chesnut CH et al. Bone mineral content of amenorrheic and eumenorrheic athletes. N Engl J Med 1984; 311: 277–281.
24. Drinkwater BL, Nilson K, Ott S et al. Bone mineral density after resumption of menses in amenorrheic athletes. JAMA 1986; 245: 380–382.
25. Nelson ME, Fisher EC, Catsos PD et al. Diet and bone status in amenorrheic runners. Am J Clin Nutr 1986; 43: 910–916.
26. Drinkwater BL, Bruemner B & Chestnut CH. Menstrual history as a determinant of current bone density in young athletes. JAMA 1990; 263: 545–548.
27. Henley K & Vaitukaitis JL. Exercise-induced menstrual dysfunction. Ann Rev Med 1988; 39: 443–451.
28. Lloyd T, Myers C, Buchanan JR et al. Collegiate women athletes with irregular menses during adolescence have decreased bone density. Obstet Gynecol 1988; 72: 639–642.
29. Ding JH, Sheckter CB, Drinkwater BL et al. High serum cortisol levels in exercise-associated amenorrhea. Ann Intern Med 1988; 108: 530–534.
30. Shangold MM, Gatz ML & Thysen B. Acute effect of exercise on plasma concentration of prolactin and testosterone in recreational women runners. Fertil Steril 1981; 35: 699–702.
31. Chang FE, Dodds WG, Sullivan M et al. The acute effects of exercise on prolactin and growth hormone secretion: comparison between sedentary women and women runners with normal and abnormal menstrual cycles. J Clin Endocrinol Metab 1986; 62: 551–556.

32. Brisson GR, Volle MA, Decarufel D et al. Exercise-induced disassociation of the blood prolactin response in young women according to their sports habits. *Horm Metab Res* 1980; **12**: 201–205.

33. Dale E, Gerlach DH & Wilhite AL. Menstrual dysfunction of distance runners. *Obstet Gynecol* 1979; **54**: 47–53.

34. Prior JC, Bigna YM, Schechter MT et al. Spinal bone loss and ovulatory disturbances. *N Engl J Med* 1990; **323**: 1221–1227.

35. Adashi EY. Ovulation induction: clomiphene citrate. In: Adashi EY, Rock JA & Rosenwaks Z, eds. *Reproductive Endocrinology, Surgery, and Technology*, 1st edn. JB Lippincott, 1996; 1181–1206.

36. Clark KM, Sowers MFR, Nichols S et al. Bone mineral density changes over two years in first-time users of depot medroxyprogesterone acetate. *Fertil Steril* 2004; **82**: 1580–1586.

37. Cromer BA, Blair JM, Mahan JD et al. A prospective comparison of bone density in adolescent girls receiving depot medroxyprogesterone acetate (Depo-Provera), levonorgestrel (Norplant) or oral contraceptives. *J Paediatr* 1996; **129**: 671–676.

38. Berenson A, Radecki C, Grady J et al. A prospective controlled study of the effects of hormonal contraception on bone mineral density. *Obstet Gynecol* 2001; **98**: 576–582.

39. Scholes D, LaCroix A, Ichikawa L et al. Injectable hormone contraception and bone density: results from a prospective study. *Epidemiology* 2002; **13**: 581–587.

40. Tang O, Tang G, Yip P et al. Further evaluation on long-term depot-medroxyprogesterone acetate use and bone mineral density: a longitudinal cohort study. *Contraception* 2000; **62**: 161–164.

41. Merki-Feld GS, Neff M & Keller PJ. A prospective study on the effects of depot medroxyprogesterone acetate on trabecular and cortical bone after attainment of peak bone mass. *Br J Obstet Gynaecol* 2000; **107**: 863–869.

42. Aitken JM, Hart DM, Lindsay R et al. Prevention of bone loss following oophorectomy in premenopausal women. *Isr J Med Sci* 1976; **12**: 607–614.

43. Alderman BW, Weiss NS, Daling JR et al. Reproductive history and postmenopausal risk of hip and forearm fracture. *Am J Epidemiol* 1986; **124**: 262–267.

44. Meema S & Meema HE. Evaluation of cortical bone mass, thickness and density by z-scores in osteopenic conditions and in relation to menopause and estrogen treatment. *Skeletal Radiol* 1982; **8**: 259–268.

45. Ohta H, Makita K, Suda Y et al. Influence of oophorectomy on serum levels of sex steroids and bone metabolism and assessment of bone mineral density in lumbar trabecular bone by QCT-c value. *J Bone Miner Res* 1992; **7**: 659–665.

46. Stepan JJ, Pospichal J, Presl J et al. Bone loss and biochemical indices of bone remodeling in surgically induced postmenopausal women. *Bone* 1987; **8**: 279–284.

47. Reeves J. Bone turnover and trabecular plate survival after artificial menopause. *BMJ* 1987; **295**: 757–760.

48. Genant HK, Cann CE, Ettinger B et al. Quantitative computed tomography of vertebral spongiosa: a sensitive method for detecting early bone loss after oophorectomy. *Ann Intern Med* 1982; **97**: 699–705.

49. Lindsay R, Hart DM, Forrest C et al. Prevention of spinal osteoporosis in oophorectomized women. *Lancet* 1980; **2**: 1151–1154.

50. Gambacciani M, Spinetti A, Cappagli B et al. Effects of ipriflavone administration on bone mass and metabolism in ovariectomized women. *J Endocrinol Invest* 1993; **16**: 333–337.

51. Mazzuoli GF, Tabolli S, Bigi F et al. Effects of salmon calcitonin on the bone loss induced by ovariectomy. *Calcif Tissue Int* 1990; **47**: 209–214.

52. Fentiman IS, Saad Z, Caleffi M et al. Tamoxifen protects against steroid-induced bone loss. *Eur J Cancer* 1992; **28**: 684–685.

53. Ward RL, Morgan G, Dalley D et al. Tamoxifen reduces bone turnover and prevents lumbar spine and proximal femoral bone loss in early postmenopausal women. *Bone Miner* 1993; **22**: 87–94.

54. Kenny AM, Prestwood KM, Pilbeam CC et al. The short term effects of tamoxifen on bone turnover in older women. *J Clin Endocrinol Metab* 1995; **80**: 3287–3291.

55. Love RR, Barden HS, Mazess RB et al. Effect of tamoxifen on lumbar spine bone mineral density in postmenopausal women after 5 years. *Arch Intern Med* 1994; **154**: 2585–2588.

56. Sowers MF, Shapiro B, Gilbraith MA et al. Health and hormonal characteristics of women with low premenopausal bone mass. *Calcif Tissue Int* 1990; **47**: 130–135.

57. Sowers MF, Corton G, Shapiro B et al. Changes in bone density with lactation. *JAMA* 1993; **269**: 3130–3135.

58. Kalkwarf H, Specker B, Bianchi D et al. The effect of calcium supplementation on bone density during lactation and after weaning. *N Engl J Med* 1997; **337**: 523–528.

59. Lees CJ, Jerome CP, Register TC et al. Changes in bone mass and bone biomarkers of cynomolgus monkeys during pregnancy and lactation. *J Clin Endocrinol Metab* 1998; **83**: 4298–4302.

60. Sowers MF, Randolph J, Shapiro B et al. A prospective study of bone density and pregnancy after an extended period of lactation with bone loss. *Obstet Gynecol* 1995; **85**: 285–289.

61. Henderson P, Sowers MF, Kutzko K et al. Bone mineral density in grand multiparous with extended lactation. *Am J Obstet Gynecol* 2000; **182**: 1371–1377.

62. Prentice A, Jarjou L, Stirling D et al. Biochemical markers of calcium and bone metabolism during 18 months of lactation in Gambian women accustomed to a low calcium intake and those consuming a calcium supplement. *J Clin Endocrinol Metab* 1998; **83**: 1059–1066.

63. Little K & Clapp J. Self-selected recreational exercise has no impact on early postpartum lactation-induced bone loss. *Med Sci Sports Exerc* 1998; **30**: 831–836.

64. Melton LJ, Bryant SC, Wahner HW et al. Influence of breastfeeding and other reproductive factors on bone mass later in life. *Osteoporosis Int* 1993; **3**: 76–83.

65. Laitinen K, Valimaki M & Keto P. Bone mineral density measured by dual-energy X-ray absorptiometry in healthy Finnish women. *Calcif Tissue Int* 1991; **48**: 224–231.

66. Walker RP, Richardson B & Walker F. The influence of numerous pregnancies and lactations on bone dimensions in South African Bantu and Caucasian mothers. *Clin Sci* 1972; **42**: 189–196.

67. Bauer DC, Browner WS, Cauley JA et al. Factors associated with appendicular bone mass in older women. *Ann Intern Med* 1993; **118**: 657–665.

68. Falch JA & Sandvik L. Perimenopausal appendicular bone loss: a 10-year prospective study. *Bone* 1990; **11**: 425–428.

69. Arlot ME, Sornay-Rendu E, Garnero P et al. Apparent pre- and post-menopausal bone loss evaluated by DEXA at different skeletal sites in women: the OFELY cohort. *J Bone Miner Res* 1997; **12**: 683–690.

70. Buchanon JR, Myers C, Lloyd T et al. Early vertebral trabecular bone loss in normal premenopausal women. *J Bone Miner Res* 1988; **3**: 583–587.

71. Block JE, Smith R, Gleuer C-C et al. Models of spinal trabecular bone loss as determined by quantitative computerized tomography. *J Bone Miner Res* 1989; **4**: 249–257.

72. Johnston CC, Hui SL, Witt RM et al. Early menopausal changes in bone mass and sex steroids. *J Clin Endocrinol Metab* 1985; **61**: 905–913.

73. Slemenda C, Hui SL, Longcope C et al. Sex steroids and bone mass. A study of changes about the time of menopause. *J Clin Invest* 1987; **80**: 1261–1269.

74. Pouilles JM, Tremollieres F & Ribot C. The effects of menopause on longitudinal bone loss from the spine. *Calcif Tissue Int* 1993; **52**: 340–343.

75. Recker RR, Lappe JM, Davies KM et al. Change in bone mass immediately before menopause. *J Bone Miner Res* 1992; **7**: 857–862.

76. Nilas L. Assessment of the physiological bone loss in women, with special emphasis on the menopausal changes. *Dan Med Bull* 1991; **38**: 317–327.

77. Riggs BL, Wahner HW, Melton LJ et al. Rates of bone loss in the appendicular and axial skeletons of women. Evidence of substantial vertebral bone loss before menopause. *J Clin Invest* 1986; **77**: 1487–1491.

78. Sowers MF, Luborsky J, Perdue C et al. Thyroid stimulating hormone (TSH) concentrations and menopausal status in women at the mid-life: SWAN. *Clin Endocrinol (Oxford)* 2003; **58**: 340–347.

79. Wada S, Kitamura H, Matsuura Y et al. Parathyroid hormone-related protein as a cause of hypercalcemia in a B-cell type malignant lymphoma. *Int Med* 1992; **31**: 968–972.

80. Sowers MF, Hollis B, Shapiro B et al. Elevated parathyroid hormone-related peptide associated with lactation and bone density loss. *JAMA* 1996; **276**: 549–554.

81. Luengo M, del Rio L, Pons F et al. Bone mineral density in asthmatic patients treated with inhaled corticosteroids: a case–control study. *Eur Respir J* 1997; **10**: 2110–2113.

82. Peel NFA, Moore DJ, Barringon NA et al. Risk of vertegral fracture and relationship to bone mineral density in steroid treated rheumatoid arthritis. *Ann Rheum Dis* 1995; **54**: 801–806.

83. Canalis E. Mechanisms of glucocorticoid action in bone: implications to glucocorticoid-induced osteoporosis. *J Clin Endocrinol Metab* 1996; **81**: 3441–3446.

84. Hsueh AJ & Erickson GF. Glucocorticoid inhibition of FSH-induced estrogen production in cultured rat granulosa cells. *Steroids* 1978; **32**: 639–648.

85. American College of Rheumatology Task Force on Osteoporosis Guidelines. Recommendations for the prevention and treatment of glucocorticoid-induced osteoporosis. *Arthritis Rheum* 1996; **39**: 1791–1801.

86. Mundy GR, Shapiro JL, Bandelin JG et al. Direct stimulation of bone resorption by thyroid hormones. *J Clin Invest* 1976; **58**: 529–534.

87. Toh SH, Claunch BC & Brown PH. Effect of hyperthyroidism and its treatment on bone mineral content. *Arch Intern Med* 1985; **145**: 883–886.

88. Faber J, Overgaard K & Jarlov AE. Bone metabolism in premenopausal women with nontoxic goiter and reduced serum thyrotropin levels. *Thyroid* 1994; **6**: 27–32.

89. Frost HM. Why do bone strength and 'mass' in aging adults become unresponsive to vigorous exercise? Insights of the Utah paradigm. *J Bone Miner Metab* 1999; **17**: 90–97.

90. Finkelstein JS, Lee MLT, Sowers MF et al. Ethnic variation in bone mineral density in pre- and early perimenopausal women: role of anthropometric and lifestyle factors. *J Clin Endocrinol Metab* 2002; **87**: 3057–3067.

91. Biering-Sorensen F, Bohr HH & Schaadt OP. Longitudinal study of bone mineral content in the lumbar spine, the forearm and the lower extremities after spinal cord injury. *Eur J Clin Invest* 1990; **20**: 330–335.

92. Bassey EJ, Rothwell MC, Littlewood JJ et al. Pre- and post-menopausal women have different bone mineral density responses to the same high-impact exercise. *J Bone Miner Res* 1998; **13**: 1805–1813.

93. Goto S, Ishima M, Shimizu M et al. A longitudinal study for femoral neck bone mineral density increases in premenopausal caddies using dual-energy X-ray absorptiometry. *J Bone Miner Metab* 2001; **19**: 125–130.

94. Winters KM & Snow CM. Detraining reverses positive effects of exercise on the musculoskeletal system in premenopausal women. *J Bone Miner Res* 2000; **15**: 2495–2503.

95. Beck BR & Snow CM. Bone health across the lifespan – exercising our options. *Exerc Sport Sci Rev* 2003; **31**: 117–122.

96. Bainbridge K, Sowers MF, Crutchfield M et al. Natural history of bone loss over 6 years among premenopausal and early postmenopausal women. *Am J Epidemiol* 2002; **156**: 410–417.

97. Hawker GA, Jamal SA, Ridout R et al. A clinical prediction rule to identify premenopausal women with low bone mass. *Osteoporosis Int* 2002; **13**: 400–406.

98. Wolff I, van Croonenborg JJ, Kemper HCG et al. The effect of exercise training programs on bone mass: a meta analysis of published controlled trials in pre- and post menopausal women. *Osteoporosis Int* 1999; **9**: 1–12.

99. Kannus P. Preventing osteoporosis, falls, and fractures among elderly people. *BMJ* 1999; **318**: 205–206.

100. Institute of Medicine. *DRI Reference Intakes for Ca, P, Mg, Vitamin D, and Fluoride*. Washington, DC: National Academy Press, 1997.

101. Flynn A. The role of dietary calcium in bone health. *Proc Nutr Soc* 2003; **62**: 851–858.

102. Martin AD, Bailey DA, McKay HA et al. Bone mineral and calcium accretion during puberty. *Am J Clin Nutr* 1997; **66**: 611–615.

103. Jackman LA, Millane SS, Martin BR et al. Calcium retention in relation to calcium intake and postmenarcheal age in adolescent females. *Am J Clin Nutr* 1997; **66**: 327–333.

104. Pettifor JM & Moodley GP. Appendicular bone mass in children with a high prevalence of low dietary calcium intakes. *J Bone Miner Res* 1997; **12**: 1824–1832.

105. Gourlay ML & Brown SA. Clinical considerations in premenopausal osteoporosis. *Arch Intern Med* 2004; **164**: 603–614.

106. Ginty F. Dietary protein and bone health. *Proc Nutr Soc* 2003; **62**: 867–876.

107. Greendale G, FitzGerald G, Huang MH et al. Dietary soy isoflavones and BMD: results from the Study of Women's Health Across the Nation (SWAN). *Am J Epidemiol* 2002; **155**: 746–754.

108. Jayo MJ, Anthony MS, Register TC et al. Dietary soy isoflavones and bone loss: a study in ovariectomized monkeys. *J Bone Miner Res* 1996; **11**(Suppl.): S228.

109. Alekel DL, St Germain A, Peterson CT et al. Isoflavone-rich soy protein isolate attenuates bone loss in the lumbar spine of perimenopausal women. *Am J Clin Nutr* 2000; **72**: 844–852.

110. Daniell HW. Osteoporosis of the slender smoker. *Arch Intern Med* 1976; **136**: 298–304.

111. Law MR & Hackshaw AK. A meta-analysis of cigarette smoking, bone mineral density and risk of hip fracture: recognition of a major effect. *BMJ* 1997; **315**: 841–846.

112. Krall EA & Dawson-Hughes B. Smoking reduces fractional calcium absorption and increases bone loss. *J Bone Miner Res* 1997; **12**(Suppl. 1): S225.

113. Clark K & Sowers MF. Alcohol dependence, smoking status, reproductive characteristics, and bone mineral density in premenopausal women. *Res Nurs Health* 1996; **19**: 399–408.

114. Chappard D, Plantard B, Petitjean M et al. Alcoholic cirrhosis and osteoporosis in men: a light and scanning electron microscopy study. *J Stud Alcohol* 1991; **52**: 269–274.

115. Clark MK, Sowers MF, Dekordi F et al. Bone mineral density and fracture among alcohol dependent women in treatment and in recovery. *Osteoporosis Int* 2003; **14**: 396–403.

116. Laitinen K, Valimaki, M, Lamberg-Allardt C et al. Deranged vitamin D metabolism but normal bone mineral density in Finnish noncirrhotic male alcoholics. *Alcohol Clin Exp Res* 1990; **14**: 551–556.

Chapter 7

Risk factors for osteoporosis and fractures in men and women

Shreyasee Amin, Richard Eastell and Jackie A. Clowes

INTRODUCTION

Osteoporosis is defined as 'an asymptomatic systemic bone disease characterized by low bone mass and microarchitectural deterioration of bone tissue, with a consequent increase in bone fragility and susceptibility to fracture'.[1] Osteoporotic fractures, especially hip fractures, are associated with substantial morbidity and mortality,[2] and prevention of fractures is thus the primary goal of osteoporosis management. While osteoporosis is a well-recognized clinical problem among post-menopausal women and the elderly, it is important to be aware that both men and women are at risk for osteoporosis, and that it can occur at any age, depending, at least in part, on the presence of clinical risk factors. Recognition of risk factors for bone loss and fracture is therefore critical, in order to target individuals at greatest risk for appropriate intervention before substantial bone loss or fractures occur, and where possible to help modify these risk factors.

Epidemiological studies have demonstrated multiple risk factors associated with the development of osteoporosis and fragility fractures. These include genetic factors, chronic medical conditions, medications, lifestyle choices, and levels of endogenous hormones and vitamins. It is important to note that risk factors vary with different fracture types.[3–5] In addition, information on risk factors in different races is limited, the majority of studies relating to Caucasian populations. Most studies have also tended to involve only women; however, there are now a growing number of studies examining risk factors in men. In this chapter, we have updated our previous review,[6] discussing some of the key clinical risk factors for osteoporosis and fragility fractures in both men and women, with attention to more recent advances in our understanding of these risk factors.

GENETIC FACTORS

Twin and family studies have suggested a strong genetic association with bone mineral density (BMD) and fracture; therefore, a positive family history of an osteoporotic fracture represents an important clinical risk factor. In a study of wrist fractures involving 6570 Caucasian female volunteer twins (age 18–80 years), there was an elevated case-wise concordance for twins compared with the population prevalence, and increased prevalence of reported maternal wrist fracture for twin pairs suffering from wrist fractures, suggesting a familial clustering.[7] The genetic influence of wrist fracture also appeared to be independent of BMD.[7]

In women, a case–control study demonstrated that a family history of osteoporotic fracture (hip and wrist) was associated with a two-fold increase in osteoporotic fractures (vertebra, hip and wrist).[8] Site-specific analysis found that a positive family history of wrist fracture was associated with a four-fold increase in prevalent wrist fracture.[8] Prospective data demonstrated that a maternal history of hip fracture doubled the risk of hip fracture independently of BMD.[9] Other maternal fractures were not associated with increased risk of hip fractures.[9] A parental history of wrist fracture increased the risk of incident wrist fractures by 70%.[10] The effect of paternal history was greater than for maternal history of wrist fracture.[10] In peri-menopausal women aged 47–51 years a history of hip fracture in the maternal grandmother was associated with a three-fold increase in self-reported appendicular fractures.[11] In the EVOS study, men with a maternal history of hip fracture had a 30% increase in vertebral fractures, but this was not seen in women.[12]

In a meta-analysis, involving 34,928 men and women followed for 134,724 person-years, a parental history of fracture was associated with a significant increased risk for fracture with a risk ratio (RR) of 1.18 (95% confidence interval (CI): 1.06–1.31) for any osteoporotic fracture and 1.49 (95% CI: 1.17–1.89) for hip fracture.[13] A parental history of hip fracture was associated with a 54% increase in risk of all osteoporotic fracture (RR: 1.54; 95% CI: 1.25–1.88) and 127% increase in risk of hip fracture (RR: 2.27; 95% CI: 1.47–3.49).[13] The risks were independent of BMD.[13]

Overall, there appears to be an important genetic contribution to osteoporosis and fracture. Findings are largely from studies in women; however, similar results have been seen in men. The available data suggest the relationship between family history and fracture may be site specific, but this has only been evaluated in a limited number of studies.

In light of these overall findings, several studies are now exploring the role of possible candidate genes in the development of skeletal geometry, bone mineral density and fractures.[14] Current evidence suggests that osteoporosis is caused by the combined effects of multiple genes, which are influenced by numerous environmental factors. Importantly, one study has suggested that genes found to be relevant for BMD may not be relevant to hip fractures, and that the relationship between BMD and risk of hip fractures appears to be primarily due to an environmental correlation.[15] There is currently no evidence to support a clinical role for the use of genetic markers in evaluating an individual's current or future risk for either osteoporosis or fracture, and these tests are not routinely measured in clinical practice at this time.

PREVALENT FRACTURES

While a family history of fracture is an important clinical risk factor for future fracture in an individual, a personal history of a previous fracture is an even more important predictor of future fractures, for both men and women. A study in perimenopausal women aged 47–51 years with a history of a previous osteoporotic fracture identified a 60% increase in subsequent self-reported fracture within 2 years.[11] A retrospective study of post-menopausal women suggested that an index ankle fracture increased the risk of a subsequent hip fracture by 60% and of vertebral fracture by 50%.[16] A previous humeral fracture increased the risk of a subsequent hip fracture two- to three-fold.[16] In a study involving over 200,000 men and women with an incident fracture during follow-up, there was a two- to three-fold increase in the risk of subsequent fractures at different skeletal sites.[17]

In women, prevalent vertebral deformities predicted a four-fold increase in risk of incident vertebral fractures, a 90% increase in risk of hip fractures, and 60% increase in non-vertebral fractures after adjusting for age and calcaneal BMD.[18] Prevalent vertebral deformities predicted a 40% increase in incident wrist fracture after adjusting for age alone; however, the study only identified women over the age of 65 years and the majority of wrist fractures occur prior to this age.[18] More than three vertebral deformities or a very severe vertebral deformity increased the risk of incident vertebral fracture by over 11-fold.[18] Similarly, in a study involving 3100 men and 3500 women followed for a mean of 3.8 years, the risk of an incident vertebral fracture increased with the number of prevalent vertebral deformities at baseline (relative risk for one prevalent deformity at baseline was 3.2 (95% CI: 2.1–4.8); 9.8 (95% CI: 6.1–15.8) for two prevalent deformities; and 23.3 (95% CI: 15.3–35.4) for three or more).[19] Relative risks also differed according to the shape of the prevalent deformity. The relative risk was 1.6 (95% CI: 0.8–3.2) if the posterior and mid-vertebral heights were reduced, but increased to 5.9 (95% CI: 4.1–8.6) if the anterior and mid-vertebral heights were reduced.[19] In a population-based study, involving 820 men and women with a history of clinically recognized vertebral fracture and 4349 person-years of follow-up, there was a 2.8-fold increase in any fracture which was greater for men than in women.[20] The estimated cumulative incidence of any fracture was 70% over 10 years.[20]

Forearm fractures also appear to increase the risk of subsequent fractures in both men and women. A retrospective population-based study of 12,162 Finnish women, using self-reported fractures, suggested that low-energy wrist fractures between the age of 20 and 34 years predicted a three-fold increase in the number of subsequent low-energy fractures and a two-fold increase in high-energy fractures in women aged 35–57 years.[21] Sixty-three per cent of the fractures occurred in pre-menopausal women.[21] In another study involving 1288 men and women with a forearm fracture, followed for 9664 person-years, the risk of a hip fracture compared to expected fracture rates in the community was increased 1.4-fold in women (95% CI: 1.1–1.8) and 2.7-fold in men (95% CI: 0.98–5.8).[22] In women with a previous forearm fracture, the risk of subsequent hip fracture differed by age. Thus, if women sustained a forearm fracture after age 70 years, there was a 1.6-fold increase (95% CI: 1.2–2.0) in the risk of a subsequent hip fracture, whereas women who sustained their first forearm fracture before age 70 years did not have a significant increase in risk.[22] By contrast, vertebral fractures were significantly increased at any age in those with a prior distal forearm fracture. Thus, there was a 5.2-fold increase (95% CI: 4.5–5.9) in subsequent vertebral fracture risk among women and a 10.7-fold increase (95% CI: 6.7–16.3) among men.[22]

Multiple studies have now demonstrated that a personal history of fracture is a strong predictor of future fracture, in both men and women. Ideally, the goal is to prevent a first fracture from occurring; however, when a fracture is identified in an individual without previous history of known osteoporosis, it should result in a clinical evaluation for modifiable risks for bone loss and fracture, as well as an opportunity for treatment intervention.[23]

IMPAIRED NEUROMUSCULAR FUNCTION AND RISK OF FALLS

Many markers of impaired physical activity, mobility and neuromuscular function have been identified as increasing the risk of falls and fractures in both men and women.[9,24,25] The risk of falls in women is twice that of men and increases two-fold between 60 and 80 years of age. In individuals who fall, over 50% fall more than twice a year. However, only 5% of falls result in a fracture, and fewer than 1% result in hip fracture.[26] A fall from a standing height or less is involved in approximately 90% of non-spinal fractures in the elderly[27] and 30% of clinically apparent vertebral fractures.[26] There is a 70% increase in the risk of a fall for every 10-year increase in age.[28] Studies have demonstrated that impaired mobility, assessed by balance, leg strength or gait, was associated with a three-fold increase in the risk of falls and a five-fold increase in risk of recurrent falls.[28]

Other risk factors include dizziness on standing, a history of stroke, poor mental state and postural hypotension.[28]

The direction and dynamics involved in a fall appear to change with ageing and influence the type of fracture observed. Previous studies have found the risk of hip fracture is increased following falls to the side and in individuals with a reduced protective arm response, decreased mobility and possibly a decreased body mass index. In addition, the ability of patients suffering a hip fracture to break their fall was absent in mentally impaired patients, and present in only 16% of lucid patients compared to 42% of controls.[29] A population-based assessment of the circumstances relating to a fall which precipitated a hip fracture suggested 13% are related to intrinsic medical problems and 40% to an environmental hazard.[30] Sedative and psychotropic medication increase the risk for falls[31,32] and therefore are another important risk factor for fracture in older individuals. The impact of intervention in fall prevention has demonstrated a reduction in the risk of falls,[33] but the effect on fracture reduction has not been well established.

CHRONIC MEDICAL CONDITIONS

Several chronic medical conditions have been associated with an increased risk of bone loss and/or fractures. For some conditions, however, conflicting results have been reported. Nevertheless, recognition that individuals with such conditions may warrant additional monitoring and preventive strategies for osteoporotic fracture is critical.

Inflammatory arthritis

There is an increased risk of generalized osteoporosis and fractures among those with an inflammatory arthritis.[34–36] The pathophysiological mechanism for this increased risk is complex and felt to be multifactorial. The unique factors which may adversely affect bone metabolism are considered to be: (i) inflammation, related to active disease; (ii) disability, with reduced physical function and mobility; and (iii) medications, particularly use of glucocorticoids.

Studies in rheumatoid arthritis have suggested that the inflammatory process, which is known to contribute to joint damage and bony erosion, may also play a direct role in the pathogenesis of generalized osteoporosis in these patients.[37,38] The role of inflammation and the immune system on bone metabolism has been an area of growing interest. There is increasing evidence that the immune system modifies bone metabolism not only in response to inflammatory conditions (e.g. rheumatoid arthritis), but also during ageing and in response to oestrogen deficiency. This involves complex interactions between circulating hormones (e.g. oestrogen, vitamin D), inflammatory cells (e.g. T- and B-lymphocytes) and proinflammatory cytokines, including tumour necrosis factor alpha (TNF-α), interleukin (IL)-1 and IL-6, among others. The majority of these factors appear to mediate their effect primarily through modulating the RANK/RANKL/OPG system.[39,40a,b] Osteoclast precursors and mature osteoclasts express a receptor

called receptor activator for NF-κB (RANK).[39] Osteoblastic cells induce osteoclastic differentiation and resorptive activity through the expression of a surface membrane protein called osteoprotegrin ligand (OPGL), also referred to as RANKL, which binds to RANK.[39] Proinflammatory cytokines in rheumatoid arthritis, for example, can stimulate bone resorption via an up-regulation of RANKL on fibroblasts and activated T-cells [39]. Osteoprotegrin (OPG) is a soluble decoy receptor for RANKL, and regulates bone resorption by blocking RANK/RANKL binding and thereby inhibiting osteoclastogenesis. In a mice transgenic model for inflammatory destructive arthritis, blocking RANKL with OPG treatment led to decreased bone destruction, but did not influence the degree of joint synovitis.[41] In inflammatory conditions, RANKL is released from cell surfaces by metalloproteases and may be a mechanism for the generalized osteoporosis seen.[42]

Osteoarthritis

In contrast to inflammatory arthritis, hip or knee osteoarthritis has been associated with higher bone mineral density in cross-sectional studies.[43–45] However, in a longitudinal study, men and women with radiographic osteoarthritis of the hip had a higher rate of bone loss at the femoral neck during 2 years of follow-up.[46] The bone loss was independent of lower limb disability.[46]

Studies involving large numbers of men and women have failed to identify a decreased risk of fracture among those with osteoarthritis, despite reports of higher BMD.[47,48] This may relate to an increased risk of falls among those with osteoarthritis. In a study involving both men and women, those with self-reported osteoarthritis had higher body sway and lower quadriceps strength.[47] In another study, women with a self-report of osteoarthritis were found to have an increased risk of falls (RR: 1.4; 95% CI: 1.2–1.5).[48] Conversely, the same study reported that women with radiographic evidence of hip osteoarthritis was associated with a 70% reduction in recurrent falls.[48] It remains possible that symptomatic arthritis, which results in greater disability and functional impairment, may increase the risk for falls, and therefore fractures, compared to those with radiographic evidence of osteoarthritis but no symptoms. While the association between osteoarthritis, osteoporosis and fractures is complex,[49] it remains important to consider a diagnosis of osteoporosis in men and women with osteoarthritis.

Endocrine disorders

Several different endocrine disorders have been associated with bone loss and increased fracture risk. A number of studies have reported that endogenous hypercortisolism or Cushing's disease is associated with increased risk of fractures[50–52] and is an important diagnosis to consider in those presenting with multiple spinal fractures or an unexplained high bone turnover state. Although rare, it is a condition especially important to consider in male and younger patients.[52] Interestingly, in a community-based cohort of over 600 men and women, a higher baseline urinary free cortisol level was significantly associated with incident fractures.[53] After adjusting for other factors, including depression, the odds ratio for an incident fracture with each quartile increase in baseline urinary free cortisol was 2.28 (95% CI: 0.91–5.77), 3.40 (95% CI: 1.33–8.69) and 5.38 (95% CI: 1.68–17.21).[53] Importantly, excluding those subjects who were using corticosteroids did not significantly change the results.[53]

In a population-based study, men and women with primary hyperparathyroidism had an increased risk of vertebral, forearm, rib and proximal femoral fractures.[54] Others have also confirmed an increased risk of fracture among men and women with hyperparathyroidism; however, the risk of fracture appeared to decrease following either surgical or non-surgical treatment.[55]

In a study in women, a previous history of hyperthyroidism was associated with an 80% increase in risk of hip fracture.[9] In a study involving 11,776 patients with hyperthyroidism (6301 patients with diffuse toxic goitre and 5475 with nodular toxic goitre) and 4473 patients with hypothyroidism, those with hyperthyroidism had a fracture risk that appeared to be significantly increased around the time of diagnosis (incidence rate ratio (IRR) between 1.26 and 2.29), but which decreased to normal levels after diagnosis.[56] Surgical treatment of hyperthyroidism was associated with a decreased fracture risk after diagnosis (RR: 0.66; 95% CI: 0.55–0.78).[56] Furthermore, in those with hypothyroidism, fracture risk was also significantly increased both before and after diagnosis, with a peak around the time of diagnosis (IRR between 2.17 and 2.35).[56] The mechanism for the increased fracture risk in untreated patients with hypothyroidism is unclear; however, it may relate to either immobility or an increased risk of falling. Importantly, overtreatment with thyroxine replacement therapy accelerates bone loss,[57] which can further increase fracture risk.

Gastrointestinal disorders

There have been several reports of gastrointestinal diseases increasing the risk for fractures in both men and women. The malabsorption of different nutrients important in bone health has a significant impact on the pathogenesis of bone disease in gastrointestinal disease. In addition, inflammatory mediators in conditions such as coeliac disease and Crohn's disease may also, at least in part, contribute to bone loss. In coeliac disease, a case–control study found a three-fold increase in peripheral fracture, with 80% of fractures occurring in patients with previously undiagnosed coeliac disease and patients who were not adherent with therapy.[58] Increased fracture risk has been reported in patients with a previous gastrectomy or a history of pernicious anaemia.[59] In Crohn's disease, a case–control study of male and female patients found a 190% increase in fracture risk in peri-menopausal females, compared to an 80% increase in fracture risk in post-menopausal women.[60] There was no increase in fracture risk in men with Crohn's disease or in any patients with ulcerative colitis.[60] Similarly, among 15,000 inflammatory bowel disease patients identified in a national hospital registry, there was an increased fracture risk of 15–20% among patients with Crohn's disease, but no increased risk for overall fracture risk was demonstrated in those with ulcerative colitis.[61] However, in recent population-based studies, fracture risk was not increased in patients with either Crohn's disease[62] or ulcerative colitis.[63]

Chronic liver diseases, including viral hepatitis, and chronic cholestatic diseases, such as primary biliary cirrhosis, also appear to be associated with lower BMD and increased fracture risk.[64–71] The mechanism may relate, at least in part, to a combination of vitamin D deficiency, vitamin K deficiency and changes in circulating cytokines related to liver inflammation.

Depression

Several studies have demonstrated an association between depression and lower BMD, increased disability and increased risk of falls. Depression is also associated with higher free urinary cortisol levels.[72] A prospective study found women with symptoms of depression had a 20% increase in non-vertebral fractures after adjusting for medication use, falls and neuromuscular function.[73] There was a 110% increase in risk of vertebral fracture and 100% increase in risk of rib fractures after adjusting for potential confounders, including prevalent vertebral fractures, hip BMD and history of falls.[73] The prevalence of depression in the elderly was 6.3%, so this may therefore represent an important potential area for targeting preventative strategies.[73]

Other medical conditions

An increasingly important secondary cause of fractures is solid organ transplantation,[74–76] with an estimated increased relative risk of five- to 34-fold depending on patient sex and the type of transplantation.[75] The effect of organ transplantation on bone metabolism is complex and multifactorial, and has been recently reviewed.[76]

The relationship between urolithiasis, the most common cause of which is hypercalciuria, and hip fracture risk is conflicting. However, there appears to be a four-fold increase in vertebral fracture risk.[77] Chronic renal disease is associated with osteoporosis and increased fracture risk,[78–80] which may relate in part to impaired activation of vitamin D, secondary hyperparathyroidism and resultant adverse effect on bone metabolism.

In a case–control study, chronic respiratory disease in women was associated with a three-fold increase in severe vertebral deformities, which remained significant despite correcting for corticosteroid use.[81] A retrospective cohort study of patients with cystic fibrosis identified a 10- to 100-fold increase in risk of vertebral and rib fractures.[82]

Patients with haemachromatosis and thalassaemia also have low BMD, which has been attributed, in part, to the loss of gonadal function that occurs with these disorders.[83,84] Limited visual acuity is associated with a doubling of the number of hip fractures.[24] There is a 40% increase in hip fractures with impaired depth perception and 20% increase with reduced contrast sensitivity.[9]

MEDICATIONS

There are a number of medications that have been shown to have an adverse effect on bone metabolism. When these medications are prescribed, preventive strategies and monitoring for osteoporosis are necessary. In contrast, several recent reports have suggested that certain commonly prescribed medications may in fact have beneficial effects on bone health.

Corticosteroids

Chronic corticosteroid use, the most common form of drug-induced osteoporosis, results in a rapid onset of bone loss within the first 3–6 months of therapy and an increased risk of fracture.[85,86] Corticosteroids decrease bone formation and also lead to increased bone resorption.[87] Bone loss and fracture risk appear to be greater in trabecular bone than cortical bone.[88] In a retrospective cohort study comprising 244,235 oral corticosteroid users and 244,235 controls, the relative risk among steroid users was 1.09 (95% CI: 1.01–1.17) for forearm fractures, 1.61 (95% CI: 1.47–1.76) for hip fractures and 2.60 (95% CI: 2.31–2.92) for vertebral fractures.[89] The risk of fracture also appeared to be dose dependent, with the greatest risk of fractures occurring at standardized daily doses of ≥7.5 mg/day of prednisolone.[89] Nevertheless, the risk for fractures, particularly vertebral fractures, was still increased at doses as low as 2.5 mg/day of prednisolone.[89] A meta-analysis comprising seven prospective cohort studies, which followed 42,500 men and women for 176,000-patient years, demonstrated that a prior exposure to corticosteroids increased the risk for osteoporotic fracture and hip fracture.[90] An increased risk was also demonstrated among current users of corticosteroids, which appeared to be independent of BMD.[90] Risks were similar for men and for women, and slightly higher at younger ages.[90]

Anticoagulants

Vitamin K deficiency results in an increased risk of osteoporotic fractures[91] and may reflect poor nutritional status or the role of osteocalcin in bone mineralization.[91,92] Oral anticoagulants inhibit vitamin K and may potentially increase fracture risk. This is supported by a case–control study that demonstrated that oral anticoagulants increased the risk of severe vertebral deformities in women three-fold.[81] In addition, a large population-based retrospective cohort study suggested treatment with oral anticoagulants for greater than 12 months was an independent predictor of vertebral, rib and all osteoporotic fractures.[93] In contrast, a prospective population-based study did not identify either lower BMD or an increase in fracture risk in those treated with warfarin; however, only 15 fractures were observed, so statistical power was limited.[94] In a meta-analysis of nine cross-sectional studies evaluating oral anticoagulants and bone density, exposure to oral anticoagulants was associated with a significantly lower BMD at the ultradistal radius only, not the distal radius, lumbar spine or femoral neck.[95]

Heparin has been demonstrated to increase bone resorption and suppress osteoblast function, although the effects of low-molecular-weight heparin are variable.[96] Long-term heparin use, including low-molecular-weight heparin, does appear to increase the risk for bone loss,[97] but the effect may be reversible with cessation of the medication. The effect of long-term heparin on fracture risk is not well established.

Antiepileptic medication

Both low BMD and osteomalacia have been reported with some antiepileptic drugs (AEDs). A population-based case–control study involving 124,655 fracture cases and 373,962 controls demonstrated an increased risk for any fracture with carbamazepine (odds ratio (OR): 1.18; 95% CI: 1.10–1.26), oxcarbazepine (OR: 1.14; 95% CI: 1.03–1.26), clonazepam (OR: 1.27; 95% CI: 1.15–1.41), phenobarbital (OR: 1.79; 95% CI: 1.64–1.95) and valproate (OR: 1.15; 95% CI: 1.05–1.26) in adjusted analyses.[98] Carbamazepine, oxcarbazepine, phenobarbital and valproate demonstrated a dose–response relationship.[98] Ethosuximide, lamotrigine, phenytoin, primidone, tiagabine, topiramate and vigabatrin were not statistically significantly associated with fracture risk after adjustment for confounders, although this may have related to a limited statistical power.[98] The increase in fracture risk was greater with liver-inducing AEDs (OR: 1.38; 95% CI: 1.31–1.45) compared with non-liver-inducing AEDs (1.19; 95% CI: 1.11–1.27).[98]

Oral contraceptive medications and hormone replacement therapy

Women using the oral contraceptive pill had a 20% reduction in the risk of hip fracture, which was especially apparent in older pre-menopausal women.[99] A reduced risk of vertebral and forearm fractures with the use of oral contraceptives has also been seen, but has not been confirmed in all studies.

The Women's Health Initiative, involving 16,608 post-menopausal women (age 50–79 years) randomized to oestrogen (0.625 mg/day) and progesterone (2.5 mg/day) replacement versus placebo, showed a protective effect of hormone replacement therapy (HRT) on hip fracture risk at 5 years of follow-up, with a hazard ratio of 0.66 (95% CI: 0.45–0.98).[100] This study was stopped prematurely due to an increased global health risk for those on HRT. This was due to an increase in the risk of pulmonary embolism, stroke, coronary artery disease and breast cancer.[100] The second trial from the Women's Health Initiative, involving 11,000 post-menopausal women who had had a hysterectomy, randomized to oestrogen replacement (0.625 mg/day) versus placebo, was also stopped prematurely due to increased health risks in the HRT group after 7 years of follow-up; however, oestrogen replacement therapy was again shown to be protective for hip fractures [hazard ratio: 0.61 (95% CI: 0.41–0.91)].[101]

Statins

Studies suggest that 3-hydroxy,3-methylglutaryl coenzyme A (HMG-CoA) reductase inhibitors (statins) may increase osteoclast apoptosis and enhance osteoblastic synthesis of bone morphogenic protein 2, a growth factor that causes osteoblastic proliferation.[102] The results of observational studies and interventional studies examining the relationship between statin use and BMD or fracture risk have, however, been conflicting, with some studies reporting increased BMD or decreased fractures with statin use, while others found no associations. A meta-analysis to determine whether statin use was associated with a reduced risk for fracture was recently performed. It included eight observational studies, four of which were large prospective studies involving women (the Study of Osteoporotic Fractures, the Fracture Intervention Trial, the Heart and Estrogen/Progestin Replacement Study and the Rotterdam Study), and two clinical trials that reported statin use and documented fracture outcomes. The pooled results from the four large prospective studies found that statin use was associated with a trend toward fewer hip fractures [relative hazards (RHs): 0.19–0.62] and, to a lesser extent, non-spine fractures (RHs: 0.49–0.95) in women, after adjustment for multiple factors, including age, body mass index and oestrogen use.[103] The meta-analysis of all eight observational studies, which involved studies of both men and women, remained consistent with these overall findings.[103] The summary odds ratio (OR) for statin use and hip fracture was 0.43 (95% CI: 0.25–0.75), whereas that for non-spine fracture was 0.69 (95% CI: 0.55–0.88).[103] In a recent prospective, population-based cohort study of 3469 men and women over the age of 55 and followed for a mean of 6.5 years, statin use was associated with a lower risk for incident vertebral fractures (RR: 0.58; 95% CI: 0.34–0.99), even though statin use was not significantly associated with lumbar spine BMD.[104] Interestingly, use of hydrophilic statins, as well as non-cholesterol-lowering drugs, was not significantly associated with vertebral fracture risk.[104]

Recently, a 1-year trial involving 82 post-menopausal women with osteopoenia randomized to simvastatin (40 mg/day) versus placebo showed no significant changes in BMD at the lumbar spine, femoral neck or total body; however, there was a significant increase in forearm BMD.[105] The meta-analysis of clinical trial results did not support a protective effect with statin use for hip fracture (summary OR: 0.87; 95% CI: 0.48–1.58) or non-spine fracture (OR: 1.02; 95% CI: 0.83–1.26).[103] Additional randomized controlled trials are required to determine the effect of statins on skeletal metabolism and fracture risk.

Thiazide diuretics and beta-blockers

There is increasing interest in the effects of commonly prescribed antihypertensive medications, thiazide diuretics and beta-blockers, on bone health. A meta-analysis of thiazide diuretics identified a 20% reduction in risk of hip fractures only in long-term users.[106] There is increasing evidence to suggest that the sympathetic nervous system may be a modulator of bone metabolism. In animal models, inactivation of the sympathetic nervous system impairs osteoclastic bone resorption and increases bone formation.[107] In a population-based study involving 569 women and 775 controls with fracture, beta-blocker use was associated with higher BMD at the total hip and ultradistal radius.[108] Beta-blocker use was also associated with a reduction in fracture risk (OR: 0.68; 95% CI: 0.49–0.96).[108] In a case–control study involving 30,601 men and women with an incident fracture and 120,819 matched controls, there was a decreased risk of fracture with current use of beta-blockers (OR: 0.77; 95% CI: 0.72–0.83) and current use of thiazide diuretics (OR: 0.80; 95% CI: 0.74–0.86).[109] Current use of both beta-blockers and thiazide diuretics was also associated with decreased risk for fracture (OR: 0.71; 95% CI: 0.64–0.79).[109]

Other medications

In a case–control study it was found that all antidepressants were associated with a 90% increase in the risk of hip fracture after adjusting for co-morbidities and concomitant drug use.[110] This may reflect a persisting effect of depression, an increased risk of falls, immobility or possibly the effects of endogenous hormones on bone metabolism. Cyclosporin and tacrolimus have been associated with an adverse effect on bone metabolism.[76,111] Methotrexate osteopathy is a recognized complication of high-dose methotrexate used in oncology, and is characterized by bone pain, low bone density and fractures.[112] The net effect on bone metabolism of long-term, low-dose methotrexate, as used in rheumatoid arthritis and other autoimmune inflammatory conditions, has been a source of debate. However, both cross-sectional[113,114] and prospective, longitudinal studies[114,115] in rheumatoid arthritis patients have failed to demonstrate lower bone density in methotrexate users compared with non-users, at least over short-term follow-up.

ANTHROPOMETRIC MEASUREMENTS

Greater height was associated with all non-vertebral fractures in men and women.[116] Morphometric vertebral fractures in both men and women are associated with greater height loss, lower weight gain, lower body mass index and lower weight in women.[117] Weight loss in middle age or old age is also important and is independent of confounding factors such as BMD, co-morbidities and health status. There are established prospective data on the association between low body weight or body mass and lower BMD[118] and an increased risk of hip fracture and non-vertebral fractures.[116,119] In a large prospective study involving 19,938 women and 19,151 men, weight loss was associated with an increase risk for hip fracture in men (RR: 2.01; 95% CI: 1.19–3.41) but not women (RR: 1.22; 95% CI: 0.88–1.69).[120] Another study reported that a 10% loss of weight was associated with a 70% increase in the number of fragility fractures of the hip, pelvis and humerus in women.[121]

LIFESTYLE CHOICES

Smoking

In men and women, current cigarette smokers have lower BMD than non- or ex-smokers.[122,123] Cigarette smoking has also been shown to predict longitudinal bone loss in men[124,125] and women.[124] The risk of cigarette smoking on fracture risk was explored in a recent meta-analysis, involving 59,232 men and women (74% women) from 10 prospective cohorts followed for a total of 250,000 person-years.[126] Current smoking was associated with an increased risk of any fracture compared to non-smokers (RR: 1.25; 95% CI: 1.15–1.36), and remained significant after adjusting for BMD (RR: 1.13).[126] Current smoking was also associated with an increased risk for osteoporotic fractures.[126] The highest risk was observed for hip fractures (RR: 1.84; 95% CI: 1.52–2.22), which was only slightly attenuated after adjusting for BMD (RR: 1.60; 95% CI: 1.27–2.02).[126] Risk ratios were significantly higher in men than in women for any fractures and for osteoporotic fractures, but not for hip fractures.[126]

Alcohol

The relationship between alcohol intake, BMD and fracture risk is conflicting. In a population-based study, men and women classified as heavy drinkers had a higher BMD than those classified as light drinkers.[127] However, in an earlier study involving this same cohort of men and women, heavy drinkers appeared to have an increased risk for incident hip fracture.[128] An effect of alcohol on bone quality, not assessed by BMD, or an effect on balance or falls may explain, at least in part, these conflicting findings.

In a study involving monozygotic female twin pairs discordant for alcohol intake, moderate alcohol intake did not appear to have an adverse effect on bone.[129] In contrast, women in treatment for alcohol addiction had BMD measures that were 7.7% ($P < 0.01$) and 6.3% ($P < 0.01$) lower at the femoral neck and lumbar spine respectively, compared to age-matched women without a history of alcohol abuse.[130] The women in treatment for alcohol addiction reported a higher lifetime prevalence of fractures ($P < 0.01$), including the period prior to the onset of alcohol abuse and during periods of sobriety.[130]

Among men, alcohol consumption has been associated with an increase risk in vertebral fractures.[131–133] In a large study from Denmark, men who drank more than 28 drinks per week were 1.8 times more likely to have a hip fracture than non-drinkers and those who drank more than 70 drinks per week were at over a five-fold increase in risk.[134] Nevertheless, while some studies indicate that heavy alcohol consumption increases the risk for hip fractures,[25,128,134,135] others have seen no association.[136,137]

Moderate alcohol intake may have a positive effect on BMD, whereas a history of alcohol abuse appears to be associated with lower BMD and increased fracture risk, although the pathogenesis for this remains unclear. Importantly, subjects categorized as heavy drinkers in some studies may not have the same characteristics as those who are classified as alcoholics. Thus, alcoholics may be more prone to nutritional deficiencies and other underlying medical conditions, including liver disease, which adversely affect bone metabolism or bone quality. In addition, alcoholics are at increased risk for fall due to imbalance and muscle weakness.[25,138] Nevertheless, it remains possible that alcohol may influence bone quality and strength independent of BMD. Those with a history of alcohol abuse require counselling to abstain regardless of their BMD or personal fracture history.

Caffeine

As caffeine can increase the urinary excretion of calcium, it has been postulated that high caffeine consumption may reduce bone mineral density (BMD) and subsequently increase the risk for osteoporotic fracture. Studies evaluating the effect of caffeine consumption on BMD or fracture risk have been somewhat conflicting, and most have evaluated women only.

Several studies have found no association between caffeine consumption and BMD[139–141] or loss in BMD.[140] Others have reported an association between high caffeine consumption and lower BMD only in older women, not younger women, suggesting that impaired calcium balance, which is more frequent in the elderly, may play a role.[142] Similarly, another study found that a lifetime caffeinated coffee intake equivalent to two cups per day was associated with decreased bone density in older women who do not drink milk on a daily basis.[143] Furthermore, another study reported that daily consumption of caffeine in amounts equal to or greater than that obtained from about two to three servings of brewed coffee may accelerate bone loss from the spine and total body in women with calcium intakes below 800 mg/day.[144]

High caffeine consumption has been associated with an increased risk for hip fracture,[9,145,146] but the risk for upper extremity fractures has been limited and conflicting.[145,147]

Physical activity

Mechanical loading of the skeleton is needed for healthy development and maintenance of bone. Weight-bearing activity during adolescence is a positive predictor of peak bone mass in men and women.[148] Immobility and decreased physical activity are important predictors of bone loss and fractures.[149] Sedentary men lose more bone density[125] and were shown to be more likely to fracture[150] than those who are physically active. Studies in women have shown that moderate to high levels of exercise reduce the risk of vertebral and hip fractures by 33% and 42% respectively,[151] and regular walking or cycling in women is protective.[152] Lower physical activity could also predispose to increased frequency of falling, from muscle weakness and deconditioning. Elderly patients living in institutions have double the risk of hip fracture which occurred despite adjusting for confounding factors that increase the risk of institutionalization or hip fractures; however, this has not been confirmed in all studies.[153]

ENDOGENOUS SEX HORMONES

Women

Premature ovarian failure and early menopause may result in an increase in fracture risk, which has been observed as early as the peri-menopause.[11] In another study, infertility resulted in a trend towards an increased risk of hip fracture, but this did not reach statistical significance.[154] However, as the median age at follow-up in this study was 55.6 years and hip fractures are more common in the elderly, this study may well have missed a significant association between infertility and hip fracture, if one was present.[154]

In a prospective study, women with a menarche after 13 years had a three-fold increase in wrist fracture.[155] Late menarche may, in fact, be a greater risk for fracture than early menopause.[156] A doubling of the number of wrist fractures was associated with a longer menstrual cycle, while a shorter bleeding cycle was protective.[155] Other studies using retrospective data on menstrual cycle and menarche have resulted in conflicting results. A prospective study in women identified a 150% increase in hip and vertebral fractures with an undetectable oestradiol level.[157] This association remained significant after adjustment for age, weight, serum oestrone, sex-hormone-binding globulin (SHBG) and calcaneal BMD.[157] Low free testosterone (<2.4 pmol/L) in women increased the risk of hip fractures 60%, although not that of vertebral fracture, after adjusting for age and weight but not BMD.[157]

High serum SHBG levels have been associated with an increase in fractures. An SHBG greater then 34.7 nmol/L and undetectable oestradiol levels (<18 pmol/L) resulted in a sevenfold increase risk of hip fracture and eight-fold increased risk of vertebral fractures.[157] In a case–control study investigating the association between endogenous sex steroid hormones and incident vertebral fractures, women in the lowest tertile of serum oestradiol (≤15.5 pmol/L) had a 2.1-fold increased risk (95% CI: 1.3–3.5) of incident vertebral fractures, independent of BMD.[158] SHBG levels in the lowest two tertiles were associated with a 50% reduction in incident vertebral fracture risk.[158] Women with a combination of both low oestradiol and high SHBG had a 7.8-fold higher risk of an incident vertebral fracture (95% CI: 2.7–22.5; P < 0.001), adjusted for age and weight.[158]

Overall, it appears that low oestradiol levels in women increase the risk for osteoporosis and fracture risk. High SHBG also increases the fracture risk in women, and may have a synergistic effect with low oestradiol levels on fracture risk.

Men

Until recently, the age-related decrease in BMD in men has frequently been attributed to low testosterone levels. However, several studies involving otherwise healthy older men have not been able to demonstrate a reliable association between low testosterone levels (either total or bioavailable measures) and low BMD.[159–163] Most studies have either demonstrated no association[159,160,162,163] or a weak one.[164] Others have reported an inverse association between testosterone levels and bone density.[161]

In contrast, there are a growing number of reports suggesting that oestrogens play a more important role than testosterone on maintenance of bone health in men. Several cross-sectional studies, including those from large population-based samples of men, have reported that low oestradiol levels are strongly associated with low bone density of men.[159,161,163–166] Low oestradiol levels have also been reported to predict bone loss better than testosterone levels among men.[167–169]

The associations previously reported between testosterone and BMD may relate to the aromatization of testosterone to oestradiol. In a study of testosterone therapy for older eugonadal men with osteoporosis, the increase in BMD was more strongly correlated with the increase in serum oestradiol rather than the increase in serum testosterone.[170] In a study of healthy older men given an aromatase inhibitor, testosterone levels increased and oestradiol levels decreased as expected, and resulted in an increase in bone resorption markers and a decrease in bone formation markers,[171] adding further evidence to the relative importance of oestrogens on bone metabolism in men. Finally, the relative contribution of testosterone and oestrogens on bone turnover in men was well studied in a group of 59 men (mean age 68 years) by first eliminating endogenous testosterone and oestradiol production using a gonadotrophic-releasing hormone agonist (which resulted in reversible hypogonadism), then blocking the conversion of androgens to oestrogens using an aromatase inhibitor and finally studying the men following physiological testosterone and oestrogen replacement.[172] Men were then randomized to withdrawing both testosterone and oestrogen, withdrawing only testosterone, withdrawing only oestrogen, or continuing both. Examining the effect on bone turnover, they found that oestrogens had a greater effect than testosterone on preventing the rise in bone resorption markers.[172] Both oestrogen and testosterone resulted in an increase in serum osteocalcin, a marker of bone formation.[172] The results suggested that oestrogen was the dominant sex steroid in regulating bone resorption in older men, whereas both oestrogen and testosterone were important for bone formation.[172]

The relative role of oestrogens and androgens on fracture occurrence in men remains understudied. Some studies have shown an association in men between hypogonadism, or low serum testosterone, and fractures.[173,174] However, it is conceivable that low oestradiol levels may have accounted for these effects, since testosterone is aromatized to oestradiol, and oestradiol was not measured in these studies. Low oestradiol levels have been associated with vertebral fractures in a large population-based study of elderly men from the Rancho-Bernardo Study.[175a] Men in the lowest quintile of total oestradiol had significantly higher odds for fracture than those in the highest quintile (OR: 4.16; 95% CI: 1.22–14.19), whereas men with low testosterone levels compatible with hypogonadism had no significant increased odds for fracture (OR: 1.24; 95% CI: 0.54–2.83).[175a] Among 793 men from the Framingham Study, followed for up to 18 years, those with low oestradiol had an increased risk for incident hip fracture (hazard ratio: 3.1; 95% CI: 1.4–6.9).[175b] Although no association was seen between low testosterone and hip fracture risk, men with both low oestradiol and low testosterone had the greatest risk for hip fracture (hazard ratio: 6.5; 95% CI: 2.9, 14.3), indicating an interaction effect.[175b]

Dehydroepiandrosterone (DHEA) and its sulphated metabolite (DHEAS) are the most abundant circulating adrenal androgens and decrease with age, leading some to speculate that these adrenal androgens may be related to bone loss in men. However, to date, most studies have shown no association between either DHEA or DHEAS and BMD in older men,[159,164,176,177] while one has seen an inverse association.[161]

Higher levels of serum SHBG have been associated with primary and secondary osteoporosis in men[178] and a two-fold increase in vertebral fracture (OR: 2.0; 95% CI: 1.2–3.5) for each one standard deviation increase in SHBG levels.[178]

In men, low oestradiol levels appear to be more strongly associated with low BMD and fractures than either low testosterone or low adrenal androgens. However, there may be a synergistic effect of low oestradiol and low testosterone on hip fracture risk. Low testosterone may lead to diminished bone strength not measurable by BMD testing or, perhaps, an increased likelihood of falling due to a decrease in muscle strength and balance. SHBG may also play an independent role on bone metabolism and fracture risk in men.

INSULIN-LIKE GROWTH FACTORS AND THEIR BINDING PROTEINS

The insulin-like growth factor (IGF) system, which includes IGF-1 and IGF-2 and six IGF binding proteins (IGFBPs), is a complex, growth-promoting regulatory system that is both growth hormone dependent and independent. IGF-1 and IGF-2 enhance osteoblastic differentiation and bone formation.[179] The IGFBPs can potentiate or inhibit the effects of IGF-1 and IGF-2, and all six IGFBPs can be synthesized by osteoblasts.[179] The IGF system is known to play an important role in skeletal modelling and growth during pubertal development of adolescent boys and girls, and appears to work synergistically with sex steroids.[180–182] The contribution of the IGF system to age-related bone loss is not as well understood, and epidemiological studies have not shown consistent associations between serum levels of the IGF/IGFBPs and BMD.

Ageing in men and women results in an apparent decrease in IGF-1, IGFBP-3 and IGFBP-5, and an increase in IGFBP-2 and IGFBP-4.[183,184] Some epidemiological studies have reported an association between lower levels of IGF-1 and lower BMD among women.[185–189] Another study reported that low IGF-1 levels were associated with bone loss, at least in post-menopausal women.[190] Others have seen no association between IGF-1 levels and bone density in either women[184,191] or men.[184,185,187,191,192] However, low IGF-1 levels have been reported in men with idiopathic osteoporosis.[193,194]

There have been reports indicating an association between low IGFBP-3 and low BMD in both men[195] and post-menopausal women.[188] Others have demonstrated only a weak association between IGFBP-3 and BMD in men, and no association in women, once the interrelation between the IGF system and sex hormones was taken into consideration.[191] In a population-based study of both men and women, spanning young and older adults, no significant associations were seen between IGFBP-3 levels with BMD, in either men or women.[184]

In contrast, in a population-based study involving men and women, IGFBP-2 was found to be the strongest, most consistent predictor of BMD.[184] Higher IGFBP-2 levels were associated with lower BMD at most sites in men and women independent of age and bioavailable sex steroids.[184] Other studies have also reported associations between high levels of IGFBP-2 and low BMD among select samples of post-menopausal women[188,196] and men.[197] These studies suggest that IGFBP-2, a known inhibitor of IGF action which increases with age in both sexes, may play a potentially deleterious role on bone metabolism with ageing.

In a study evaluating serum levels of IGFBP-4 and IGFBP-5 in a cohort of older men and women, IGFBP-5, not IGFBP-4, was found to be positively associated with femoral neck BMD, but not lumbar spine BMD, in post-menopausal women.[183] No association was seen with either IGFBP-4 or IGFBP-5 with BMD in men.[183]

In vitro studies and some epidemiological studies do suggest a potential role of the IGF/IGFBP system in regulating bone metabolism in ageing men and women. The influence of the IGF/IGFBPs on fracture risk remains unclear. Further understanding on how the IGF/IGFBPs influence bone health with ageing may assist with risk stratification or help identify targets for pharmacological manipulation in the management of osteoporosis.

VITAMINS AND MICRONUTRIENTS

Calcium and vitamin D

Calcium and vitamin D are essential for bone health. Low vitamin D levels can lead to alterations in calcium and phosphorus homeostasis, and secondary hyperparathyroidism, thereby increasing the risk for bone loss, osteoporosis and fractures. A low fractional absorption of calcium was associated with a 24% increase risk in hip fractures, and increased to 150% in those women with a dietary calcium intake of less than 400 mg per day.[198] No relationship between low fractional absorption of calcium and non-hip fractures was observed.[198] In prospective population-based studies of post-menopausal women, measurement of parathyroid hormone and 25-hydroxyvitamin D did not predict either hip fracture[157,199] or vertebral fracture.[157] The risk of hip fracture in women was increased by 110% with a low 1,25-dihydroxyvitamin D level (<55 pmol/L) after adjusting for age and weight but not BMD, however no association with vertebral fractures was seen.[157] In men, those with hip fractures were more likely to have lower 25-hydroxyvitamin D levels compared with controls.[200] Subclinical vitamin D deficiency (<50 nmol/L) was also seen more frequently among those with hip fractures than controls (OR: 3.9; 95% CI: 1.74–8.78).[200]

A recent meta-analysis has shown that oral vitamin D supplementation between 700 and 800 IU/day appeared to reduce the risk of hip and non-vertebral fractures in ambulatory and institutionalized elderly persons, whereas vitamin D doses of 400 IU/day were not sufficient to prevent fracture.[201] And yet, a more recent randomized, placebo-controlled trial of oral calcium (1000 mg/day) and vitamin D supplementation (800 IU/day) found no beneficial effect on fracture prevention among over 5000 men and women over the age of 70 years.[202] However, the baseline vitamin D level of the majority of participants was unknown.[202] Vitamin D supplementation, at least for those who are vitamin D deficient, is likely to have the most beneficial effect on fracture prevention.

Vitamin A

Vitamin A is a fat-soluble vitamin important for vision, but it has been suggested that vitamin A in excess of 1500 μg/day may be associated with a two-fold increased risk of hip fracture.[203] In addition, in a population-based longitudinal cohort study involving men, the risk of any fracture was increased by 64% (RR: 1.64; 95% CI: 1.12–2.41) and the risk of hip fracture was increased by 147% (RR: 2.47; 95% CI: 1.15–5.28) in men with the highest quintile for serum retinol [>75.62 µg/dL (>2.64 µmol/L)].[204] The level of serum beta-carotene was not associated with the risk of fracture.[204]

In a population-based study of post-menopausal women, using a semiquantitative food frequency questionnaire to determine baseline levels of vitamin A and retinol intake, the users of supplements containing vitamin A had a borderline significant 18% increase in the risk of incident hip fractures (RR: 1.18; 95% CI: 0.99–1.41).[205] There was no evidence of an increase in risk of all fractures, nor was there evidence of a dose–response relationship in hip fracture risk with increasing amounts of vitamin A or retinol from supplements.[205] In another study there was no association between intake of vitamin A and BMD at the femoral neck or lumbar spine, nor was there an association with fracture risk in peri-menopausal women.[206] Furthermore, in a nested case–control study involving older women, serum retinol, retinyl palmitate and beta-carotene were not associated with increased fracture risk, and multivitamin or cod liver oil supplementation was actually associated with a significantly lower risk of any fracture.[207]

Vitamin B$_{12}$

Patients with pernicious anaemia have been shown to have a greater risk for osteoporosis and fractures.[59,208] Patients diagnosed with pernicious anaemia were 1.9 times more likely to have a proximal femur fracture, 1.8 times more likely to have a vertebral fracture and 2.9 times more likely to have a distal forearm fracture, relative to the general community.[208] In population-based studies, low serum B$_{12}$ levels have been associated with low bone density among women[209–211] and men.[211] While the mechanism of action remains somewhat unclear, vitamin B$_{12}$ has been associated with osteoblast activation and bone formation,[212,213] and so may have a direct effect on bone metabolism. Vitamin B$_{12}$ deficiency is a common and correctable condition, so represents an important potentially modifiable risk factor for osteoporosis.

Homocysteine

There is an increased risk of osteoporosis among people with homocystinuria, a rare autosomal recessive biochemical abnormality, characterized by elevated levels of plasma homocysteine.[214] Two large population-based studies have recently reported an increased risk of fractures among those with the highest homocysteine levels.[215,216] In one study involving 825 men and 1174 women, the hazard ratio for hip fracture was 3.84 (95% CI: 1.38–10.70) among men in the highest quartile of homocysteine levels (>15 µmol/L) and 1.92 (95% CI: 1.18–3.92) for women in the highest quartile of homocysteine levels (>13.5 µmol/L).[215] The other study, involving 2406 men and women, followed for 11,253 person-years, reported a rela-

tive risk of 1.9 (95% CI: 1.4–2.6) for any osteoporotic fracture among those with the highest quartile of homocysteine.[216] The mechanism of action for this increased risk of fracture is unclear but could be the result of inhibition of collagen crosslinking by high homocysteine levels. It may also relate to other associated nutritional deficiencies or, possibly, associated oestrogen deficiency.[217]

In a 2-year, double-blind, randomized controlled study of 628 consecutive patients aged 65 years or older with residual hemiplegia at least 1 year following first ischaemic stroke, in those assigned to daily oral treatment with 5 mg of folate and 1500 µg of mecobalamin, plasma homocysteine level decreased by 38%, whereas it increased by 31% in the placebo group (P < 0.001).[218] The number of hip fractures per 1000 patient-years was 10 and 43 for the treatment and placebo groups respectively (P < 0.001).[218] The adjusted relative risk, absolute risk reduction and the number needed to treat for hip fractures in the treatment versus placebo groups were 0.20 (95% CI: 0.08–0.50), 7.1% (95% CI: 3.6–10.8%) and 14 (95% CI: 9–28) respectively.[218] No significant adverse effects were reported.

CLINICAL ROLE OF RISK FACTORS

Investigation and identification of clinical risk factors for osteoporosis and fractures is important in order to target high-risk individuals for further management. Addressing modifiable risk factors may also lead to a reduction in risk of fracture. BMD is an integral component of bone strength and fracture risk.[219] Measurement of BMD enables an assessment of the net effect of historical and current risk factors for bone loss in an individual and is thus a strong predictor of future fracture risk. Multiple risk factors combined with a low BMD can significantly increase the risk of fracture. One study found the incidence of hip fracture was increased 17-fold in the 15% of women with greater than five risk factors and increased to 27-fold in those women with a BMD in the lowest third for their age.[9] Others have reported similar findings.[24] The combination of BMD with a previous history of fracture increased the gradient of risk/standard deviation (SD) compared to BMD alone. Furthermore, if multiple tests with a moderate gradient of risk (RR = 2.0/SD) were used to screen women aged 65 years or to target 25% of the population it would save up to 23% of all fractures in women over the subsequent 10 years.[220]

Risk factors can be used clinically to adjust the thresholds for intervention when interpreting BMD results and, in combination with BMD, provide a clinical assessment of the relative fracture risk for an individual. Many of the models developed have been used to assess relative risk.[221] However, the determination of absolute fracture risk rather than relative risk is more appropriate in the management of individuals requiring long-term interventions for fracture prevention.

Models need to be developed to assess the absolute risk of fracture based on combinations of readily ascertainable risk factors and BMD.[222,223] One model based on absolute risk of first hip fracture identified that combining risk factors and BMD can increase the sensitivity without loss of specificity.[222] It remains unclear whether such models can be generalized to different populations, sexes, age groups and fracture types. The role of risk factors in the interpretation of BMD results, determination of intervention thresholds for pharmacological and non-pharmacological therapies, and the clinical evaluation of an individual patient's fracture risk require further study. Currently, the use of BMD and risk factors is being developed formally by a working party of the World Health Organization in order to establish absolute fracture risk. This approach is likely to be widely adopted for the identification of patients at risk for osteoporosis.

SUMMARY

There is an increasing depth of knowledge on the risk factors for osteoporotic fractures. It is, however, important to recognize that not all risk factors are modifiable, the impact of any change may only be minor, and risk factors may not be sensitive in discriminating between individuals at high risk of osteoporosis or fracture. The assessment of individuals to identify those at high risk of falls and therefore fracture may enable the correction of certain pathologies or the targeting of resources for fracture prevention. Ideally, risk assessment should involve evaluation of absolute rather than relative risk, target modifiable risk factors and involve appropriate models that integrate clinical risk factors and bone densitometry.

PRACTICE POINTS

- Epidemiological studies in both men and women have demonstrated multiple risk factors associated with the development of osteoporosis and fragility fractures, many of which may be modifiable.

- Bone mineral density measurement is a useful predictor of future fracture risk as it reflects the cumulative effect on bone tissue of an individual's historical and current risk factors for bone loss.

- Prior fragility fracture is a strong predictor of future fracture.

- The optimal prevention of osteoporotic fractures involves identification of an individual's clinical risk factors in order to modify the risks where possible and, in conjunction with bone density results, determine an appropriate threshold for intervention.

RESEARCH AGENDA

- Models need to be developed to assess the absolute risk of fracture for an individual based on combinations of readily ascertainable risk factors and bone density results.

- Currently, the use of bone density results and clinical risk factors is being developed formally by a working party of the World Health Organization in order to establish absolute fracture risk.

- The determination of intervention thresholds for pharmacological and non-pharmacological therapies based on both clinical risk factors and bone density results requires further study.

REFERENCES

1. Anonymous. Consensus development conference: diagnosis, prophylaxis, and treatment of osteoporosis. *Am J Med* 1993; **94**: 646–650.
2. Center JR, Nguyen TV, Schneider D et al. Mortality after all major types of osteoporotic fracture in men and women: an observational study. *Lancet* 1999; **353**: 878–882.
3. Honkanen R, Tuppurainen M, Kroger H et al. Relationships between risk factors and fractures differ by type of fracture: a population-based study of 12,192 perimenopausal women. *Osteoporosis Int* 1998; **8**: 25–31.
4. Kelsey JL, Browner WS, Seeley DG et al. Risk factors for fractures of the distal forearm and proximal humerus. The Study of Osteoporotic Fractures Research Group [erratum appears in *Am J Epidemiol* 1992; **135**(10): 1183]. *Am J Epidemiol* 1992; **135**: 477–489.
5. Mallmin H, Ljunghall S, Persson I et al. Risk factors for fractures of the distal forearm: a population-based case–control study. *Osteoporosis Int* 1994; **4**: 298–304.
6. Clowes JA & Eastell R. The role of bone turnover markers and risk factors in the assessment of osteoporosis and fracture risk. *Best Pract Res Clin Endocrinol Metab* 2000; **14**: 213–232.
7. Andrew T, Antionades L, Scurrah KJ et al. Risk of wrist fracture in women is heritable and is influenced by genes that are largely independent of those influencing BMD. *J Bone Miner Res* 2005; **20**: 67–74.
8. Keen RW, Hart DJ, Arden NK et al. Family history of appendicular fracture and risk of osteoporosis: a population-based study. *Osteoporosis Int* 1999; **10**: 161–166.
9. Cummings SR, Nevitt MC, Browner WS et al. Risk factors for hip fracture in white women. Study of Osteoporotic Fractures Research Group [see comment]. *N Engl J Med* 1995; **332**: 767–773.
10. Fox KM, Cummings SR, Powell-Threets K et al. Family history and risk of osteoporotic fracture. Study of Osteoporotic Fractures Research Group. *Osteoporosis Int* 1998; **8**: 557–562.
11. Torgerson DJ, Campbell MK, Thomas RE et al. Prediction of perimenopausal fractures by bone mineral density and other risk factors. *J Bone Miner Res* 1996; **11**: 293–297.
12. Diaz MN, O'Neill TW & Silman AJ. The influence of family history of hip fracture on the risk of vertebral deformity in men and women: the European Vertebral Osteoporosis Study. *Bone* 1997; **20**: 145–149.
13. Kanis JA, Johansson H, Oden A et al. A family history of fracture and fracture risk: a meta-analysis. *Bone* 2004; **35**: 1029–1037.
14. Albagha OM & Ralston SH. Genetic determinants of susceptibility to osteoporosis. *Endocrinol Metab Clin North Am* 2003; **32**: 65–81.
15. Deng HW, Mahaney MC, Williams JT et al. Relevance of the genes for bone mass variation to susceptibility to osteoporotic fractures and its implications to gene search for complex human diseases. *Genet Epidemiol* 2002; **22**: 12–25.
16. Gunnes M, Mellstrom D & Johnell O. How well can a previous fracture indicate a new fracture? A questionnaire study of 29,802 postmenopausal women. *Acta Orthop Scand* 1998; **69**: 508–512.
17. Van Staa TP, Leufkens HG & Cooper C. Does a fracture at one site predict later fractures at other sites? A British cohort study. *Osteoporosis Int* 2002; **13**: 624–629.

18. Black DM, Arden NK, Palermo L et al. Prevalent vertebral deformities predict hip fractures and new vertebral deformities but not wrist fractures. Study of Osteoporotic Fractures Research Group. *J Bone Miner Res* 1999; **14**: 821–828.

19. Lunt M, O'Neill TW, Felsenberg D et al. Characteristics of a prevalent vertebral deformity predict subsequent vertebral fracture: results from the European Prospective Osteoporosis Study (EPOS). *Bone* 2003; **33**: 505–513.

20. Melton LJ III, Atkinson EJ, Cooper C et al. Vertebral fractures predict subsequent fractures. *Osteoporosis Int* 1999; **10**: 214–221.

21. Honkanen R, Tuppurainen M, Kroger H et al. Associations of early premenopausal fractures with subsequent fractures vary by sites and mechanisms of fractures. *Calcif Tissue Int* 1997; **60**: 327–331.

22. Cuddihy MT, Gabriel SE, Crowson CS et al. Forearm fractures as predictors of subsequent osteoporotic fractures. *Osteoporosis Int* 1999; **9**: 469–475.

23. Eastell R, Reid DM, Compston J et al. Secondary prevention of osteoporosis: when should a non-vertebral fracture be a trigger for action? *QJ Med* 2001; **94**: 575–597.

24. Dargent-Molina P, Favier F, Grandjean H et al. Fall-related factors and risk of hip fracture: the EPIDOS prospective study [erratum appears in Lancet 1996; **348**(9024): 416]. *Lancet* 1996; **348**: 145–149.

25. Poor G, Atkinson EJ, O'Fallon WM et al. Predictors of hip fractures in elderly men. *J Bone Miner Res* 1995; **10**: 1900–1907.

26. Nevitt MC. Osteoporosis and fragility fractures in the elderly. In: Rosen C, Glowacki J, Bilezikian J, eds. *The Aging Skeleton*. Academic Press, San Diego, 1999; 349–357.

27. Ross PD. Risk factors for osteoporotic fracture. *Endocrinol Metab Clin North Am* 1998; **27**: 289–301.

28. Graafmans WC, Ooms ME, Hofstee HM et al. Falls in the elderly: a prospective study of risk factors and risk profiles. *Am J Epidemiol* 1996; **143**: 1129–1136.

29. Parkkari J, Kannus P, Palvanen M et al. Majority of hip fractures occur as a result of a fall and impact on the greater trochanter of the femur: a prospective controlled hip fracture study with 206 consecutive patients. *Calcif Tissue Int* 1999; **65**: 183–187.

30. Norton R, Campbell AJ, Lee-Joe T et al. Circumstances of falls resulting in hip fractures among older people. *J Am Geriatr Soc* 1997; **45**: 1108–1112.

31. Tinetti ME, Speechley M & Ginter SF. Risk factors for falls among elderly persons living in the community. *N Engl J Med* 1988; **319**: 1701–1707.

32. Nevitt MC, Cummings SR, Kidd S et al. Risk factors for recurrent nonsyncopal falls. A prospective study. *JAMA* 1989; **261**: 2663–2668.

33. Tinetti ME, Baker DI, McAvay G et al. A multifactorial intervention to reduce the risk of falling among elderly people living in the community [see comments]. *N Engl J Med* 1994; **331**: 821–827.

34. Cooper C, Carbone L, Michet CJ et al. Fracture risk in patients with ankylosing spondylitis: a population based study. *J Rheumatol* 1994; **21**: 1877–1882.

35. Segal LG & Lane NE. Osteoporosis and systemic lupus erythematosus: etiology and treatment strategies. *Ann Med Intern* 1996; **147**: 281–289.

36. Hooyman JR, Melton LJ III, Nelson AM et al. Fractures after rheumatoid arthritis. A population-based study. *Arthritis Rheum* 1984; **27**: 1353–1361.

37. Shenstone BD, Mahmoud A, Woodward R et al. Longitudinal bone mineral density changes in early rheumatoid arthritis. *Br J Rheumatol* 1994; **33**: 541–545.

38. Gough AK, Lilley J, Eyre S et al. Generalised bone loss in patients with early rheumatoid arthritis [see comment]. *Lancet* 1994; **344**: 23–27.

39. Jones DH, Kong YY & Penninger JM. Role of RANKL and RANK in bone loss and arthritis. *Ann Rheum Dis* 2002; **61**: 32–39.

40a. Kong YY, Feige U, Sarosi I et al. Activated T cells regulate bone loss and joint destruction in adjuvant arthritis through osteoprotegerin ligand. *Nature* 1999; **402**: 304–309.

40b. Clowes JA, Riggs BL, Khosla S. The role of the immune system in the pathophysiology of osteoporosis. *Immunol Rev* 2005; **208**: 207–227.

41. Redlich K, Hayer S, Maier A et al. Tumor necrosis factor alpha-mediated joint destruction is inhibited by targeting osteoclasts with osteoprotegerin. *Arthritis Rheum* 2002; **46**: 785–792.

42. Green MJ & Deodhar AA. Bone changes in early rheumatoid arthritis. *Best Pract Res Clin Rheumatol* 2001; **15**: 105–123.

43. Cooper C, Cook PL, Osmond C et al. Osteoarthritis of the hip and osteoporosis of the proximal femur. *Ann Rheum Dis* 1991; **50**: 540–542.

44. Hannan MT, Anderson JJ, Zhang Y et al. Bone mineral density and knee osteoarthritis in elderly men and women. The Framingham Study. *Arthritis Rheum* 1993; **36**: 1671–1680.

45. Nevitt MC, Lane NE, Scott JC et al. Radiographic osteoarthritis of the hip and bone mineral density. The Study of Osteoporotic Fractures Research Group. *Arthritis Rheum* 1995; **38**: 907–916.

46. Burger H, van Daele PL, Odding E et al. Association of radiographically evident osteoarthritis with higher bone mineral density and increased bone loss with age. The Rotterdam Study. *Arthritis Rheum* 1996; **39**: 81–86.

47. Jones G, Nguyen T, Sambrook PN et al. Osteoarthritis, bone density, postural stability, and osteoporotic fractures: a population based study. *J Rheumatol* 1995; **22**: 921–925.

48. Arden NK, Nevitt MC, Lane NE et al. Osteoarthritis and risk of falls, rates of bone loss, and osteoporotic fractures. Study of Osteoporotic Fractures Research Group. *Arthritis Rheum* 1999; **42**: 1378–1385.

49. Amin S. Osteoarthritis and bone mineral density: what is the relation and why does it matter? *J Rheumatol* 2002; **29**: 1348–1349.

50. Shaker JL & Lukert BP. Osteoporosis associated with excess glucocorticoids. *Endocrinol Metab Clin North Am* 2005; **34**: 341–356.

51. Vestergaard P, Lindholm J, Jorgensen JO et al. Increased risk of osteoporotic fractures in patients with Cushing's syndrome. *Eur J Endocrinol* 2002; **146**: 51–56.

52. Freehill AK & Lenke LG. Severe kyphosis secondary to glucocorticoid-induced osteoporosis in a young adult with Cushing's disease. A case report and literature review. *Spine* 1999; **24**: 189–193.

53. Greendale GA, Unger JB, Rowe JW et al. The relation between cortisol excretion and fractures in healthy older people: results from the MacArthur studies-Mac. *J Am Geriatr Soc* 1999; **47**: 799–803.

54. Khosla S, Melton LJ III, Wermers RA et al. Primary hyperparathyroidism and the risk of fracture: a population-based study [see comment]. *J Bone Miner Res* 1999; **14**: 1700–1707.

55. Vestergaard P & Mosekilde L. Fractures in patients with primary hyperparathyroidism: nationwide follow-up study of 1201 patients. *World J Surg* 2003; **27**: 343–349.

56. Vestergaard P & Mosekilde L. Fractures in patients with hyperthyroidism and hypothyroidism: a nationwide follow-up study in 16,249 patients. *Thyroid* 2002; **12**: 411–419.

57. Stall GM, Harris S, Sokoll LJ et al. Accelerated bone loss in hypothyroid patients overtreated with L-thyroxine [see comment]. *Ann Intern Med* 1990; **113**: 265–269.

58. Vasquez H, Mazure R, Gonzalez D et al. Risk of fractures in celiac disease patients: a cross-sectional, case–control study. *Am J Gastroenterol* 2000; **95**: 183–189.

59. Eastell R, Vieira NE, Yergey AL et al. Pernicious anaemia as a risk factor for osteoporosis. *Clin Sci* 1992; **82**: 681–685.

60. Vestergaard P, Krogh K, Rejnmark L et al. Fracture risk is increased in Crohn's disease, but not in ulcerative colitis. *Gut* 2000; **46**: 176–181.

61. Vestergaard P & Mosekilde L. Fracture risk in patients with celiac disease, Crohn's disease, and ulcerative colitis: a nationwide follow-up study of 16,416 patients in Denmark. *Am J Epidemiol* 2002; **156**: 1–10.

62. Loftus EV Jr, Crowson CS, Sandborn WJ et al. Long-term fracture risk in patients with Crohn's disease: a population-based study in Olmsted County, Minnesota. *Gastroenterology* 2002; **123**: 468–475.

63. Loftus EV Jr, Achenbach SJ, Sandborn WJ et al. Risk of fracture in ulcerative colitis: a population-based study from Olmsted County, Minnesota. *Clin Gastroenterol Hepatol* 2003; **1**: 465–473.

64. Diamond T, Stiel D, Lunzer M et al. Osteoporosis and skeletal fractures in chronic liver disease. *Gut* 1990; **31**: 82–87.

65. Idilman R, de Maria N, Uzunalimoglu O et al. Hepatic osteodystrophy: a review. *Hepatol Gastroenterol* 1997; **44**: 574–581.

66. Isaia G, Di Stefano M, Roggia C et al. Bone disorders in cholestatic liver diseases. *Forum* 1998; **8**: 28–38.

67. Ormarsdottir S, Ljunggren O, Mallmin H et al. Increased rate of bone loss at the femoral neck in patients with chronic liver disease. *Eur J Gastroenterol Hepatol* 2002; **14**: 43–48.

68. Crosbie OM, Freaney R, McKenna MJ et al. Bone density, vitamin D status, and disordered bone remodeling in end-stage chronic liver disease. *Calcif Tissue Int* 1999; **64**: 295–300.

69. Guichelaar MM, Malinchoc M, Sibonga J et al. Bone metabolism in advanced cholestatic liver disease: analysis by bone histomorphometry. *Hepatology* 2002; **36**: 895–903.

70. Le Gars L. Bone involvement in patients with chronic cholestasis. Joint, bone, spine. *Rev Rhumat* 2002; **69**: 373–378.

71. Carey E & Balan V. Metabolic bone disease in patients with liver disease. *Curr Gastroenterol Rep* 2003; **5**: 71–77.

72. Carroll BJ, Curtis GC & Mendels J. Cerebrospinal fluid and plasma free cortisol concentrations in depression. *Psychol Med* 1976; **6**: 235–244.

73. Whooley MA, Kip KE, Cauley JA et al. Depression, falls, and risk of fracture in older women. Study of Osteoporotic Fractures Research Group. *Arch Intern Med* 1999; **159**: 484–490.

74. Vautour LM, Melton LJ III, Clarke BL et al. Long-term fracture risk following renal transplantation: a population-based study. *Osteoporosis Int* 2004; **15**: 160–167.

75. Ramsey-Goldman R, Dunn JE, Dunlop DD et al. Increased risk of fracture in patients receiving solid organ transplants. *J Bone Miner Res* 1999; **14**: 456–463.

76. Cohen A, Sambrook P & Shane E. Management of bone loss after organ transplantation. *J Bone Miner Res* 2004; **19**: 1919–1932.

77. Melton LJ III, Crowson CS, Khosla S et al. Fracture risk among patients with urolithiasis: a population-based cohort study. *Kidney Int* 1998; **53**: 459–464.

78. Cunningham J, Sprague SM, Cannata-Andia J et al. Osteoporosis in chronic kidney disease. *Am J Kidney Dis* 2004; **43**: 566–571.

79. Drueke TB & Moe SM. Disturbances of bone and mineral metabolism in chronic kidney disease: an international initiative to improve diagnosis and treatment. *Nephrol Dial Transplant* 2004; **19**: 534–536.

80. Stehman-Breen C. Osteoporosis and chronic kidney disease. *Semin Nephrol* 2004; **24**: 78–81.

81. Melton LJ III, Atkinson EJ, Khosla S et al. Secondary osteoporosis and the risk of vertebral deformities in women. *Bone* 1999; **24**: 49–55.

82. Aris RM, Renner JB, Winders AD et al. Increased rate of fractures and severe kyphosis: sequelae of living into adulthood with cystic fibrosis. *Ann Intern Med* 1998; **128**: 186–193.

83. Anapliotou ML, Kastanias IT, Psara P et al. The contribution of hypogonadism to the development of osteoporosis in thalassaemia major: new therapeutic approaches. *Clin Endocrinol* 1995; **42**: 279–287.

84. Diamond T, Stiel D & Posen S. Osteoporosis in hemochromatosis: iron excess, gonadal deficiency, or other factors? *Ann Intern Med* 1989; **110**: 430–436.

85. LoCascio V, Bonucci E, Imbimbo B et al. Bone loss in response to long-term glucocorticoid therapy. *Bone Miner* 1990; **8**: 39–51.

86. Lukert BP & Raisz LG. Glucocorticoid-induced osteoporosis: pathogenesis and management [see comments]. *Ann Intern Med* 1990; **112**: 352–364.

87. Canalis E. Clinical review 83. Mechanisms of glucocorticoid action in bone: implications to glucocorticoid-induced osteoporosis. *J Clin Endocrinol Metab* 1996; **81**: 3441–3447.

88. Dykman TR, Gluck OS, Murphy WA et al. Evaluation of factors associated with glucocorticoid-induced osteopenia in patients with rheumatic diseases. *Arthritis Rheum* 1985; **28**: 361–368.

89. Van Staa TP, Leufkens HGM, Abenhaim L et al. Use of oral corticosteroids and risk of fractures. *J Bone Miner Res* 2000; **15**: 993–1000.

90. Kanis JA, Johansson H, Oden A et al. A meta-analysis of prior corticosteroid use and fracture risk. *J Bone Miner Res* 2004; **19**: 893–899.

91. Iwamoto J, Takeda T & Sato Y. Effects of vitamin K2 on osteoporosis. *Curr Pharm Des* 2004; **10**: 2557–2576.

92. Vergnaud P, Garnero P, Meunier PJ et al. Undercarboxylated osteocalcin measured with a specific immunoassay predicts hip fracture in elderly women: the EPIDOS Study [see comment]. *J Clin Endocrinol Metab* 1997; **82**: 719–724.

93. Caraballo PJ, Heit JA, Atkinson EJ et al. Long-term use of oral anticoagulants and the risk of fracture. *Arch Intern Med* 1999; **159**: 1750–1756.

94. Jamal SA, Browner WS, Bauer DC et al. Warfarin use and risk for osteoporosis in elderly women. Study of Osteoporotic Fractures Research Group. *Ann Intern Med* 1998; **128**: 829–832.

95. Caraballo PJ, Gabriel SE, Castro MR et al. Changes in bone density after exposure to oral anticoagulants: a meta-analysis. *Osteoporosis Int* 1999; **9**: 441–448.

96. Handschin AE, Trentz OA, Hoerstrup SP et al. Effect of low molecular weight heparin (dalteparin) and fondaparinux (Arixtra) on human osteoblasts in vitro. *Br J Surg* 2005; **92**: 177–183.

97. Wawrzynska L, Tomkowski WZ, Przedlacki J et al. Changes in bone density during long-term administration of low-molecular-weight heparins or acenocoumarol for secondary prophylaxis of venous thromboembolism. *Pathophysiol Haemostas Thromb* 2003; **33**: 64–67.

98. Vestergaard P, Rejnmark L & Mosekilde L. Fracture risk associated with use of antiepileptic drugs. *Epilepsia* 2004; **45**: 1330–1337.

99. Michaelsson K, Baron JA, Farahmand BY et al. Oral-contraceptive use and risk of hip fracture: a case–control study [see comment]. *Lancet* 1999; **353**: 1481–1484.

100. Rossouw JE, Anderson GL, Prentice RL et al. Risks and benefits of estrogen plus progestin in healthy postmenopausal women: principal results from the Women's Health Initiative randomized controlled trial [see comment]. *JAMA* 2002; **288**: 321–333.

101. Anderson GL, Limacher M, Assaf AR et al. Effects of conjugated equine estrogen in postmenopausal women with hysterectomy: the Women's Health Initiative randomized controlled trial. *JAMA* 2004; **291**(14): 1701–1712.

102. Mundy G, Garrett R, Harris S et al. Stimulation of bone formation in vitro and in rodents by statins [see comment]. *Science* 1999; **286**: 1946–1949.

103. Bauer DC, Mundy GR, Jamal SA et al. Use of statins and fracture: results of 4 prospective studies and cumulative meta-analysis of observational studies and controlled trials. *Arch Intern Med* 2004; **164**: 146–152.

104. Schoofs MW, Sturkenboom MC, van der Klift M et al. HMG-CoA reductase inhibitors and the risk of vertebral fracture. *J Bone Miner Res* 2004; **19**: 1525–1530.

105. Rejnmark L, Buus NH, Vestergaard P et al. Effects of simvastatin on bone turnover and BMD: a 1-year randomized controlled trial in postmenopausal osteopenic women. *J Bone Miner Res* 2004; **19**: 737–744.

106. Jones G, Nguyen T, Sambrook PN et al. Thiazide diuretics and fractures: can meta-analysis help? *J Bone Miner Res* 1995; **10**: 106–111.

107. Cherruau M, Facchienetti P, Baroukh B et al. Chemical sympathectomy impairs bone resorption in rats: a role for the sympathetic nervous system on bone metabolism. *Bone* 1999; **25**: 545–551.

108. Pasco JA, Henry MJ, Sanders KM et al. Beta-adrenergic blockers reduce the risk of fracture partly by increasing bone mineral density: Geelong Osteoporosis Study. *J Bone Miner Res* 2004; **19**: 19–24.

109. Schlienger RG, Kraenzlin ME, Jick SS et al. Use of beta-blockers and risk of fractures. *JAMA* 2004; **292**: 1326–1332.

110. Liu B, Anderson G, Mittmann N et al. Use of selective serotonin-reuptake inhibitors of tricyclic antidepressants and risk of hip fractures in elderly people [see comment]. *Lancet* 1998; **351**: 1303–1307.

111. Epstein S, Shane E, Bilezikian JP. Organ transplantation and osteoporosis. *Curr Opin Rheumatol* 1995; **7**: 255–261.

112. Ragab AH, Frech RS & Vietti TJ. Osteoporotic fractures secondary to methotrexate therapy of acute leukemia in remission. *Cancer* 1970; **25**: 580–585.

113. Carbone LD, Kaeley G, McKown KM et al. Effects of long-term administration of methotrexate on bone mineral density in rheumatoid arthritis. *Calcif Tissue Int* 1999; **64**: 100–101.

114. Cranney AB, McKendry RJ, Wells GA et al. The effect of low dose methotrexate on bone density. *J Rheumatol* 2001; **28**: 2395–2399.

115. Mazzantini M, Di Munno O, Incerti-Vecchi L et al. Vertebral bone mineral density changes in female rheumatoid arthritis patients treated with low-dose methotrexate. *Clin Exp Rheumatol* 2000; **18**: 327–331.

116. Joakimsen RM, Fonnebo V, Magnus JH et al. The Tromso Study: body height, body mass index and fractures. *Osteoporosis Int* 1998; **8**: 436–442.

117. Johnell O, O'Neill T, Felsenberg D et al. Anthropometric measurements and vertebral deformities. European Vertebral Osteoporosis Study (EVOS) Group. *Am J Epidemiol* 1997; **146**: 287–293.

118. Felson DT, Zhang Y, Hannan MT et al. Effects of weight and body mass index on bone mineral density in men and women: the Framingham study. *J Bone Miner Res* 1993; **8**: 567–573.

119. Cumming RG, Nevitt MC & Cummings SR. Epidemiology of hip fractures. *Epidemiol Rev* 1997; **19**: 244–257.

120. Meyer HE, Tverdal A & Selmer R. Weight variability, weight change and the incidence of hip fracture: a prospective study of 39,000 middle-aged Norwegians. *Osteoporosis Int* 1998; **8**: 373–378.

121. Ensrud KE, Cauley J, Lipschutz R et al. Weight change and fractures in older women. Study of Osteoporotic Fractures Research Group. *Arch Intern Med* 1997; **157**: 857–863.

122. Egger P, Duggleby S, Hobbs R et al. Cigarette smoking and bone mineral density in the elderly. *J Epidemiol Community Health* 1996; **50**: 47–50.

123. Kiel DP, Zhang Y, Hannan MT et al. The effect of smoking at different life stages on bone mineral density in elderly men and women. *Osteoporosis Int* 1996; **6**: 240–248.

124. Burger H, de Laet CE, van Daele PL et al. Risk factors for increased bone loss in an elderly population: the Rotterdam Study. *Am J Epidemiol* 1998; **147**: 871–879.

125. Hannan MT, Felson DT, Dawson-Hughes B et al. Risk factors for longitudinal bone loss in elderly men and women: the Framingham Osteoporosis Study. *J Bone Miner Res* 2000; **15**: 710–720.

126. Kanis JA, Johnell O, Oden A et al. Smoking and fracture risk: a meta-analysis. *Osteoporosis Int* 2005; **16**: 155–162.

127. Felson DT, Zhang Y, Hannan MT et al. Alcohol intake and bone mineral density in elderly men and women. The Framingham Study. *Am J Epidemiol* 1995; **142**: 485–492.

128. Felson DT, Kiel DP, Anderson JJ et al. Alcohol consumption and hip fractures: the Framingham Study. *Am J Epidemiol* 1988; **128**: 1102–1110.

129. Williams FM, Cherkas LF, Spector TD et al. The effect of moderate alcohol consumption on bone mineral density: a study of female twins. *Ann Rheum Dis* 2005; **64**: 309–310.

130. Clark MK, Sowers MF, Dekordi F et al. Bone mineral density and fractures among alcohol-dependent women in treatment and in recovery. *Osteoporosis Int* 2003; **14**: 396–403.

131. Scane AC, Francis RM, Sutcliffe AM et al. Case–control study of the pathogenesis and sequelae of symptomatic vertebral fractures in men. *Osteoporosis Int* 1999; **9**: 91–97.

132. Seeman E, Melton LJ III, O'Fallon WM et al. Risk factors for spinal osteoporosis in men. *Am J Med* 1983; **75**: 977–983.

133. Lau EMC, Chan YH, Chan M et al. Vertebral deformity in Chinese men: Prevalence, risk factors, bone mineral density, and body composition measurements. *Calcif Tissue Int* 2000; **66**: 47–52.

134. Hoidrup S, Gronbaek M, Gottschau A et al. Alcohol intake, beverage preference, and risk of hip fracture in men and women. Copenhagen Centre for Prospective Population Studies. *Am J Epidemiol* 1999; **149**: 993–1001.

135. Kanis J, Johnell O, Gullberg B et al. Risk factors for hip fracture in men from southern Europe: the MEDOS study. Mediterranean Osteoporosis Study. *Osteoporosis Int* 1999; **9**: 45–54.

136. Mussolino ME, Looker AC, Madans JH et al. Risk factors for hip fracture in white men: the NHANES I Epidemiologic Follow-up Study. *J Bone Miner Res* 1998; **13**: 918–924.

137. Grisso JA, Kelsey JL, LA OB et al. Risk factors for hip fracture in men. Hip Fracture Study Group. *Am J Epidemiol* 1997; **145**: 786–793.

138. Laitinen K & Valimaki M. Alcohol and bone. *Calcif Tissue Int* 1991; **49**: S70–S73.

139. Conlisk AJ & Galuska DA. Is caffeine associated with bone mineral density in young adult women? *Prev Med* 2000; **31**: 562–568.

140. Lloyd T, Johnson-Rollings N, Eggli DF et al. Bone status among postmenopausal women with different habitual caffeine intakes: a longitudinal investigation. *J Am Coll Nutr* 2000; **19**: 256–261.

141. Grainge MJ, Coupland CA, Cliffe SJ et al. Cigarette smoking, alcohol and caffeine consumption, and bone mineral density in postmenopausal women. The Nottingham EPIC Study Group. *Osteoporosis Int* 1998; **8**: 355–363.

142. Cooper C, Atkinson EJ, Wahner HW et al. Is caffeine consumption a risk factor for osteoporosis? *J Bone Miner Res* 1992; **7**: 465–471.

143. Barrett-Connor E, Chang JC & Edelstein SL. Coffee-associated osteoporosis offset by daily milk consumption. The Rancho Bernardo Study. *JAMA* 1994; **271**: 280–283.

144. Harris SS & Dawson-Hughes B. Caffeine and bone loss in healthy postmenopausal women. *Am J Clin Nutr* 1994; **60**: 573–578.

145. Hernandez-Avila M, Colditz GA, Stampfer MJ et al. Caffeine, moderate alcohol intake, and risk of fractures of the hip and forearm in middle-aged women. *Am J Clin Nutr* 1991; **54**: 157–163.

146. Kiel DP, Felson DT, Hannan MT et al. Caffeine and the risk of hip fracture: the Framingham Study [see comment]. *Am J Epidemiol* 1990; **132**: 675–684.

147. Hansen SA, Folsom AR, Kushi LH et al. Association of fractures with caffeine and alcohol in postmenopausal women: the Iowa Women's Health Study. *Public Health Nutr* 2000; **3**: 253–261.

148. Welten DC, Kemper HC, Post GB et al. Weight-bearing activity during youth is a more important factor for peak bone mass than calcium intake [see comments]. *J Bone Miner Res* 1994; **9**: 1089–1096.

149. Smith EL & Gilligan C. Physical activity effects on bone metabolism. *Calcif Tissue Int* 1991; **49**: S50–S54.

150. Kujala UM, Kaprio J, Kannus P et al. Physical activity and osteoporotic hip fracture risk in men. *Arch Intern Med* 2000; **160**: 705–708.

151. Gregg EW, Cauley JA, Seeley DG et al. Physical activity and osteoporotic fracture risk in older women. Study of Osteoporotic Fractures Research Group [see comment]. *Ann Intern Med* 1998; **129**: 81–88.

152. Silman AJ, O'Neill TW, Cooper C et al. Influence of physical activity on vertebral deformity in men and women: results from the European Vertebral Osteoporosis Study. *J Bone Miner Res* 1997; **12**: 813–819.

153. Norton R, Campbell AJ, Reid IR et al. Residential status and risk of hip fracture. *Age Ageing* 1999; **28**: 135–139.

154. Hesdorffer DC, Melton LJ III, Malkasian GD et al. Hip fractures among infertile women. *Am J Epidemiol* 1999; **149**: 810–813.

155. Cooper GS & Sandler DP. Long-term effects of reproductive-age menstrual cycle patterns on peri- and postmenopausal fracture risk. *Am J Epidemiol* 1997; **145**: 804–809.

156. Eastell R. Role of oestrogen in the regulation of bone turnover at the menarche. *J Endocrinol* 2005; **185**: 223–234.

157. Cummings SR, Browner WS, Bauer D et al. Endogenous hormones and the risk of hip and vertebral fractures among older women. Study of Osteoporotic Fractures Research Group [see comment]. *N Engl J Med* 1998; **339**: 733–738.

158. Goderie-Plomp HW, van der Klift M, de Ronde W et al. Endogenous sex hormones, sex hormone-binding globulin, and the risk of incident vertebral fractures in elderly men and women: the Rotterdam Study. *J Clin Endocrinol Metab* 2004; **89**: 3261–3269.

159. Khosla S, Melton LJ III, Atkinson EJ et al. Relationship of serum sex steroid levels and bone turnover markers with bone mineral density in men and women: a key role for bioavailable estrogen. *J Clin Endocrinol Metab* 1998; **83**: 2266–2274.

160. Rapado A, Hawkins F, Sobrinho L et al. Bone mineral density and androgen levels in elderly males. *Calcif Tissue Int* 1999; **65**: 417–421.

161. Slemenda CW, Longcope C, Zhou L et al. Sex steroids and bone mass in older men. Positive associations with serum estrogens and negative associations with androgens. *J Clin Invest* 1997; **100**: 1755–1759.

162. Taaffe DR, Cooper CS, Holloway L et al. Lack of association of anabolic hormone status and muscle strength with regional and whole body bone mineral density in healthy men aged 60–79 years. *Aging (Milan)* 1999; **11**: 4–11.

163. Amin S, Zhang Y, Sawin CT et al. Association of hypogonadism and estradiol levels with bone mineral density in elderly men from the Framingham study [comment]. *Ann Intern Med* 2000; **133**: 951–963.

164. Greendale GA, Edelstein S & Barrett-Connor E. Endogenous sex steroids and bone mineral density in older women and men: the Rancho Bernardo Study. *J Bone Miner Res* 1997; **12**: 1833–1843.

165. Szulc P, Munoz F, Claustrat B et al. Bioavailable estradiol may be an important determinant of osteoporosis in men: the MINOS study. *J Clin Endocrinol Metab* 2001; **86**: 192–199.

166. Center JR, Nguyen TV, Sambrook PN et al. Hormonal and biochemical parameters in the determination of osteoporosis in elderly men. *J Clin Endocrinol Metab* 1999; **84**: 3626–3635.

167. Gennari L, Merlotti D, Martini G et al. Longitudinal association between sex hormone levels, bone loss, and bone turnover in elderly men. *J Clin Endocrinol Metab* 2003; **88**: 5327–5333.

168. Van Pottelbergh I, Goemaere S & Kaufman JM. Bioavailable estradiol and an aromatase gene polymorphism are determinants of bone mineral density changes in men over 70 years of age. *J Clin Endocrinol Metab* 2003; **88**: 3075–3081.

169. Khosla S, Melton LJ III, Atkinson EJ et al. Relationship of serum sex steroid levels to longitudinal changes in bone density in young versus elderly men. *J Clin Endocrinol Metab* 2001; **86**: 3555–3561.

170. Anderson FH, Francis RM, Peaston RT et al. Androgen supplementation in eugonadal men with osteoporosis: effects of six months' treatment on markers of bone formation and resorption. *J Bone Miner Res* 1997; **12**: 472–478.

171. Taxel P, Kennedy DG, Fall PM et al. The effect of aromatase inhibition on sex steroids, gonadotropins, and markers of bone turnover in older men. *J Clin Endocrinol Metab* 2001; **86**: 2869–2874.

172. Falahati-Nini A, Riggs BL, Atkinson EJ et al. Relative contributions of testosterone and estrogen in regulating bone resorption and formation in normal elderly men. *J Clin Invest* 2000; **106**: 1553–1560.

173. Baillie SP, Davison CE, Johnson FJ et al. Pathogenesis of vertebral crush fractures in men. *Age Ageing* 1992; **21**: 139–141.

174. Stanley HL, Schmitt BP, Poses RM et al. Does hypogonadism contribute to the occurrence of a minimal trauma hip fracture in elderly men? [see comment]. *J Am Geriatr Soc* 1991; **39**: 766–771.

175a. Barrett-Connor E, Mueller JE, von Muhlen DG et al. Low levels of estradiol are associated with vertebral fractures in older men, but not women: the Rancho Bernardo Study. *J Clin Endocrinol Metab* 2000; **85**: 219–223.

175b. Amin S, Zhang Y, Felson DT et al. Estradiol, testosterone, and the risk for hip fractures in elderly men from the Framingham Study. *Am J Med*, in press.

176. Barrett-Connor E, Kritz-Silverstein D & Edelstein SL. A prospective study of dehydroepiandrosterone sulfate (DHEAS) and bone mineral density in older men and women. *Am J Epidemiol* 1993; **137**: 201–206.

177. Murphy S, Khaw KT, Cassidy A et al. Sex hormones and bone mineral density in elderly men. *Bone Miner* 1993; **20**: 133–140.

178. Legrand E, Hedde C, Gallois Y et al. Osteoporosis in men: a potential role for the sex hormone binding globulin. *Bone* 2001; **29**: 90–95.

179. Conover CA & Rosen C. The role of insulin-like growth factors and binding proteins in bone cell biology. In: Bilezikian JP, Raisz LG & Rodan GA, eds. *Principles of Bone Biology*, Vol. 1. San Diego, CA: Academic Press, 2002; 801–815.

180. Rajaram S, Baylink DJ & Mohan S. Insulin-like growth factor-binding proteins in serum and other biological fluids: regulation and functions. *Endocr Rev* 1997; **18**: 801–831.

181. Rogol AD. Growth and growth hormone secretion at puberty: the role of gonadal steroid hormones. *Acta Paediatr Suppl* 1992; **383**: 15–20; discussion 21.

182. Van Wyk JJ & Smith EP. Insulin-like growth factors and skeletal growth: possibilities for therapeutic interventions. *J Clin Endocrinol Metab* 1999; **84**: 4349–4354.

183. Karasik D, Rosen CJ, Hannan MT et al. Insulin-like growth factor binding proteins 4 and 5 and bone mineral density in elderly men and women. *Calcif Tissue Int* 2002; **71**: 323–328.

184. Amin S, Riggs BL, Atkinson EJ et al. A potentially deleterious role of IGFBP-2 on bone density in aging men and women. *J Bone Miner Res* 2004; **19**: 1075–1083.

185. Barrett-Connor E & Goodman-Gruen D. Gender differences in insulin-like growth factor and bone mineral density association in old age: the Rancho Bernardo Study. *J Bone Miner Res* 1998; **13**: 1343–1349.

186. Boonen S, Lesaffre E, Dequeker J et al. Relationship between baseline insulin like growth factor-I (IGF-I) and femoral bone density in women aged over 70 years: potential implications for the prevention of age-related bone loss. *J Am Geriatr Soc* 1996; **44**: 1301–1306.

187. Langlois JA, Rosen CJ, Visser M et al. Association between insulin-like growth factor I and bone mineral density in older women and men: the Framingham Heart Study [see comments]. *J Clin Endocrinol Metab* 1998; **83**: 4257–4262.

188. Sugimoto T, Nishiyama K, Kuribayashi F et al. Serum levels of insulin-like growth factor (IGF) I, IGF-binding protein (IGFBP)-2, and IGFBP-3 in osteoporotic patients with and without spinal fractures. *J Bone Miner Res* 1997; **12**: 1272–1279.

189. Nakaoka D, Sugimoto T, Kaji H et al. Determinants of bone mineral density and spinal fracture risk in postmenopausal Japanese women. *Osteoporosis Int* 2001; **12**: 548–554.

190. Seck T, Scheidt-Nave C, Leidig-Bruckner G et al. Low serum concentrations of insulin-like growth factor I are associated with femoral bone loss in a population-based sample of postmenopausal women. *Clin Endocrinol* 2001; **55**: 101–106.

191. Pfeilschifter J, Scheidt-Nave C, Leidig-Bruckner G et al. Relationship between circulating insulin-like growth factor components and sex hormones in a population-based sample of 50- to 80-year-old men and women. *J Clin Endocrinol Metab* 1996; **81**: 2534–2540.

192. Rudman D, Drinka PJ, Wilson CR et al. Relations of endogenous anabolic hormones and physical activity to bone mineral density and lean body mass in elderly men. *Clin Endocrinol* 1994; **40**: 653–661.

193. Kurland ES, Rosen CJ, Cosman F et al. Insulin-like growth factor-I in men with idiopathic osteoporosis [comment]. *J Clin Endocrinol Metab* 1997; **82**: 2799–2805.

194. Ljunghall S, Johansson AG, Burman P et al. Low plasma levels of insulin-like growth factor 1 (IGF-1) in male patients with idiopathic osteoporosis. *J Intern Med* 1992; **232**: 59–64.

195. Johansson AG, Forslund A, Hambraeus L et al. Growth hormone-dependent insulin-like growth factor binding protein is a major determinant of bone mineral density in healthy men. *J Bone Miner Res* 1994; **9**: 915–921.

196. Kim JG & Lee JY. Serum insulin-like growth factor binding protein profiles in postmenopausal women: their correlation with bone mineral density. *Am J Obstet Gynecol* 1996; **174**: 1511–1517.

197. Gillberg P, Olofsson H, Mallmin H et al. Bone mineral density in femoral neck is positively correlated to circulating insulin-like growth factor (IGF)-I and IGF-binding protein (IGFBP)-3 in Swedish men. *Calcif Tissue Int* 2002; **70**: 22–29.

198. Ensrud KE, Duong T, Cauley JA et al. Low fractional calcium absorption increases the risk for hip fracture in women with low calcium intake. Study of Osteoporotic Fractures Research Group. *Ann Intern Med* 2000; **132**: 345–353.

199. Garnero P, Hausherr E, Chapuy MC et al. Markers of bone resorption predict hip fracture in elderly women: the EPIDOS Prospective Study. *J Bone Miner Res* 1996; **11**: 1531–1538.

200. Diamond T, Smerdely P, Kormas N et al. Hip fracture in elderly men: the importance of subclinical vitamin D deficiency and hypogonadism. *Med J Aust* 1998; **169**: 138–141.

201. Bischoff-Ferrari HA, Willett WC, Wong JB et al. Fracture prevention with vitamin D supplementation: a meta-analysis of randomized controlled trials. *JAMA* 2005; **293**: 2257–2264.

202. Grant AM, Avenell A, Campbell MK et al. Oral vitamin D3 and calcium for secondary prevention of low-trauma fractures in elderly people (Randomised Evaluation of Calcium Or vitamin D, RECORD): a randomised placebo-controlled trial [see comment]. *Lancet* 2005; **365**: 1621–1628.

203. Melhus H, Michaelsson K, Kindmark A et al. Excessive dietary intake of vitamin A is associated with reduced bone mineral density and increased risk for hip fracture [see comment]. *Ann Intern Med* 1998; **129**: 770–778.

204. Michaelsson K, Lithell H, Vessby B et al. Serum retinol levels and the risk of fracture [see comment]. *N Engl J Med* 2003; **348**: 287–294.

205. Lim LS, Harnack LJ, Lazovich D et al. Vitamin A intake and the risk of hip fracture in postmenopausal women: the Iowa Women's Health Study. *Osteoporosis Int* 2004; **15**: 552–559.

206. Rejnmark L, Vestergaard P, Charles P et al. No effect of vitamin A intake on bone mineral density and fracture risk in perimenopausal women. *Osteoporosis Int* 2004; **15**: 872–880.

207. Barker ME, McCloskey E, Saha S et al. Serum retinoids and beta-carotene as predictors of hip and other fractures in elderly women. *J Bone Miner Res* 2005; **20**: 913–920.

208. Goerss JB, Kim CH, Atkinson EJ et al. Risk of fractures in patients with pernicious anemia. *J Bone Miner Res* 1992; **7**: 573–579.

209. Dhonukshe-Rutten RA, Lips M, de Jong N et al. Vitamin B-12 status is associated with bone mineral content and bone mineral density in frail elderly women but not in men. *J Nutr* 2003; **133**: 801–807.

210. Stone KL, Bauer DC, Sellmeyer D et al. Low serum vitamin B-12 levels are associated with increased hip bone loss in older women: a prospective study [see comment]. *J Clin Endocrinol Metab* 2004; **89**: 1217–1221.

211. Tucker KL, Hannan MT, Qiao N et al. Low plasma vitamin B12 is associated with lower BMD: the Framingham Osteoporosis Study. *J Bone Miner Res* 2005; **20**: 152–158.

212. Kim GS, Kim CH, Park JY et al. Effects of vitamin B12 on cell proliferation and cellular alkaline phosphatase activity in human bone marrow stromal osteoprogenitor cells and UMR106 osteoblastic cells. *Metab: Clin Exp* 1996; **45**: 1443–1446.

213. Carmel R, Lau KH, Baylink DJ et al. Cobalamin and osteoblast-specific proteins. *N Engl J Med* 1988; **319**: 70–75.

214. Mudd SH, Skovby F, Levy HL et al. The natural history of homocystinuria due to cystathionine beta-synthase deficiency. *Am J Hum Genet* 1985; **37**: 1–31.

215. McLean RR, Jacques PF, Selhub J et al. Homocysteine as a predictive factor for hip fracture in older persons [see comment]. *N Engl J Med* 2004; **350**: 2042–2049.

216. Van Meurs JB, Dhonukshe-Rutten RA, Pluijm SM et al. Homocysteine levels and the risk of osteoporotic fracture [see comment]. *N Engl J Med* 2004; **350**: 2033–2041.

217. Raisz LG. Homocysteine and osteoporotic fractures – culprit or bystander? [see comment]. *N Engl J Med* 2004; **350**: 2089–2090.

218. Sato Y, Honda Y, Iwamoto J et al. Effect of folate and mecobalamin on hip fractures in patients with stroke: a randomized controlled trial [see comment]. *JAMA* 2005; **293**: 1082–1088.

219. Marshall D, Johnell O & Wedel H. Meta-analysis of how well measures of bone mineral density predict occurrence of osteoporotic fractures [see comment]. *BMJ* 1996; **312**: 1254–1259.

220. Kanis JA, Johnell O, Oden A et al. Ten-year risk of osteoporotic fracture and the effect of risk factors on screening strategies. *Bone* 2002; **30**: 251–258.

221. Tromp AM, Ooms ME, Popp-Snijders C et al. Predictors of fractures in elderly women. *Osteoporosis Int* 2000; **11**: 134–140.

222. Kanis JA, Johnell O, Oden A et al. Risk of hip fracture derived from relative risks: an analysis applied to the population of Sweden. *Osteoporosis Int* 2000; **11**: 120–127.

223. Burger H, de Laet CE, Weel AE et al. Added value of bone mineral density in hip fracture risk scores. *Bone* 1999; **25**: 369–374.

Chapter 8

The use of bone densitometry in clinical practice

Claus-C. Glüer

Bone densitometry is an established method for the assessment of osteoporosis.[1] The information provided about skeletal status is key to the appropriate management of the osteoporotic patient. More than 25 years of development have provided a wealth of experience and data for this approach, and meta-analyses have confirmed its utility for the assessment of osteoporotic fracture risk.[2] Despite all these achievements, there is an ongoing debate about the strengths and limitations of bone densitometry. Both technique-inherent limitations and the potential for misuse need to be acknowledged. Like virtually all other diagnostic approaches, bone densitometry can provide misleading information if it is not applied appropriately.

In this chapter, an attempt is made to provide guidance for the appropriate use of bone densitometry in the clinical management of osteoporotic patients by a discussion of its strong and weak points. A detailed overview of the technical performance features of densitometric approaches can be found in many articles in the literature, and only a number of key aspects will be covered in this chapter. For further information, the reader is directed to recent review articles and published books covering this subject.[1,3,4]

OVERVIEW OF BONE DENSITOMETRY TECHNOLOGIES

A variety of different bone densitometry approaches has been developed over the past 25 years. In this chapter, only a brief overview is provided, with references for detailed review articles and book chapters that provide a more in-depth coverage of the technology and the performance of these approaches.

Dual X-ray absorptiometry

Dual X-ray absorptiometry (DXA) is the most widely used bone densitometry technique today.[4] The assessment of the proximal femur, specifically the bone mineral density (BMD) of the total femur region, probably represents the most important single diagnostic assessment of osteoporosis and fracture risk. A large body of evidence from prospective studies documents the strong gradient of risk that allows the best assessment of hip fracture risk and an estimation of risk for other fractures that is comparable to that of other techniques. The measurement of BMD in the postero-anterior lumbar spine is also of value, particularly in early post-menopausal women, in whom changes in cancellous bone are of particular importance. Later in life, degenerative changes obscure the result and lead to a falsely elevated BMD level.

Nevertheless, postero-anterior spine measurements are sensitive to treatment changes and thus represent the most widely used technique for monitoring purposes. Lateral spinal DXA techniques further improve the responsiveness but at the expense of precision.

Peripheral DXA

As a successor to previous single X-ray absorptiometry (SXA) approaches, peripheral DXA (pDXA) techniques enable the measurement of BMD in the periphery, specifically at the radius and the calcaneus.[4] Both sites have been shown to provide a good estimate of global osteoporotic fracture risk, but they do not quite match the performance of central DXA measurements in assessing spine or hip fractures, and they have limitations in assessing treatment efficacy.

Quantitative computed tomography

Quantitative computed tomography (QCT) enables the selective assessment of the skeletal status of cancellous bone of the vertebral bodies of the lower thoracic and the lumbar spine. QCT is the most sensitive technique for the assessment of early post-menopausal skeletal change.[5] Correspondingly, cross-sectional studies have generally shown a better discrimination of fractured and unfractured subjects using QCT compared with DXA. Because of the lack of prospective studies and limited information on measurements at the proximal femur, the data that support the use of QCT are not quite as convincing and comprehensive as those for DXA.

An advantage over other techniques can be expected if the change mostly occurs in cancellous bone and also if size effects or overlying structures obscure DXA measurements. QCT enables the clear separation of abnormal BMD values from size-related deviations that are difficult to discriminate using technologies such as DXA, which assesses areal BMD, or quantitative ultrasound (QUS). While this is of particular importance in paediatric studies, the QCT radiation level is somewhat higher than that of DXA, which is of particular concern in children. For adult studies, radiation exposure is less problematic; the radiation dose of QCT is smaller by a factor of 40–50 than that required for spinal X-rays.[6]

Peripheral QCT

Peripheral QCT (pQCT) measurements are typically obtained at the radius or the tibia.[7,8] Again, cancellous bone can be evaluated selectively, but this translates into high longitudinal sensitivity only if a small precision error level is achieved. Technologically, devices of different complexity and performance have been developed. The lack of prospective studies limits the ability to evaluate the performance of pQCT for the assessment of fracture risk. Promising results for monitoring bisphosphonate treatment have recently been reported, which is of particular interest since negative results have been reported with DXA measurements performed at the radius. Thus, volumetric technology may offer some advantage over planar measurements, an observation that needs to be confirmed by independent studies.

pQCT, as in the case of QCT, provides three-dimensional information on bone morphology, particularly when performed in a multislice or spiral scan fashion. This enables a calculation of the biomechanically relevant properties of bone, such as the areal moment of inertia, a measurement that should provide a better assessment of bone strength than BMD or other bone mass estimates.[9] Whether the application of this refinement at a peripheral measurement site will also provide an improvement in the assessment of spine or hip fracture risk remains to be seen.

Quantitative ultrasound approaches

There are a variety of QUS approaches, some of which show a substantial difference in performance.[10,11] Both transverse and axial transmission techniques are used.[12] Clinical QUS devices measure speed of sound (SOS) and broadband ultrasound attenuation (BUA) at the calcaneus, phalanges, radius, tibia and other peripheral measurement sites.

SOS and BUA mostly reflect a change in bone mineral density.[10,12] In experimental settings, it has been shown that structural aspects of bone also affect QUS parameters independently of bone mineral density.[13] Further research is required to establish whether bone structure can be directly assessed using QUS approaches. QUS is second only to DXA in terms of providing a large body of evidence supporting its predictive power for assessing future fracture risk. In general, QUS performs almost as well as DXA, with the possible exception of DXA of the hip, for assessing hip fracture risk. Further research is required to determine how QUS approaches can be used to diagnose osteoporosis and monitor treatment.

Digital X-ray radiogrammetry

Standard radiographs of the forearm that include the radius and the metacarpals provide the basis for digital X-ray radiogrammetry (DXR).[14] Automated image-processing techniques are used to measure cortical bone width plus a variety of structure-related features. Mathematical modelling allows the estimation of (areal) BMD level and possibly some aspects of bone structure (e.g. cortical porosity or endosteal trabecularization). The assessment of the clinical utility of this new approach is ongoing.

Other techniques

A variety of other bone densitometry techniques have been used in the past, and new ones are currently being developed. Older approaches such as radiographic absorptiometry (RA) showed a strong predictive power in a limited number of studies.[15] Sophisticated innovative approaches for assessing bone structure include high-resolution CT (HRCT)[16] and high-resolution magnetic resonance (HRMR).[17] However, these are not currently widely used in the clinical setting. It remains to be seen whether they will enable an improvement in the assessment of fracture risk, particularly for subjects undergoing treatment.

BONE DENSITOMETRY FOR THE DIAGNOSIS OF OSTEOPOROSIS

According to the current definition, osteoporosis is 'a systemic skeletal disease characterized by low bone mass and microarchitectural deterioration of bone tissue, with a consequent increase in bone fragility and susceptibility to fracture'.[18] According to this definition, the diagnostic approach could follow two different strategies. On the one hand, the technique could aim to assess the reduction in bone mass and/or the impairment of bone structure. Alternatively, the technique might enable the consequences of such a change in bone mass and bone structure, i.e. the reduction in bone strength, to be assessed.

The first approach aims at the direct diagnostic assessment of those properties which characterize osteoporosis, whereas the second is focused on the principal consequence of osteoporosis – the enhanced fracture risk. It is obvious that an approach that has been validated according to the second strategy can only be used in a diagnostic setting if it is complemented by other diagnostic approaches that allow proper differential diagnostic assessments. Only if this complementary information is available can the results be used for therapy decisions.

Assessing bone mass and density

The quantitative assessment of bone mass should provide a result that is as close as possible to the true status. *Accuracy errors* describe the deviation of measured results obtained by bone densitometry from the true finding. In the case of bone mass, the true value can only be approximated in vitro by comparing the results of bone densitometry with those of ashing techniques. In vivo the situation is more complex, and correspondingly the accuracy error can be estimated from in situ studies carried out on cadavers. It is reasonable to assume that the accuracy error for measurements in vivo would be somewhat higher. Studies reported in the literature list accuracy errors in the range of 2–15% for most densitometric approaches.[3] This is somewhat smaller than one standard deviation of the population variance. Hence bone densitometry enables the assessment of the bone mass status of a patient compared with the normal reference population with reasonable accuracy, but it is not possible to define a threshold value above which the level of bone mass is considered normal and below which it is to be considered osteoporotic. Instead, it is necessary to recognize the intrinsic error sources and limits of accuracy in determining bone mass.

In the definition of osteoporosis, reference is made to *bone mass*, but the technique for its assessment is referred to as *bone densitometry*. This raises the question of whether it is preferable to assess bone mass or bone density. The answer is not straightforward. It is clear that body size is reflected in bone size, which in turn affects bone mass. An assessment of volumetric BMD would correct for this size effect. On the other hand, larger people are heavier, and they need bigger and stronger bones to support this weight. Fractures commonly occur as a result of a fall or another larger force impacting on the bone. Bones with equal volumetric density but of different size would not show equal strength against such forces. Areal BMD techniques only partially adjust for the effect of body size. While this introduces an additional component of accuracy errors in certain situations, it may work in the 'right' direction: subjects with bigger bones have a larger areal BMD, and because of the larger cross-sectional area, these bones are also stronger.

So from a theoretical point of view it is difficult to judge which is the optimum measure to assess bone strength. Empirically, areal BMD measurements have been found to be a slightly stronger predictor of future fracture risk compared with direct measurements of bone mass. In cross-sectional studies, volumetric measures of BMD usually show a better discrimination between subjects with and without vertebral fractures compared with techniques that measure areal BMD.[19,20] However, whether this results from the different measurement approach or from the fact that such techniques selectively measure the highly responsive cancellous bone is difficult to assess. In situations in which a large variation in bone size is common, an assessment of volumetric BMD may be advantageous. This is particularly so in paediatric studies, in which the increase seen in areal BMD with increasing age is almost totally due to the increase in bone size and reflects to only a small degree a real increase in volumetric density.[21,22]

Assessing bone structure

The performance of bone densitometry techniques in assessing bone architecture is more difficult to characterize.[3] Unlike bone mass, bone architecture cannot be represented by a single number. Instead, a variety of aspects contribute, including trabecular spacing, trabecular anisotropy, connectivity, and trabecular and cortical thickness.[23] There is no consensus on which of these aspects is most important with regard to the diagnostic assessment of osteoporosis. The definition given above implies that architectural deterioration is not simply a by-product of bone loss but that there is a component independently affecting bone strength. While a few papers have indeed demonstrated an independent contribution of bone structure to bone strength,[24,25] the magnitude of this independent contribution remains controversial. A large number of techniques are currently being developed that will allow a more accurate assessment of bone structure. Once these techniques have found an application in clinical practice, the relevance of the assessment of bone structure in addition to bone mass and density will become clearer.

With current bone densitometry techniques, only a very few aspects of bone structure can be measured in vivo. Most of them relate to bone macrostructure or geometry, i.e. aspects that are not addressed in the current definition of osteoporosis, although it has been shown that geometric aspects (for example, hip axis length[26] and other measures of bone size[27]) are related to fracture risk. Some aspects of inhomogeneity of the distribution of bone mass within the region imaged can be assessed by several bone densitometry techniques. In addition, the assessment of bone texture is possible with some of the newer bone densitometry approaches (and on radiographs).[1,3] Tomographic techniques such as HRCT[16] and HRMR[17] provide the best spatial information and enable quantitation of some aspects of cancellous and cortical bone structure. However, none of these techniques is currently used in clinical practice.

Assessing bone strength

Biomechanical studies have revealed that BMD may explain between 10% and 80% of bone strength.[28] This is based on destructive biomechanical testing studies carried out in vitro. The large range of values points to certain caveats that need to be noted in this context. The percentage depends on the range of BMD values in the group of specimens tested. Even with a correlation coefficient as high as 0.9, a large and unexplained variability may occur in some individuals, a limitation that is important in clinical practice.

Moreover, the correlation typically deteriorates substantially if the measurement site and the fracture site are not identical. Bone strength is quite variable across different measurement sites, and the observation may in part be explained by a variation in bone structure that is not reflected in bone densitometry measurements.[29] Consequently, it is understandable that the best results for fracture risk assessment have usually been obtained for technologies that assess BMD at the prospective fracture site. Only if the accuracy error of a given technique is very large might assessment at a distant site be preferable. One example is the presence of degenerative changes in the lumbar spine, which can result in a substantial overestimation of BMD values for planar densitometry techniques.[30] In subjects with such degenerative changes, a better assessment, even for vertebral fracture risk, may be obtained by measurements at the hip or at a peripheral measurement site.[31]

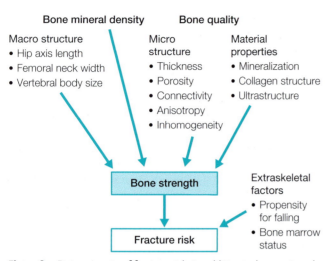

Figure 8.1. Determinants of fracture risk. In addition to bone mineral density, a number of other factors, both skeletal and extraskeletal, affect fracture risk. The individual factors listed represent examples rather than a complete set of influencing variables.

As stated above, bone strength depends not only on BMD and bone structure, but also on other skeletal characteristics. Figure 8.1 shows a schematic representation of the factors that affect bone strength and fracture risk. The large number of non-BMD-related factors might lead to the conclusion that the assessment of BMD is of only limited value for assessing bone strength, but this interpretation would be wrong. In osteoporosis, a change in the material properties of the bone tissue has not been demonstrated. Moreover, as long as bone structure and BMD change in parallel, the impact on bone strength could be completely explained as a (non-linear) function of BMD alone. All these observations explain why, in some situations, BMD is almost a perfect surrogate marker of bone strength, although in other settings, a discrepancy between BMD and bone strength can be observed. (Such a deviation is even more likely if the patient is receiving medication, an effect that will be discussed below in the section on monitoring.)

Clinical consequences

What are the clinical consequences of the observations discussed above? Most importantly, it has to be recognized that bone densitometry cannot provide an accurate diagnostic assessment of osteoporosis if performed and interpreted in isolation, as it should be considered in conjunction with other diagnostic methods. In the clinical setting, these include:[32]

1. A comprehensive physical examination.
2. An assessment of the risk factor profile of the patient.
3. An assessment of fracture history and fracture status and severity.
4. Tests to rule out secondary osteoporosis.

Bone densitometry can be regarded as the single most important factor that contributes to the diagnosis of osteoporosis,

because it is the only approach that directly and quantitatively assesses the fundamental characteristic of osteoporosis, i.e. reduced bone mass.

Diagnostic criteria

In 1994, a working group of the World Health Organization (WHO) proposed criteria that have been largely, albeit not universally, accepted. According to these criteria, osteopoenia is defined as a BMD below a T-score of −1 (the T-score reflecting the deviation from the young population mean in units of standard deviations of the population variance of the young reference population), whereas osteoporosis is defined as a BMD level below a T-score of −2.5.[33] The number of subjects diagnosed as osteoporotic by these criteria, based on DXA measurements of the lumbar spine, femoral neck or forearm, approximately equals the 30% lifetime risk of fracture in post-menopausal women.

The WHO definition has been widely implemented and has in general been helpful in the clinical management of osteoporotic patients. Limitations of the approach have, however, become more apparent in recent years.[34] Besides the problem that osteoporosis cannot be defined solely on the BMD value, the disparity in the BMD level at different measurement sites has become a source of increasing confusion. Although the agreement between assessments at different DXA measurement sites is in general fairly good (typically fewer than 3–10% of subjects who are defined as normal at one site being ranked as osteoporotic at another[34]), the discrepancy is larger for peripheral measurement approaches.

QUS measurements of the calcaneus, phalanges, radius and other peripheral bones, as well as a variety of DXA and other X-ray-based peripheral measurement techniques (such as DXR, RA or pDXA of the calcaneus), have recently found widespread clinical use.[10] The pattern of age-related decline of bone loss defined by these approaches, even when standardized as a T-score, varies substantially,[34,35] as illustrated in Figure 8.2.

The age-related decline of bone loss shown by QCT of the spine is much more rapid than for some of the QUS measurements of the calcaneus. Consequently, the uniform application of a threshold level of T equal to −2.5 results in the classification of a varying number of subjects as osteoporotic, with a range from 10% to more than 40%. Moreover, the WHO definition has been developed only for women, and it is unclear which thresholds should be used for men.

There is currently some debate over how to replace the system of T-score-based diagnostic criteria.[34] Different techniques have a different sensitivity and specificity, and thus no uniform criterion can be derived.[34] Equivalent T-scores could be calculated based either on equal prevalence (i.e. the number of subjects determined to be osteoporotic would be very similar for all techniques) or on equivalent estimates of fracture risk. The first approach is not acceptable because it would ignore differences in performance of different bone densitometry techniques. Risk-based T-scores or direct estimates of absolute risk would be preferable and would provide information about the magnitude of fracture risk. Efforts are

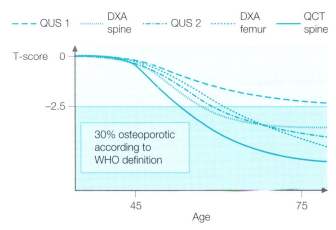

Figure 8.2. A schematic drawing demonstrating the different age dependency of various bone densitometry and quantitative ultrasound (QUS) techniques. It is obvious that the number of subjects falling below the threshold of T = −2.5 would greatly vary between techniques, inconsistent with the concept of a given number of osteoporotic subjects within a population that can be estimated from epidemiological studies. DXA, dual X-ray absorptiometry; QCT, quantitative computed tomography.

currently underway to calculate these figures for the various bone densitometry approaches.

Even if this approach were established, however, the issue of discordant findings at different measurement sites would remain. Consequently, it has been proposed that diagnostic criteria should be limited to central bone density measures and possibly restricted to DXA measurements of the total proximal femur.[34] This technique has been shown to yield the highest gradient of risk for the most severe outcome of osteoporosis, that of hip fracture.[2] Moreover, it is less susceptible to the accuracy errors that limit the utility of DXA of the lumbar spine in elderly subjects with degenerative changes of the spine. Following this strategy, all approaches other than DXA of the total proximal femur would be used for fracture risk assessment rather than for the diagnostic assessment of osteoporosis per se. While this would, by definition, eliminate the site dependency problem, it would also limit the role of techniques that are particularly sensitive in detecting the risk of vertebral fractures, most notably QCT of the spine. Therefore, the choice of DXA of the total proximal femur as the 'gold standard' may unnecessarily limit the sensitivity of bone densitometry approaches in detecting early bone loss caused by osteoporosis, thereby reducing the potential for preventive measures. This is clearly an area of ongoing discussion, and WHO criteria should be used with caution until a consensus on an alternative approach is reached.

BONE DENSITOMETRY FOR THE ASSESSMENT OF FRACTURE RISK

The key strength of bone densitometry lies in its ability to provide an accurate estimate of future fracture risk. Numerous prospective studies have demonstrated the association between a decease in BMD and an increase in fracture risk. The gradient of risk ranges from a relative risk of about 1.2–1.5 for peripheral fractures up to 2.5–3.0 for hip fractures for each standard deviation decrease in BMD.[1,2] When comparing the ability of central and peripheral techniques to predict an osteoporotic fracture at any site (global fracture risk), the risk ratio is around 1.5 per standard deviation decrease.[36]

For the prediction of a specific fracture, a site-matched assessment of BMD usually provides superior predictive power compared with measurements at other sites. Most notably, the gradient of risk for hip fractures predicted by measurements at the proximal femur using DXA is of the order of 2.5–3.0 per standard deviation decrease in BMD. QUS techniques also perform very well (Figure 8.3).

For vertebral fractures, the situation is not quite as clear. Spinal DXA results can be falsely elevated by degenerative calcification in the spine. In cross-sectional studies, however, a site-matched measurement using QCT has generally proved superior to any other technology tested.[19,20] Since there are only limited prospective data for QCT, it has not been firmly established whether QCT of the spine is the best predictor of vertebral fractures.

Colles fractures can be well predicted by measurements at the forearm, which are at least as predictive as measurements at other sites.[36] The reason for these differences in performance can be found in the variability of the pattern of bone loss at different anatomical sites.

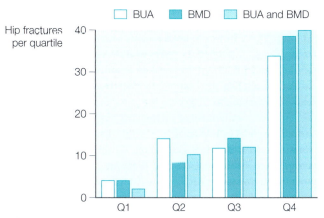

Figure 8.3. Gradient of risk for broadband ultrasound attenuation (BUA) of the calcaneus, bone mineral density (BMD), measured by dual X-ray absorptiometry (DXA), of the femoral neck and a combination of both. Subjects were grouped in quartiles according to their age-adjusted hip fracture risk, the number of hip fractures occurring during about 2–3 years of follow-up being plotted for each quartile (Q1, lowest estimated risk; Q4, highest estimated risk). Results demonstrate comparable gradients of risk, with a slight advantage of DXA over BUA and a minimal advantage of combinations of DXA and BUA over DXA alone. Data from the Study of Osteoporotic Fractures.[10]

Interpretation of fracture risk

An assessment of fracture risk can never be expected to predict with absolute certainty whether or not a fracture will occur. This in part explains why, in cross-sectional studies, there is a substantial overlap in BMD level between those individuals who have and those who have not sustained a fracture. Those with a very low BMD level are likely to suffer from a fracture in the future, so this overlap must be interpreted with caution. Wasnich and colleagues[37,38] have repeatedly pointed out that cross-sectional studies are inappropriate as a means of characterizing the ability of bone densitometry to assess osteoporotic fracture risk. Moreover, the magnitude of overlap in BMD value depends strongly on the disease status of the patients: the more severe the osteoporotic fracture status, the smaller the overlap will be. On the other hand, carefully designed cross-sectional studies can, if interpreted with caution, provide a significant insight into the performance of competing techniques.

The gradients of fracture risk observed for bone densitometry are at least as strong as those for a number of well-established risk predictors, including blood pressure or cholesterol level in the prediction of stroke or coronary heart disease.[33] In principle, therefore, bone densitometry has the potential to be used to identify individuals who will benefit from preventive intervention, and it may thus have a potential role in screening. Cost-efficiency analyses are, however, required to determine the value and benefit of such programmes. Some analyses have shown cost-efficiency for certain strategies – for example, performing bone densitometry on all women above the age of 65.[40] At present, however, there is no consensus on these issues, and further analyses need to be performed.

The software currently implemented on bone densitometers does not provide an output that specifies the relative or absolute risk for the individual examined. The need for such an output has, however, been recognized, and software is currently being developed. In order to allow for a straightforward clinical interpretation, the level of absolute risk is preferable to that of relative risk. Moreover, the absolute risk estimates should describe the risk over the next 5 or 10 years.[34] There are, however, only limited prospective data that cover such a time range. Therefore, the uncertainty of the estimate increases with increasing duration. Given the relatively slow progression of the disease and the time required to reach a sustained improvement in bone status with treatment, the absolute risk level for a very short time period is inappropriate. Second, other clinical risk factors should be considered,[1] especially the number and severity of prevalent osteoporotic fractures, which have a strong impact on the estimate of future fracture risk.[41] Thus, any programme that calculates the absolute risk level needs to be based on a multifactorial model that includes bone densitometry as well as other relevant risk factors. Given the recent evidence that bone turnover may also be an independent predictor of fracture risk, it may also be useful to incorporate measurements of markers of bone turnover.[42]

BONE DENSITOMETRY FOR MAKING TREATMENT DECISIONS

In order to make responsible treatment decisions, an accurate knowledge of BMD status is required. Bone densitometry is relevant for treatment decisions for two reasons. First, the strong association between decreased BMD and the risk of a future fracture enables the identification of those subjects who are at highest risk of fracture[2] and thus most urgently require treatment. As stated above, such a decision must also take into account the information obtained from a clinical assessment of the patient, the risk factor profile and the number and severity of osteoporotic fractures. In addition, bone-related fragility should be clearly differentiated from fall-related problems.

The second reason why BMD is important for making treatment decisions has only recently been established. It has been shown that, among subjects with prevalent vertebral fractures, those individuals with a lower BMD may gain more from anti-resorptive treatment than those with a higher BMD.[43] Similarly, it has been reported that among those who have not yet suffered a vertebral fracture, only individuals who are in the osteoporotic range will benefit from anti-resorptive treatment.[44] Subjects with a normal BMD, on the other hand, did not benefit. Interestingly, clinical risk factors appear to be of limited use in this decision-making process. This is probably related to the fact that clinical risk factors do not necessarily differentiate between fall-related and bone-related fracture risk. An improvement in the selection of clinical risk factors may in the future enable their use in addition to BMD to identify those subjects who will benefit most from treatment. Much less information is available for the identification of subjects who will benefit most from bone-forming treatments, and more research is required in this area.

BONE DENSITOMETRY FOR MONITORING SKELETAL CHANGES

Comparing longitudinal sensitivity

In order to study the progression of disease or the efficacy of treatment, an accurate assessment of changes in bone mass and bone structure, analogous to the definition of osteoporosis, is desirable. Currently, however, only changes in BMD can be measured with reasonable accuracy. In order to judge the ability of a technique to monitor skeletal changes, the reproducibility of a measurement, typically characterized by the precision error, is of critical importance. Since the monitoring of skeletal changes has to be performed over the time course of several years, long-term precision errors are the most relevant. Precision errors alone are not, however, sufficient to characterize a technique's ability to monitor skeletal changes. The response rate, i.e. the typical change in BMD per annum, is of equal importance.[45] Longitudinal sensitivity – the ability of a technique to monitor skeletal change – can be defined as the ratio of the response rate to the precision error. For example, a technique with a response rate twice that of another technique

Table 8.1. Example of the calculation of least significant change (LSC) and monitoring time interval (MTI).

Technique	Long-term precision error (%)	Response per annum (%)	LSC (%)	MTI (years)
DXA spine	1.5	4.0	4.2	1.1
DXA femur	2.0	2.8	5.6	2.0
Speed of sound	0.15	0.2	0.42	2.1
Broadband ultrasound attenuation	1.5	2.0	4.2	2.1

The numbers given do not represent actual data but are taken from the ranges reported for dual X-ray absorptiometry (DXA) and quantitative ultrasound devices. They illustrate the impact of precision errors on LSC and both precision errors and response rates on MTI. It becomes obvious that a low precision error does not necessarily translate into a shorter MTI (i.e. a better ability to monitor skeletal change).

can afford a precision error twice as high and still maintain the same level of longitudinal sensitivity.

For a comparison of the longitudinal sensitivity of different diagnostic techniques, the concept of standardized precision errors has been introduced. Among various definitions proposed, the following appears to be most appropriate for monitoring purposes:[45]

$$sPE = PE \times \frac{\text{Response rate (reference technique)}}{\text{Response rate (technique studied)}}$$

where PE is the uncorrected precision error and sPE the standardized precision error of the technique that is being studied. The ideal reference technique is postero-anterior DXA of the lumbar spine. Using this definition, the uncorrected precision errors are all re-scaled to the level for postero-anterior DXA of the spine, so techniques with good longitudinal sensitivity, which would be those with sPE of about 1% (like postero-anterior DXA of the spine), can be identified.

Interpretation of measured changes

While the standardized precision error is most suited to the comparison of different techniques, two other concepts may be more relevant in the clinical setting: the least significant change (LSC) and the monitoring time interval (MTI).[45] The LSC is given by:

$$LSC = 2.8 \times PE$$

and represents the magnitude of measured change that could be interpreted as reflecting true change with 95% confidence. The time interval required to see a significant change in the majority of patients is given by the MTI, defined as:

$$MTI = \frac{LSC}{\text{Response rate}}$$

For a technique with a precision error of 1.5%, for example, the LSC would amount to 4.2%, and the MTI for a group of subjects

in their first year of bisphosphonate treatment (during which a 4% change can be expected) would be $4.2 \div 4 = 1.1$ years, or a little more than 13 months (Table 8.1). Note that it may be acceptable to compare the measured change to the expected bone loss (if that individual had not started treatment) as opposed to comparing the measured change to a stable reading.

The concepts of LSC and MTI can also be helpful for the identification of fast losers of bone. As a first step, one should calculate the MTI required to show a significant normal bone loss in the majority of subjects. For a technique with a 1% precision error and an expected loss of bone of 1% per annum, for example, the monitoring time interval would be 2.8 years. If one were to define fast losers as those individuals who lose bone at twice the normal rate, it would also take 2.8 years for the majority of fast losers to show a bone loss significantly greater than the average normal bone loss (specifically 5.6% instead of the normal loss of 2.8% during this time interval). Thus, only subjects with a substantially higher rate of bone loss can be identified over a reasonably short time period using bone densitometry.

Another topic that has recently gained substantial attention is the so-called 'regression to the mean' effect.[46] A subject that has demonstrated a particularly high bone mineral gain in the first year after starting treatment is likely to show a reduced increase or perhaps even a decrease in BMD in the second year. Similarly, a subject who has lost an unexpectedly large amount of bone after the first year of treatment is likely to show less of a loss, or even a gain, in the second year. Over a longer period of time (with multiple measurements), the extremes will be less deviant from the mean because some of the errors of repeated measurements will smooth the results. Consequently, it is quite difficult to predict the change in year 2 based on the results of year 1. However, those subjects who showed a large increase in BMD in the first year are still likely to show a net gain over 2 years that is larger than the average gain of the group, despite a loss or reduced gain in year 2. This effect demonstrates the difficulty of interpreting data on changes in BMD over a short time period and with a limited number of repeat measurements.

BMD changes versus changes in fracture risk

So far, we have discussed only the ability of bone densitometry techniques to assess a change in BMD. Perhaps even more important is their ability to monitor the effect of treatment on fracture risk. Recent studies using a variety of different anti-resorptive agents have more or less consistently found that the fracture rate can be reduced by about 50% (the range around this mean depends on the severity of fracture status and, to a lesser extent, on the type of treatment).[47] However, the change in BMD (compared with placebo) ranged from virtually zero to an annual increase of more than 4%.[48] This demonstrates that the beneficial effect of these treatments with regard to reducing the risk to fracture cannot be completely explained by the increase induced in the BMD. In fact, only about one-third of the effect can be thus explained (Figure 8.4). A possible explanation is that the small amount of bone that is added in response to treatment is formed in the weaker parts of the trabecular network or the cortex, thus producing a disproportionately large effect on bone strength.

While this highlights some limitations of BMD as a surrogate marker of bone strength in a treatment setting, it does not mean that the change in BMD is not important in achieving a reduction in fracture risk. Nor should it lead to the conclusion that it is not important to monitor the changes in BMD when assessing the efficacy of treatment. It has been shown that those subjects who gain less than average under treatment will also show a smaller than expected beneficial effect in reducing fracture incidence.[43] Thus, while the relationship of BMD to fracture risk may be weaker during treatment compared with bone loss in untreated primary osteoporosis, there is still a relevant relationship that can be used to identify non-responders, albeit over a relatively long time period of 1 or more years.

SUMMARY

Bone densitometry is a mature technology that is indispensable in the assessment of osteoporosis. In the areas of diagnosis, fracture risk assessment, the identification of subjects to treat and the monitoring of treatment, bone densitometry can provide valuable information not attainable by other diagnostic approaches. Both the technique-specific and the generic strengths and limitations of bone densitometry approaches need to be recognized. If used appropriately by trained responsible operators and physicians, and if a rigorous quality assurance programme is implemented, an accurate and precise assessment of bone mass can be achieved, providing the single most important component for assessing skeletal status in osteoporosis. Further research is warranted to investigate the ability of other technologies to provide information on bone structure and quality in order to further improve diagnosis, risk assessment and monitoring. Specifically, the development of better surrogate markers for bone strength in subjects undergoing treatment warrants further investigation.

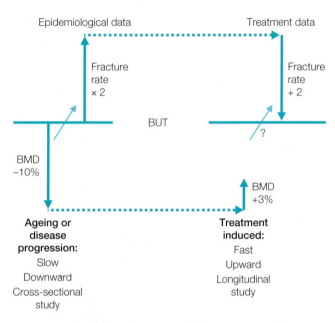

Figure 8.4. Relationship of bone mineral density (BMD) to fracture risk. Epidemiological data show that a reduction in BMD of 10% (which is close to one standard deviation of the population variance for dual X-ray absorptiometry and would occur over a time period of 5–10 years) is associated with a doubling in fracture risk. However, it only takes an increase of perhaps about 3% (varying, depending on the type of treatment, from close to zero to 6%, which can be achieved in about 1–2 years) to reduce the risk of fracture by 50%. Thus, the fracture risk is back to the initial level, whereas the BMD is still substantially reduced.

PRACTICE POINTS

Strengths of bone densitometry

- BMD is a valid surrogate marker of bone strength. Biomechanical studies have shown that BMD explains up to 80% of bone strength, and fracture risk increases by 1.5–2.5 per standard deviation decrease in BMD.

- Bone densitometry techniques are accurate and precise. The accuracy error for assessing bone mineral content is in the range of ±5%, and the (standardized) long-term precision error is about 1–2%.

- The ability to predict fractures is similar or stronger when compared with other well-accepted risk factors for other disorders.

- BMD enables the identification of subjects that are likely to benefit most from treatment. A lower BMD level indicates the highest fracture risk and the largest probability of benefiting from anti-resorptive treatment.

- There is potential for the early prediction of fracture risk: long-term studies have shown a predictive power over longer than 15 years.

- BMD results cannot be replaced by clinical risk factors: both affect fracture risk independently.

- Bone densitometry is a mature technology. The results for spinal and femoral measurements have been standardized across different manufacturers, and a consensus on normative data has been reached. Quality assurance measures have been developed and validated in multicentre studies.

- Radiation exposure is minimal. DXA assessments expose patients to a radiation dose lower by a factor of 1000 than the annual natural radiation exposure.

- The cost of diagnosis is substantially smaller than the cost of treatment. Appropriately performed bone densitometry can thus avoid misguided therapy decisions at a reasonable cost level.

- Despite technical limitations, the quantitative nature of bone densitometry makes it less susceptible to misuse compared with, for example, the subjective assessment of clinical risk factors: no consistent set of risk factors could be identified across various large epidemiological studies that showed a consistent relationship between BMD and fracture risk.

Caveats and limitations

- The WHO definition of osteoporosis is only appropriate for DXA assessments in women. It should perhaps be limited to DXA of the proximal femur, and further research is required to confirm its validity for the assessment of osteoporosis in men.

- There is no evidence for a fracture threshold. The relationship between BMD and fracture incidence is represented by an exponential gradient of risk and is further diluted by accuracy errors. There may, however, be a BMD cut-off level below which it is very difficult to re-establish a strong trabecular network using current therapy options.

- The WHO definition reflects only a diagnostic criterion rather than a criterion for therapy, and it should only be applied in conjunction with other (differential) diagnostic approaches.

- Precision errors are meaningless on their own. Only when they are interpreted in the light of the typical response rate in the subject group investigated can the ability of a technique to monitor skeletal change be judged. QUS approaches, for example, have a precision error level for SOS measurements that is far below the 1% level without reaching the longitudinal sensitivity of postero-anterior DXA of the spine.

- Fundamental as well as technological differences between different bone densitometry approaches should be recognized. A similar performance cannot be assumed for methods that assess cortical instead of cancellous bone, peripheral sites instead of central sites, volumetric instead of areal BMD or ultrasound instead of X-ray interaction. The small magnitude of changes in bone imposes a high demand on the technological performance of bone densitometry.

- Rigorous quality assurance measures that include the appropriate training of the operator and physician, as well as the technical monitoring and maintenance of the equipment, are required to achieve the level of performance described in this chapter.[49,50] Therefore, great emphasis has to be put on the rigorous implementation of quality control procedures and standardized, internationally harmonized training and perhaps even certification.

RESEARCH AGENDA

Further assessment is needed of:

- The role of quantitative ultrasound in assessing bone structure, diagnosing osteoporosis and monitoring treatment.

- Clinical utility of digital X-ray radiogrammetry.

- Areal bone mineral density measurements versus volumetric measures of bone mineral density as predictors of fracture risk.

- Role of bone microarchitecture in bone strength and methods to assess it.

- Relative strengths and interactions of risk factors for osteoporosis and fracture in different populations.

- Ways of predicting absolute 10-year risk versus relative lifetime risk of fracture.

- Cost-effectiveness analysis of case-finding strategies in different populations.

REFERENCES

1. Genant HK, Guglielmi G & Jergas M. *Bone Densitometry and Osteoporosis*. Berlin: Springer, 1998.

2. Marshall D, Johnell O & Wedel H. Meta-analysis of how well measures on bone mineral density predict occurrence of osteoporotic fractures. *BMJ* 1996; **312**: 1254–1259.

3. Genant HK, Engelke K, Fuerst T et al. Noninvasive assessment of bone mineral and structure: state of the art. *J Bone Miner Res* 1996; **11**: 707–730.

4. Blake GM, Wahner HW, Lang TF et al. *The Evaluation of Osteoporosis: Dual X-ray Absorptiometry and Ultrasound in Clinical Practice*. London: Martin Dunitz, 1999.

5. Guglielmi G et al. Quantitative computed tomography at the axial skeleton. In: Genant HK, Guglielmi G & Jergas M, eds. *Bone Densitometry and Osteoporosis*. Berlin: Springer, 1998; 335–347.

6. Kalender WA. Effective dose values in bone mineral measurements by photon absorptiometry and computed tomography. *Osteoporosis Int* 1992; **2**: 82–87.

7. Rüegsegger P, Elsasser U, Anliker M et al. A quantification of bone mineralization using computed tomography. *Radiology* 1976; **121**: 93–97.

8. Schneider P & Reiners C. Peripheral quantitative computed tomography. In: Genant HK, Guglielmi G & Jergas M, eds. *Bone Densitometry and Osteoporosis*. Berlin: Springer, 1998; 349–363.

9. Feretti JL. Perspectives of pQCT technology associated to biomechanical studies in skeletal research employing rat models. *Bone* 1995; **17**: 353–364.

10. Glüer CC & the International Quantitative Ultrasound Consensus Group. Quantitative ultrasound techniques for the assessment of osteoporosis: expert agreement on current status. *J Bone Miner Res* 1997; **12**: 1280–1288.

11. Njeh CF, Boivin CM & Langton CM. The role of ultrasound in the assessment of osteoporosis: a review. *Osteoporosis Int* 1997; **7**: 7–22.

12. Barkmann R, Heller M & Glüer CC. Methoden der in vivo-Ultraschallmesstechnik am Skelett: Grundlagen und technische Realisierung. *J Mineralstoff* 1999; **6**: 22–27.

13. Glüer CC, Wu CY, Jergas M et al. Three quantitative ultrasound parameters reflect bone structure. *Calcif Tissue Int* 1994; **55**: 46–52.

14. Rosholm A, Hyldstrup L, Baelesgaard L et al. BDM from digital X-ray radiogrammetry: correlation to DEXA and in vivo reproducibility. *J Bone Miner Res* 1999; **14**(Suppl. 1): S368.

15. Huang C, Ross PD, Yates AJ et al. Prediction of fracture risk by radiographic absorptiometry and quantitative ultrasound: a prospective study. *Calcif Tissue Int* 1998; **63**: 380–384.

16. Durand EP & Rüegsegger P. High-contrast resolution of CT images for bone structure analysis. *Med Phys* 1992; **19**: 569–573.

17. Majumdar S, Genant HK, Grampp S et al. Correlation of trabecular bone structure with age, bone mineral density, and osteoporotic status: in vivo studies in the distal radius using high resolution magnetic resonance imaging. *J Bone Miner Res* 1997; **12**: 111–118.

18. Anonymous. Consensus Development Conference: diagnosis, prophylaxis, and treatment of osteoporosis. *Am J Med* 1993; **94**: 646–650.

19. Heuck A, Block J, Glüer CC et al. Mild versus definite osteoporosis: comparison of bone densitometry techniques using different statistical models. *J Bone Miner Res* 1989; **4**(6): 891–900.

20. Yu W, Glüer CC, Grampp S et al. Spinal bone mineral assessment in postmenopausal women: a comparison between dual X-ray absorptiometry and quantitative computed tomography. *Osteoporosis Int* 1995; **5**: 433–439.

21. Schönau E, Wentzlik U, Michalk D et al. Is there an increase of bone density in children? [letter]. *Lancet* 1993; **342**: 689–690.

22. Gilsanz V, Boechat MI, Roe TF et al. Gender differences in vertebral body sizes in children and adolescents. *Radiology* 1994; **190**: 673–677.

23. Odgaard A. Three-dimensional methods for quantification of cancellous bone architecture. *Bone* 1997; **20**: 315–328.

24. Kleerekoper M, Villanueva AA, Stancin J et al. The role of three-dimensional trabecular microstructure in the pathogenesis of vertebral compression fractures. *Calcif Tissue Int* 1998; **37**: 594–597.

25. Goldstein SA, Goulet R & McCubbrey D. Measurement and significance of three-dimensional architecture in the mechanical integrity of trabecular bone. *Calcif Tissue Int* 1993; **53**: 127–133.

26. Faulkner KG, McClung M & Cummings SR. Automated evaluation of hip axis length for predicting hip fracture. *J Bone Miner Res* 1997; **9**: 1065–1070.

27. Glüer CC, Cummings SR, Pressman A et al. Prediction of hip fractures from pelvic radiographs: the study of osteoporotic fractures. *J Bone Miner Res* 1994; **9**: 671–677.

28. Bouxsein ML & Augat P. Biomechanics of bone. In: Njeh CF, Hans D, Fuerst T et al., eds. *Quantitative Ultrasound: Assessment of Osteoporosis and Bone Status*. London: Martin Dunitz, 1999; 21–46.

29. Grampp S, Genant HK, Mathur A et al. Comparisons of noninvasive bone mineral measurements in assessing age-related loss, fracture discrimination, and diagnostic classification. *J Bone Miner Res* 1997; **12**: 697–711.

30. Yu W, Glüer CC, Fuerst T et al. Influence of degenerative joint disease on spinal bone mineral measurements in post menopausal women. *Calcif Tissue Int* 1995; **57**: 169–174.

31. Svendsen OL, Hassager C, Skødt V et al. Impact of soft tissue on in vivo accuracy of bone mineral measurements in the spine, hip and forearm: a human cadaver study. *J Bone Miner Res* 1995; **10**: 868–873.

32. Meunier PJ, ed. *Osteoporosis: Diagnosis and Management*. London: Martin Dunitz, 1998.

33. Kanis JA, for the WHO Study Group. Assessment of fracture risk and its application to screening for postmenopausal osteoporosis: synopsis of a WHO report. *Osteoporosis Int* 1994; **4**: 368–381.

34. Kanis J & Glüer CC, for the Committee of Scientific Advisors of the IOF. An update on the diagnosis and assessment of osteoporosis with densitometry. *Osteoporosis Int* 2000; **11**: 192–202.

35. Greenspan SL, Maitland-Ramsey L & Myers E. Classification of osteoporosis in the elderly is dependent on site-specific analysis. *Calcif Tissue Int* 1998; **58**: 409–414.

36. Jergas M & Genant HK. Contributions of bone mass measurements by densitometry in the definition and diagnosis of osteoporosis. In: Meunier PJ, ed. *Osteoporosis: Diagnosis and Management*. London: Martin Dunitz, 1998; 37–57.

37. Wasnich RD. Does current bone mass predict future fractures? In: Christiansen C & Overgaard K, eds. *Osteoporosis*. Copenhagen: Osteopress, 1990; 442–445.

38. Ross PD, Heilbrun LK, Wasnich RD et al. Perspectives: methodologic issues evaluating risk factors for osteoporotic fractures. *J Bone Miner Res* 1989; **4**: 649–656.

39. Gaerdsell P, Johnell O & Nilsson BE. The predictive value of bone loss for fragility fractures in women: a longitudinal study over 15 years. *Calcif Tissue Int* 1991; **49**: 90–94.

40. National Osteoporosis Foundation. Analysis of the cost-effectiveness and cost of screening and treatment strategies for osteoporosis: a basis for development of practice guidelines. *Osteoporosis Int* 1998; **8**(Suppl. 4): 1–88.

41. Ross PD, Genant HK, Davis JW et al. Predicting vertebral fracture incidence from prevalent fractures and bone density among non-black, osteoporotic women. *Osteoporosis Int* 1993; **3**: 120–126.

42. Garnero P & Delmas PD. Clinical usefulness of markers of bone remodeling in osteoporosis. In: Meunier PJ, ed. *Osteoporosis: Diagnosis and Management*. London: Martin Dunitz, 1998; 79–101.

43. Hochberg MC, Ross PD, Black D et al. Larger increases in bone mineral density during alendronate therapy are associated with a lower risk of new vertebral fractures in women with postmenopausal osteoporosis. Fracture Intervention Trial Research Group. *Arthritis Rheum* 1999; **42**: 1246–1254.

44. Cummings SR, Black DM, Thompson DE et al. Effect of alendronate on risk of fracture in women with low bone density but without vertebral fractures: results from the Fracture Intervention Trial [see comments]. *JAMA* 1998; **280**: 2077–2082.

45. Glüer CC. Monitoring skeletal changes by radiological techniques. *J Bone Miner Res* 1999; **14**: 1952–1962.

46. Cummings SR, Palermo L, Browner W et al. Monitoring osteoporosis therapy with bone densitometry: misleading changes and regression to the mean. Fracture Intervention Trial Research Group [in process citation]. *JAMA* 2000; **283**: 1318–1321.

47. Eastell R. Treatment of postmenopausal osteoporosis [see comments]. *N Engl J Med* 1998; **338**: 736–746.

48. Black DM, Cummings SR, Karpf DB et al. Randomised trial of effect of alendronate on risk of fracture in women with existing vertebral fractures. *Lancet* 1996; **348**: 1535–1541.

49. Glüer CC, Faulkner KG, Estilo MJ et al. Quality assurance for bone densitometry research studies: concept and impact. *Osteoporosis Int* 1993; **3**: 227–235.

50. Faulkner KG & McClung MR. Quality control of DXA instruments in multicenter trials. *Osteoporosis Int* 1995; **5**: 218–227.

Chapter 9
Role of biochemical markers in the management of osteoporosis

Peter R. Ebeling and Kristina Åkesson

INTRODUCTION

Osteoporosis is one of the most common and serious diseases of the musculoskeletal system. The lifetime fracture risk of a female aged 60 years is 56%, compared with 29% in a man of the same age. As a result of fragility fractures, the individual experiences pain, decreased mobility and a reduced quality of life. The onset of the disease is silent and insidious, with the diagnosis often only being made after there is irreversible damage resulting from a fragility fracture. Thus, it would be highly desirable to develop sensitive and reliable methods for the early diagnosis and monitoring of treatment for this debilitating disease. The effective monitoring of treatment efficacy might also aid in long-term compliance with anti-osteoporotic therapy.

Advances in bone biochemistry and physiology have provided important insights into the pathogenesis of osteoporosis. Both post-menopausal and age-related bone loss are due to increased bone turnover, with a relative imbalance between bone formation and bone resorption, favouring the latter. The goal of the majority of the currently available treatments for osteoporosis is to normalize the increased bone turnover and to stabilize or increase bone mineral density (BMD), reducing the risk of subsequent fragility fractures.

Early biochemical changes in osteoporosis include the increased release of bone collagen degradation products by the action of osteoclasts and also the increased production of molecules released from either osteoblasts or by the bone matrix. The rate of release of these products of bone cells or their actions indicates abnormalities of bone and mineral metabolism. Biochemical assays for these molecules may be used to detect increased bone turnover and to monitor treatment efficacy. A number of biochemical assays readily detect these molecules released from the bone matrix and bone collagen degradation in both serum and urine. Several of these biochemical markers of bone turnover have the potential to serve as both aids in the decision to treat patients with low bone density and as effective and early indicators of the response to anti-osteoporotic therapy.

In this chapter, we will discuss the potential utility of biochemical markers of bone turnover in the management of patients with osteoporosis. To facilitate the understanding of the rationale and the value of biochemical bone turnover markers in osteoporosis management, a summary of the biochemistry of bone turnover and the markers currently available will be included.

BIOCHEMICAL CONSIDERATIONS IN OSTEOPOROSIS

Previously, the only way to accurately assess bone turnover was by bone histomorphometry following double labelling using tetracycline.[1,2] However, this technique is invasive and expensive and may not reflect bone turnover rates at other skeletal sites. Nevertheless, it does provide information regarding static and dynamic rates of bone formation and bone resorption, and the percentage of the bone undergoing active bone formation and bone resorption. Using this technique, the overall normal skeletal bone turnover rate is relatively low and estimated to be about 10% per year, on average, with a higher rate in trabecular bone (15–20% per year) and a lower rate in cortical bone (3–5% per year).[3] Bone tissue is very vascular and susceptible to systemic regulation by factors that include hormones. Bone remodelling is activated by factors such as parathyroid hormone (PTH), 1,25-dihydroxyvitamin D, growth factors, cytokines, mechanical loading and bone micro-trauma.

Bone resorption relies on osteoclasts creating a suitable environment by locally increasing the acidity of the bone surface as well as secreting proteinases. Calcium and phosphorus are liberated during the process, and the osteoclasts continue to digest bone type I collagen (Figure 9.1), which is released as a series of peptides that can be measured in the serum and urine to quantify the bone resorption rate of the entire skeleton. Similarly, new bone formation leads to the production of collagen cleavage products and other bone matrix proteins that are released during different stages of osteoblast differentiation (Figure 9.2).

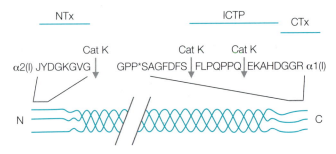

Figure 9.1. The cathepsin K (Cat K) proteolytic sites and bone marker epitopes at the N- and C-termini of type I bone collagen. NTx, N-telopeptide cross-links; CTx, C-telopeptide cross-links; ICTP, pyridinoline cross-linked carboxy-terminal telopeptide of type I collagen. Reproduced with permission from: Nishi Y et al. *J Bone Miner Res* 1999; **14**(11): 1902–1908.[19]

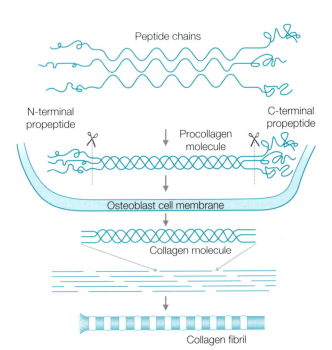

Figure 9.2. Schematic illustration of collagen formation.

METABOLISM OF TYPE I COLLAGEN IN BONE

Type I collagen is formed in bone from the combination of two α-1 and one α-2 collagen polypeptides containing hydroxylated proline and lysine residues. This structure is known as procollagen. As procollagen is secreted from the osteoblast, the amino-terminal and carboxy-terminal regions are cleaved. These propeptides are released into the extracellular fluid,

although a proportion of the amino-terminal propeptide is also incorporated into bone. Type I collagen is helical and the non-helical domains at the amino- and carboxy-termini are known as the N-telopeptide and the C-telopeptide regions.

The side chains of three hydroxylysine residues from different type I collagen molecules condense to form a pyridinium ring so that pyridinium cross-links are formed connecting three different collagen molecules and stabilizing the structure of type I collagen. Pyridinoline cross-links result from the combination of three hydroxylysine side chains (hydroxylysylpyridinoline),[4] while deoxypyridinoline cross-links result from the combination of two hydroxylysine side chains with one lysine side chain (lysylpyridinoline).[5]

The pyridinium cross-link in the N-telopeptide region (NTx) joins α-1 type I collagen polypeptides to α-2 type I collagen polypeptides.[6] By contrast, pyridinium cross-links in other tissues join α-1 type I collagen polypeptides to α-1 type I collagen polypeptides (e.g. C-telopeptide). This makes the N-telopeptide relatively bone-specific. In addition, two-thirds of deoxypyridinoline cross-links in bone type I collagen are N-telopeptide cross-links and only one-third are C-telopeptide cross-links. Assuming that bone turnover under normal circumstances remains at a fairly steady state, products released during bone resorption could be used as markers for the catabolic events. Similarly, during the anabolic phase osteoblasts are actively producing collagen and other proteins to be incorporated in the newly synthesized matrix. Surplus products or fragments released into serum may then be used as markers of bone formation. In disease states, alterations of marker levels should preferably provide insight into the metabolic disturbances in a particular bone disorder.

In the following section, each one of the potentially useful markers for bone will be separately reviewed (Table 9.1) and the current utility of these bone markers in osteoporosis management will be discussed.

BONE FORMATION MARKERS

The predominant product of osteoblasts is type I collagen, which comprises 95% of the extracellular non-mineral bone matrix. Other proteins such as osteopontin, osteonectin and osteocalcin are also secreted to form the osteoid or organic substrate in which mineralization occurs. Osteoblasts stain positively for the enzyme alkaline phosphatase, which is attached to their cell membranes. This alkaline phosphatase is functionally similar but antigenically different to hepatic, intestinal or placental alkaline phosphatases.[7]

Osteocalcin

Osteocalcin is one of the most abundant non-collagenous proteins of bone matrix, synthesized by osteoblasts.[8] The serum concentration of osteocalcin reflects the rate of osteoblast synthesis of osteocalcin. However, only approximately 50% of newly synthesized osteocalcin is released into the circulation, while the remaining 50% is incorporated into hydroxyapatite.

Table 9.1. Potential biochemical markers of bone turnover in osteoporosis.

Bone formation	Bone resorption

Serum
    Osteocalcin
    Bone-specific alkaline phosphatase
    Procollagen type I C-/N-extension peptide
    (PICP, PINP)
	Serum
	    Pyridinoline cross-linking telopeptides
	    (C- and N-telopeptides, CTx, NTx, ICTP)
	    Free pyridinoline and deoxypyridinoline
	    Tartrate-resistant acid phosphatase
	    Bone sialoprotein
	
	Urine
	    Pyridinoline cross-links:
	        Pyridinoline
	        Deoxypyridinoline
	        Pyridinoline cross-linking telopeptides
	        (C- and N-telopeptides, CTx, NTx)

Osteocalcin is regarded as bone-specific, since the small amount present in dentine is negligible, but its precise function remains unknown. Osteocalcin contains three γ-carboxylated glutamic acid residues and the degree of carboxylation (i.e. number of residues carboxylated) seems to influence mineralization. Osteocalcin in serum is susceptible to rapid enzymatic cleavage and, subsequently, both intact and fragmented osteocalcin, including a large N-mid-molecular fragment, are detectable in serum at any given time. In addition, this degradation occurs most rapidly at room temperature, which means that specimens should be frozen as soon as possible after collection. For these reasons, assays providing a combined measure of intact and N-mid-fragment are more robust and may improve the sensitivity of the assay; furthermore, novel assays relying on different osteocalcin fragments may provide additional information.[9,10]

Serum bone alkaline phosphatase

The skeletal isoform of alkaline phosphatase (ALP) is a membrane-bound protein with enzymatic activity. Despite this, its release mechanism from osteoblasts remains to be elucidated. However, ALP plays an important role in bone mineralization. Serum ALP exists in several isomeric forms depending on its tissue origin. In children and adolescents, up to 80% of ALP measurable in serum is derived from bone, mirroring bone growth. In adults, only about 50% is bone-derived, while the remainder mostly emanates from liver tissue. Recently developed immunoradiometric or enzyme immunoassays have facilitated the determination of serum levels of bone ALP.[11] Despite a residual and significant cross-reactivity with the liver isoenzyme, bone ALP provides a higher specificity for bone than the other bone formation markers.

Carboxy-terminal propeptide of type I procollagen

During the synthesis of type I collagen by the osteoblasts, the amino- (N-) and carboxy- (C-) terminal extension propeptides are cleaved. The intact terminal fragment is released into the circulation in its entirety prior to extracellular fibril formation.[12]

The serum concentration of the carboxy-terminal propeptide of type I collagen (PICP) reflects changes in the synthesis of new collagen, both by osteoblasts in bone and by fibroblasts in other connective tissues.[13] Theoretically, utilization of the propeptides as markers of bone formation is appealing, since their synthesis should be directly proportional to the amount of type I collagen produced. However, PICP appears to lack sensitivity for identifying subtle alterations in bone turnover.[14]

Amino-terminal propeptide of type I procollagen

The serum concentration of the amino-terminal propeptide of type I collagen (PINP) also reflects changes in the synthesis of new collagen, both by osteoblasts in bone and by fibroblasts in other connective tissues.[15,16] However, unlike PICP, a proportion is also incorporated into bone as non-dialysable hydroxyproline and thus a component of the measured fragments might represent bone resorption. Nevertheless, PINP appears to be a more dynamic and sensitive marker of changes in bone formation than PICP, but there has been less clinical evaluation of PINP. Early changes in PINP and PICP have recently been shown to be the best predictors of spinal BMD increases with teriparatide therapy.[17]

BONE RESORPTION MARKERS

Bone resorption is initiated by osteoclasts, which contain acid phosphatase.[1] Although acid phosphatase activity is present in other tissues such as the prostate gland and blood cells, the type 5b enzyme is specific to osteoclasts. Osteoclasts attach to the bone surface and secrete acid and hydrolytic enzymes that resorb bone, releasing bone minerals and collagen fragments. The N-telopeptide epitope is preferentially liberated from type I collagen in bone by osteoclastic hydrolysis with cathepsin K.[18] Cathepsin K is located in osteoclast intracellular vacuoles and in the subosteoclastic space. Within type I collagen telopeptide domains there are three proteolytic sites for cathepsin K. In addition, both serum NTx and C-telopeptide cross-link (CTx) concentrations are reduced in pycnodyostosis, a disorder of reduced cathepsin K activity, while serum pyridinoline cross-linked carboxyterminal telopeptide of type I collagen (ICTP) levels and urine free deoxypyridinoline (Dpd) excretion are elevated in this disorder.[19] This interesting observation has been further clarified and distinct enzymatic pathways have been described, with metalloproteinases involved in the ICTP collagenolytic pathway.[20]

N-telopeptide cross-links may be degraded further in the liver and kidney in particular, where free Dpd may be generated. Serum NTx concentrations are elevated in chronic renal failure. Some of the collagen is completely digested by osteoclasts to its smallest units, free pyridinoline and Dpd residues, which are excreted in the urine. The majority, however, appears to be incompletely digested, resulting in the formation of pyridinium cross-links bound to fragments of the NTx α-1 and α-2 polypeptides; peptide-bound cross-links are also excreted in the urine.[6,21]

Hydroxypyridinium cross-links

Urinary excretion of the hydroxypyridinium cross-links of type I collagen reflects osteoclastic bone resorption, and not dietary calcium or collagen intake. Thus, it is a more precise indicator of bone resorption than urinary calcium or hydroxyproline excretion. The distribution of hydroxypyridinium cross-links varies depending on tissue type; pyridinoline is primarily present in cartilage, but also in bone collagen, while Dpd is predominantly found in bone and dentine.[5,22] Theoretically, Dpd is the preferred marker of bone resorption and it correlates positively with other indices of bone resorption, and inversely with bone mass in osteoporosis.[23] Although Dpd is also found in relatively high concentrations in vascular tissue (such as the aorta) and in skeletal muscle, the metabolic turnover rate of these tissues is far lower than that of bone. As a result these tissues contribute little to the circulating pool of Dpd. Free Dpd can be measured in the urine or serum.

Peptide-bound N-telopeptide and C-telopeptide cross-link assays

Recently, the cross-linking telopeptide regions, C-telopeptide to helix and N-telopeptide to helix, have emerged as potential markers of bone resorption, measurable either in serum or urine by immunoassays. These particular markers have been widely employed in studies of osteoporosis, including therapeutic trials, and are currently considered to be the preferred markers of bone resorption because of their convenience and dynamic response to therapeutic intervention. Peptide-bound NTx can be measured in the urine by an immunoassay[6] and CTx can be measured in serum by two immunoassays.[24,25] Only the β-isomer of the CTx is measured in the serum assays, while both the α- and β-isomers of CTx are measured in the urine assay. The serum CTx assays are affected by the non-fasting state, whereas the urine assay is not. The CTx immunoassay does not measure cross-links, but measures a sequence (octapeptide) of the C-telopeptide region of the α-1 chain of type I collagen in the urine.[25] The NTx immunoassay has also been automated and modified to measure the same epitope in serum.

Bone sialoprotein

Bone sialoprotein (BSP) is a phosphorylated glycoprotein, containing sialic acid, which has cell adhesive properties. Bone sialoprotein is specific for bone and it is enriched in the immediate subchondral bone. Serum BSP is increased in states of high bone turnover and correlates well with other bone resorption markers.[26]

Tartrate-resistant acid phosphatase

Osteoclasts produce acid to dissolve the mineral phase of bone and various enzymes to degrade the matrix. Tartrate-resistant acid phosphatase (TRAP) is produced by osteoclasts during bone resorption and the type 5b isoform has been identified as a potential marker of osteoclast activity through recently developed assays using two-site monoclonal antibodies.[27] It may provide different information from the pyridium cross-links that measure osteoclast action, rather than cellular activity of osteoclasts.

VALIDATION AND LIMITATIONS IN THE USE OF BIOCHEMICAL BONE MARKERS

Three major criteria need to be satisfied before a biochemical test can be established as a biological marker of bone turnover. Firstly, the marker must change in parallel with changes in bone turnover measured by bone histomorphometry or calcium kinetics.[2] Secondly, the serum concentration or urinary excretion of the substance must be high in conditions characterized by high bone turnover, such as Paget's disease of bone. Finally, the serum concentration or urinary excretion of the substance must be low in conditions characterized by low bone turnover, e.g. after the administration of anti-resorptive drugs.

In the early phase of bone marker development, high analytical variability was a major problem. Improved analytical techniques, from high-pressure liquid chromatography (HPLC) to fully automated immunoassays and the addition of serum versus urine assays, have substantially diminished these problems. However, a continuing major concern limiting their wider clinical use relates instead to the relatively high intra-individual variability. This biological variability, together with the residual analytical variability, limits the interpretation of results for the individual patient both at baseline and during monitoring of treatment. The intra-individual variation is related to factors that can at large be categorized as either non-modifiable or potentially modifiable or controllable. Factors that are non-modifiable include age, with high values during childhood and growth and high values again after the menopause in women. The larger skeleton of men may increase bone marker variability. Biological variability is also increased in women with postmenopausal osteoporosis.

Fractures also confound the interpretation of biochemical bone turnover marker results. Hip and other peripheral fractures cause a rapid increase in bone turnover that can last for up to a year.[28–30] The impact of vertebral fractures on bone turnover is uncertain, but could be considerable given the generally higher turnover of trabecular bone. Physical inactivity or immobility because of fracture, illness or for other reasons also lead to rapid increases in bone resorption as seen in studies of bed rest;[31] however, physical activity prior to sampling may also influence the results.[32–34]

In addition, bone turnover is subject to a circadian variability, with peak values in the early morning and with a nadir in the early afternoon and evening.[35] Moreover, the degree of variation is not uniform for all markers, but is most pronounced for serum bone resorption markers, i.e. CTx, reaching 20–50% depending on the time of day. To this the intra-individual day-to-day variability should be added. Seasonal changes with increased bone resorption have also been described, with a corresponding pattern of PTH with an inverse curve for 25-hydroxyvitamin D.[36,37] The seasonal interference may be greater in Northern latitudes with fewer hours of daylight and sun exposure during winter. Although previously it was believed only hydroxyproline was influenced by diet, it has been shown that the combined effect of time of day and diet may also signifi-

cantly influence other biochemical markers, particularly serum beta-CTx.[38] In general bone resorption markers, including serum beta-CTx, decrease more than bone formation markers after an oral nutrient load. Pancreatic and enteric hormones may regulate the responses of bone turnover markers to nutrients[39] (Figure 9.3).

In order to minimize these fluctuations, the timing of sample collection is critical and should be similar for each patient and at each time point. Urine samples for measurements of bone turnover markers can be collected either as random, non-fasting, 2-h post-voiding or as 24-h urine collections. The results in 2-h early morning post-voiding samples correlate well with those in 24-h samples and rates of bone loss correlate with 2-h urinary Dpd values better than with values from 24-h urine collections.[40] Short-term variability of 2-h post-voiding cross-link excretion (9–13%) is less than that of 24-h collections (26%), but differences in long-term variability may be lower. Similarly, awareness of collection times needs to be taken regarding serum assays since, for example, both serum NTx and CTx may be more sensitive to diurnal variation than urine assays. When ordering these tests through a local laboratory, it is important that samples are collected according to their instructions so that results can be compared with the normal reference ranges established by that laboratory. Exposure of the sample to ultraviolet light should be avoided. Standardized curves adjusted for age and sex should also be developed to facilitate and improve the interpretation of the result by the manufacturer. The treating physician needs to be aware of the limitations of bone marker assays to be able to accurately interpret the results.

A

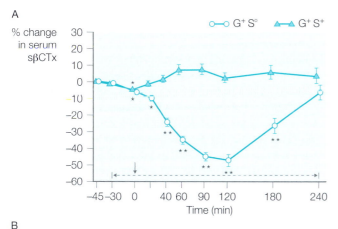

B

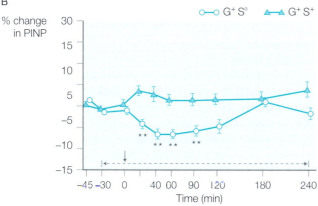

Figure 9.3. Percentage change from baseline for: (A) the bone turnover marker serum β-CTx and (B) PINP to oral glucose (G⁺ S°) and oral glucose with intravenous octreotide (G⁺ S⁺). The horizontal arrows indicate the onset (←: time –30 min) and completion (→: time 240 min) of the octreotide or saline infusion, and the vertical arrow (↓: time 0 min) indicates oral ingestion of either glucose or distilled water. *$P < 0.05$, **$P < 0.01$ comparison with fasting baseline (time –45 to –30 min) after adjustment for multiple comparisons ($n = 8$). Copyright © 2003 The Endocrine Society. Source: Clowes JA, Allen HC, Prentis DM et al. Octreotide abolishes the acute decrease in bone turnover in response to oral glucose. *J Clin Endocrinol Metab* 2003; **88**(10): 4867–4873.[39] Reproduced with permission.

BONE MARKERS IN THE MANAGEMENT OF OSTEOPOROSIS

Biochemical bone turnover markers do not replace dual-energy absorptiometry (DEXA) for the diagnosis of osteoporosis. However, bone markers may give some additional indication about the future risk for bone loss and fractures. They may also be useful in monitoring the efficacy of anti-resorptive therapy in patients with osteoporosis. Biochemical indicators of disease are available in several disease areas. The most successful markers identify patients at risk or in the early stages of disease, thereby enabling the final outcome of the condition to be altered by therapeutic intervention.

Enhancement of prediction of future risk of bone loss

Although advancing age is the strongest predictor for low bone mass and fracture, a patient's current bone mineral density (BMD) is an important predictor of fracture risk.[41] However, a single measurement indicates only current BMD, not the anticipated rate of bone loss. Thus, patients with a BMD value corresponding to osteopoenia may have a greater risk of osteoporosis and fracture if they are losing bone at a rapid rate.

Recent studies have demonstrated that markers of bone turnover may be useful in predicting rates of future bone loss and may therefore provide independent information about fracture risk beyond that available from BMD measurements alone. However, the diagnostic utility of a single bone turnover measurement is limited because individuals with low levels of bone turnover have rates of bone loss that range from 0 to 10%/year;[42] the test therefore has a low specificity. Nevertheless, a person with a high value for a bone turnover marker is generally at greater risk of bone loss than a person with a low value.

In most studies there is a highly significant correlation between bone turnover markers and subsequent rates of bone loss.[43-47] The rate of bone turnover explains up to 50% of the variance in bone mass in 80-year-old women.[23] After the age of 30, women with high bone turnover have bone mass values at the hip, spine or forearm that are 6–11% lower that those of women with a low bone turnover as measured using osteocalcin and CTx.[48] In post-menopausal women the differences in bone mass between those with high versus low turnover were larger (8–14%). In women aged 67 years or more, an increased value for all bone resorption markers was associated with an increased rate of bone loss from the hip after 4 years.[49] In women with a yearly femoral neck bone loss of 85% above average, 56–73% of the resorption marker levels were above the median; however, significant overlap occurred.

Bone markers are not usually adjusted for age, sex, height or weight; thus, the pre-menopausal mean is often used as a reference value. Post-menopausal women with a bone turnover rate that is 2 SD above the pre-menopausal mean lose two to six times more bone in the distal forearm over a 4-year period, depending on the marker chosen.[50] Bone turnover increases at the time of menopause and it has been suggested that some women are more susceptible to metabolic changes related to oestrogen deficiency than others. However, it remains uncertain whether bone markers measured early in the menopause predict post-menopausal bone loss in the individual patient.[47,51]

Taken together, it would seem reasonable to measure BMD at menopause if preventive therapy is being contemplated for women at risk for osteoporosis. If the BMD is in the osteopaenic range, the finding of a urine or serum bone turnover marker that is elevated above the upper limit of normal for pre-menopausal women would add further impetus to the recommendation for preventative therapy.

Bone markers in fracture prediction

Identification of prospective fracture patients is a key goal in osteoporosis. Ideally, the bone marker should predict all types of fracture, or at least major fractures such as hip fracture. Retrospective studies have suggested that there is a difference in bone marker levels between fracture patients and controls. However, because the fracture preceded the bone marker measurement, it is uncertain whether the difference in turnover was caused by the fracture or existed prior to the fracture.[52]

Prospective population-based studies using a nested case–control design, despite a low number of fractures even in large studies, have shown consistent relationships between resorption markers, alone or in combination with BMD, and fracture risk. In the EPIDOS study, urine free Dpd and CTx

independently predicted hip fracture (odds ratio = 1.9–2.5).[53] Their predictive value increased when combined with low bone mass to a more than four-fold fracture risk in these women (odds ratio = 4.1–5.2). In the Rotterdam study, high urinary free Dpd was associated with an increased risk of hip fracture over 4 years. However, the number of women with fractures was low (n = 17), the women were generally more disabled and the marker levels were affected by the subsequent immobility.[54] Women in early menopause with high bone turnover had a doubled risk of sustaining vertebral or peripheral fractures during 15 years of follow-up, compared with women having normal early menopausal bone turnover.[55] In the population-based Malmö OPRA cohort of elderly women followed over almost 5 years, TRAP 5b, serum CTx and osteocalcin fragments were significantly higher in those women prospectively sustaining a fracture. The resorption markers, TRAP 5b and urine osteocalcin, were predictive of vertebral fractures (odds ratio = 2.02–2.25), indicating a doubling of risk independent of BMD[56] (Figure 9.4).

The predictive value of bone markers has been evaluated to a much lesser extent in men; however, in one study ICTP is equally predictive of fracture as BMD in elderly men.[57]

The degree of vitamin K-dependent γ-carboxylation of osteocalcin may affect hydroxyapatite binding and bone mineralization. Because the degree of γ-carboxylation is reduced with ageing,[58] impaired γ-carboxylation may increase the risk of low BMD and fracture. High serum levels of under-carboxylated osteocalcin are associated with an increased risk of hip fracture, independent of BMD, while adding BMD enhanced its predictive ability.[59,60] In a community-based study of women and men over the age of 70, low levels of carboxylated osteocalcin or a low carboxylated-to-total osteocalcin ratio conferred a high risk for any type of fracture, including hip fracture [relative risk = 5.32 (3.26–8.68)]. The relative risk was greatest in persons over 80 years and the increased risk persisted for 3 years out of a 5-year follow-up period.[61]

Increased levels of bone resorption markers and possibly decreased level of carboxylated osteocalcin or osteocalcin fragments have the potential to allow for the estimation of fracture risk, in the elderly, over at least 3–5 years. In combination with BMD measurements, the fracture risk prediction is further strengthened. The fracture risk predictions for other peripheral fractures or vertebral fractures are similar. Therefore, bone markers, particularly bone resorption markers, may have a role in the clinical evaluation of the individual woman with osteoporosis together with other risk factors for fracture, in particular BMD.

Bone markers and monitoring of treatment

Because the skeletal bone turnover rate is low, with less than one-tenth of the skeleton exchanged per year, the impact of alterations in bone turnover, i.e. change in bone mass, is only evident after 1–2 years, at the earliest, using DEXA to measure BMD. Given that the precision of spine DEXA is between 1% and 2%, the smallest change in BMD required for a $P < 0.05$ level of significance would be 2.77–5.54%. In the individual

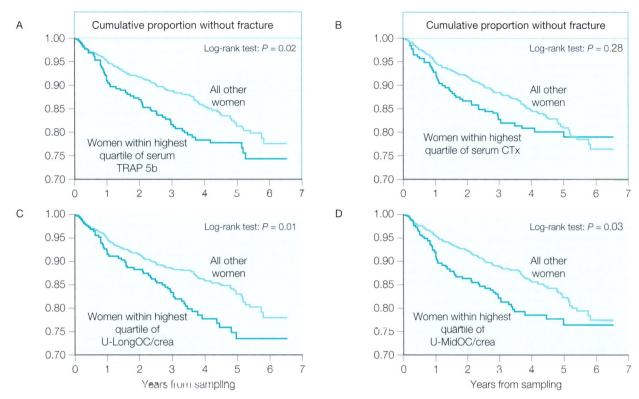

Figure 9.4. Proportion of subjects without any prospective fracture (Kaplan–Meier). Women within the highest quartile of serum TRAP 5b (A), serum CTx (B). Long osteocalcin fragment (U-LongOC/crea; C) or mid-molecular osteocalcin fragment (U-MidOC/crea; D) are compared with all other women. *P* values for log-rank tests are shown. Reproduced with permission from: Gerdhem P et al. *J Bone Miner Res* 2004; **19**(3): 386 – 393.[56]

patient, BMD measurement is a surrogate for assessing the anti-fracture efficacy of currently used anti-osteoporotic drugs. Until recently the majority of fracture-reducing pharmacological interventions have targeted osteoclasts to induce an anti-resorptive effect, whereas bone anabolic agents have been accessible for clinical use only during the past few years.

Anti-resorptive agents are currently regarded as the cornerstones of osteoporosis treatment, with bisphosphonates of varying potency regularly producing significant changes in BMD within this time. For other treatments, such as selective oestrogen receptor-modulating drugs (SERMs) and intranasal calcitonin, the change in bone mass may be borderline for detection in the individual within this timeframe, despite a demonstrated fracture-sparing effect in clinical trials. Bone anabolic agents, on the other hand, specifically parathyroid hormone, produce incremental changes in BMD over short time periods below 2 years.

The evaluation of efficacy of pharmacotherapy and the monitoring of response in the individual patient is of equal importance, particularly within a future perspective of pharmacological intervention involving sequential treatments. The possibilities to conveniently evaluate bone turnover status will provide a basis for decision-making of treatment modification.

Treatment efficacy involves two main factors: biological response or non-response and adherence-related response.

Biological non-response to bisphosphonates is estimated to 10–15%; however, lack of response is more commonly caused by poor adherence to therapy, either from not taking the medication according to instructions or from lacking persistence. Hence, there is a need for a more rapid tool to evaluate the treatment response in the individual patient.

In a clinical setting, an alternative to using BMD measurements alone for assessing early therapeutic efficacy would be to also measure a bone marker. In all clinical trials of anti-osteoporotic drugs, bone markers have been used as intermediate end-points. Bone markers indicate early treatment effects on bone metabolism. A decrease in bone resorption markers occurs within 6 weeks to 3 months after initiation of anti-resorptive therapy, while the nadir in bone formation markers is delayed until 6 months. After this time, bone turnover is stabilized at a lower level. Effects on bone resorption markers have been of greater interest, since the therapeutic agents act on osteoclast number and activity. The effect on bone formation is secondary and related to the coupling effect, which also explains the delayed response. The absolute percentage change from baseline is variable depending on the specific properties of each individual biochemical bone marker. Treatment with bone anabolic agents shows a different pattern, with a rapid increase in bone formation markers and a slightly delayed increase in bone resorption.

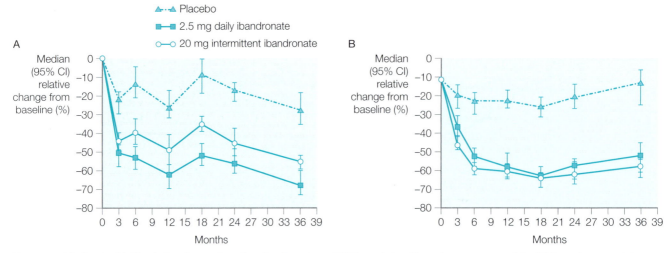

Figure 9.5. Median (95% CI) relative change from baseline for urinary NTX/creatinine (A) and serum osteocalcin (B) in patients receiving placebo, oral daily and oral intermittent ibandronate over 3 years (PP). Reproduced with permission from: Delmas PD et al. *Osteoporosis Int* 2004; **15**(10): 792–798.[70]

Prediction of BMD response

Women with the highest bone turnover appear to derive the greatest benefit from anti-resorptive therapy with alendronate,[62] oestrogen,[46] calcium[46] or calcitonin,[63] while by comparison, women with the baseline urinary N-telopeptide values in the lowest quartile are no less likely to lose bone than those on placebo.[46] Bisphosphonates induce marked, dose-related decreases in bone resorption; alendronate decreases NTx by 50–65% and CTx by 70–75%, risedronate decreases NTx by 30–40% and CTx by 50–55% after 3 months of therapy.[62,64,65] Bone formation is decreased to a lesser extent: BALP by 20–30% and PINP by 40–50%.[65] The decrease in NTx level at 6 months correlates with the change in BMD at 2 years at all sites after alendronate treatment. In addition, the subgroup of women with the largest percentage initial decrease in bone resorption showed the largest gain in bone mass after 2.5 years of treatment. The responsiveness of TRAP 5b, a novel marker of osteoclast proteolytic action, to detect early effects of alendronate has been tested in postmenopausal women.[66] The change in spine BMD at 12 months correlated with the changes in TRAP 5b and CTx at 3 months, indicating that the decrease in direct cellular action in the early phase of treatment is of importance for bone density outcome. Further studies have shown similar correlations between short-term decreases in other bone markers following alendronate treatment and the change in bone mass at 2 years, including NTx.[67,68] By comparison, Dpd decreases by 10–30% during alendronate treatment. Extending the dosing interval to 1 week produces similar decreases in bone turnover, suggesting equivalent anti-resorptive effects.[69]

Because of the specificity for bone and the accumulation in bone tissue, bisphosphonates with still higher potency allow for lengthening of the dosing interval even further, a possibility utilized in the treatment with ibandronate. Despite increasing the dosing interval to more than 2 months, the effect on bone markers was similar to that of daily dosing[70] (Figure 9.5).

Ibandronate may also be administered intravenously every other or every third month. Ibandronate given intravenously rapidly decreased bone turnover, an effect that is, as expected, most pronounced for bone resorption (–90%). However, as early as 2 weeks after administration bone resorption starts to increase and continue to do so until the next drug administration and prior to the second injection, being about –20%.[71] Bone formation (osteocalcin) decreased at a slower rate and the rebound increase was not as prominent.

Selective oestrogen modulators are alternative anti-resorptives and the corresponding changes seen after 6–9 months of raloxifene treatment are a 20–30% and a 30–40% decrease in osteocalcin and CTx respectively.[72] By comparison, calcium supplementation alone decreases bone turnover by 5–15%.

Parathyroid hormone induces large changes in spinal BMD over relatively short time periods of time, but with lower levels of change in hip BMD, and is commonly reserved for those with most pronounced risk of fracture. As expected from the difference in cellular targets, the response pattern in bone turnover is distinctly different from that of anti-resorptive agents. Bone formation increases rapidly and significantly within 6 weeks of treatment using the recommended 20 μg teriparatide dose, whereas bone resorption increases somewhat later, at 3 months, and remains elevated.[17] The early change in bone formation markers correlated with spine BMD at 18 months, a relationship that was stronger than that of the response rate in hip BMD (Figure 9.6).

Strontium ranelate has a different mode of action, with an apparent simultaneous increase in bone formation and decrease in bone resorption, leading to an increase in bone mass and reduction in vertebral and non-vertebral fractures.[73,74] Consequently, a divergent pattern is observed in bone marker response; alkaline phosphatase peaks at 3 months whereas CTx reaches an inverse peak and then each plateaus out until the end of treatment.

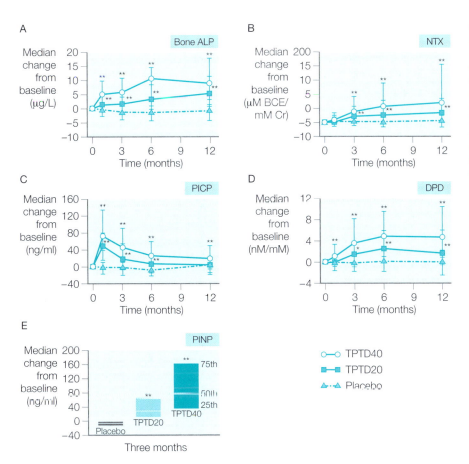

Figure 9.6. Median absolute changes for serum bone ALP (A), urinary NTx (B), serum PICP (C) and urinary free Dpd (D) from baseline at 1, 3, 6 and 12 months. Bars represent the 25th and 75th percentiles. Absolute changes of serum PINP at 3 months are represented in E. The 75th percentile is represented by the top of the bar graph, the median by the white line and the 25th percentile by the bottom of the bar graph. TPTD20, teriparatide, 20 µg/day; TPTD40, teriparatide, 40 µg/day ($*P < 0.05$, $**P < 0.01$ vs. placebo). Reproduced with permission from: Chen P et al. *J Bone Miner Res* 2005; **20**(6): 962–970.[17]

Prediction of anti-fracture efficacy

A number of recent studies have tried to estimate if the change in bone turnover can be translated into a fracture-sparing effect. In a meta-analysis based on randomized controlled trials of anti-resorptive agents, a 70% reduction in bone resorption markers reduced the risk of non-vertebral fractures by 40% and a 50% reduction in bone formation markers reduced the risk by 44%, suggesting that a substantial decrease in bone turnover is necessary to produce a fracture-sparing effect on non-vertebral fractures.[75] Based on the risedronate trial, 3 or 6 months change in bone marker levels, urinary CTx and NTx, were predictive of a reduction in vertebral fracture over 3 years of treatment (75% over 1 year, 50% over 3 years).[76] CTx and NTx accounted for about half (55% and 49%) of the anti-fracture effect. The change in bone markers was also predictive of the reduction in non-vertebral fractures. It was also estimated that the maximum benefit on vertebral fracture risk reduction was obtained, decreases of 55–60% for CTx and 35–40% for NTx, with no benefit from further suppressing bone turnover. When using baseline Dpd as an index of pretreatment bone resorption, elevated pretreatment Dpd (above the young adult mean) was more common in women with vertebral fracture after 12 months.[77] However, pretreatment urine Dpd levels did not predict the BMD response over 3 years. These findings are interesting because bone markers may indicate other properties of bone resistance to fracture,

not mediated through bone density. Similar findings are evident with alendronate treatment using BALP, PINP and CTx.[78] In women treated with raloxifene, the 1-year change in osteocalcin was a better predictor of 3-year decrease in vertebral fracture risk than the 1-year increase in femoral neck BMD.[79]

Response rate and adherence to therapy

The identification of responders versus non-responders to treatment remains problematic. One approach is to calculate the least significant change (LSC) based on the known marker variability. The LSC for bone resorption markers was 46–72% and 30–62% for formation markers in the oestrogen/progestin intervention trial, indicating that large changes in markers are necessary and that predictive values in study populations may include significant overlap in individual values.[80] However, it should be noted that when expressed as the expected change over long-term variability, the predictive power of BMD and biochemical bone markers is similar and with certain treatments even higher than BMD. The fact that bone markers are independently predictive of both fracture and anti-fracture effect during treatment indicates that bone markers are conveying different information on bone quality that is not encompassed by simply measuring BMD. This qualitative property is further emphasized by the knowledge that BMD only explains 4–28% of the reduction in vertebral fracture risk during anti-resorptive treatment.[81]

The question of responders and non-responders is also relevant in the context of adherence. Bone turnover markers are well suited to detecting responders and non-responders due to their rapid rates of change, an advantageous property allowing for early feedback of treatment effect to the patient and thereby enhancing adherence to therapy, which is crucial in obtaining the ultimate fracture reduction. However, it needs to be kept in mind that adherence is most likely influenced by a number of additional factors, with continuous nurse contact being one of the most important, increasing adherence by 57%.[82] Adding a marker may rather serve as a useful secondary indicator of good adherence, since the early change is prognostic of a later increase in BMD.

Based on currently available evidence, it seems likely that bone markers, especially bone resorption markers, can predict the BMD response to treatment for up to 3 years reasonably well. Encouragingly, early changes in bone markers also seem to indicate reduced fracture risk, particularly vertebral fracture risk, for up to 3 years. Further improvements in analytical techniques, including automation, together with careful measures for minimizing sample handling differences, may reduce marker variability and optimize the predictive power of these tests. In addition, this will decrease the cost of each test, which should improve cost-effective assessment of the individual patient. Using bone densitometry it would seem prudent to wait 2 years before changing therapy. It is hoped that by using biochemical bone markers and, in particular, bone resorption markers during anti-resorptive therapy, this decision can be made before further bone is lost. Bone markers will also fill an essential gap in evaluating bone anabolic therapies, which require closer monitoring, especially when anabolic therapy becomes integrated in a sequential treatment plan with anti-resorptive therapy.

SUMMARY

An understanding of the underlying cellular processes of bone turnover in osteoporosis and other bone metabolic diseases has led to the development of biochemical markers of bone resorption and formation that can be measured in the serum and urine. Previously, bone turnover could only be assessed by invasive and expensive bone histomorphometry or nuclear techniques. Regarding osteoporosis, we have reached a stage where there are strong indications that biochemical bone markers, particularly bone resorption markers, may add an independent, predictive value to the assessment of bone loss and fracture risk. There are also potential advantages for monitoring anti-osteoporotic treatment in addition to bone mass measurements – for example, to identify non-responders or non-compliance. Despite the rapid advances in the use of biochemical markers in the assessment of disorders of bone metabolism, including

osteoporosis, bone markers are currently mainly used as very useful research tools. However, their transition into everyday clinical practice is fast approaching, particularly with the advent of more complex treatment regimens requiring closer monitoring in the near future.

PRACTICE POINTS

- Bone markers, in particular high levels of resorption markers, may indicate progressive bone loss and, in addition to bone mass measurement in post-menopausal women, may strengthen the indication for treatment.

- Bone markers, in particular high levels of resorption markers and under-carboxylated osteocalcin, in combination with bone mass measurement, may enhance fracture prediction, particularly in the elderly.

- Changes in bone marker levels may indicate a response to both anti-resorptive and bone anabolic treatment, and in terms of BMD change for up to 3 years.

- Changes in bone marker levels may indicate a prospective treatment-related reduction of vertebral fracture risk over up to 3 years but, because of limitations related to intra-individual variation, bone markers are not yet an established method for evaluating treatment efficacy in the individual patient.

- Changes in bone marker levels is an additional tool in evaluating adherence to therapy in the individual patient.

RESEARCH AGENDA

- Development of tools to enhance the utility of markers in the management of the individual patient, including normality curves for each marker related to age and BMD to facilitate interpretation of values.

- Long-term evaluation (up to 10 years) of the association between bone markers, BMD and fracture, to determine the duration of the predictive ability of bone markers for bone loss and fracture.

- Prospective studies aimed at determining treatment response by bone markers as an intermediate end-point for various treatment modalities in order to assign cut-off levels that would be usable in individual patients.

- Bone markers are at present mainly evaluated in post-menopausal women. Future research needs to further evaluate bone markers in relation to bone loss and fracture in men and in patients with other skeletal disorders.

REFERENCES

1. Calvo MS, Eyre DR & Gundberg CM. Molecular basis and clinical application of biological markers of bone turnover. *Endocr Rev* 1996; **17**(4): 333–368.

2. Parfitt AM, Drezner MK, Glorieux FH et al. Bone histomorphometry: standardization of nomenclature, symbols, and units. Report of the ASBMR Histomorphometry Nomenclature Committee. *J Bone Miner Res* 1987; **2**(6): 595–610.

3. Parfitt AM. The physiological and clinical significance of bone histomorphometric data. In: Recker R, ed. *Bone Histomorphometry. Techniques and Interpretations.* Boca Raton: CRC Press; 1993; 143–223.

4. Horgan DJ, King NL, Kurth LB et al. Collagen crosslinks and their relationship to the thermal properties of calf tendons. *Arch Biochem Biophys* 1990; **281**(1): 21–26.

5. Eyre DR, Koob TJ & Van Ness KP. Quantitation of hydroxypyridinium crosslinks in collagen by high-performance liquid chromatography. *Analyt Biochem* 1984; **137**(2): 380–388.

6. Hanson DA, Weis MA, Bollen AM et al. A specific immunoassay for monitoring human bone resorption: quantitation of type I collagen cross-linked N-telopeptides in urine. *J Bone Miner Res* 1992; **7**(11): 1251–1258.

7. Gomez B Jr, Ardakani S, Ju J et al. Monoclonal antibody assay for measuring bone-specific alkaline phosphatase activity in serum. *Clin Chem* 1995; **41**(11): 1560–1566.

8. Price PA. Vitamin K-dependent formation of bone Gla protein (osteocalcin) and its function. *Vitam Horm* 1985; **42**: 65–108.

9. Kakonen SM, Hellman J, Karp M et al. Development and evaluation of three immunofluorometric assays that measure different forms of osteocalcin in serum. *Clin Chem* 2000; **46**(3): 332–337.

10. Ivaska KK, Hellman J, Likojarvi J et al. Identification of novel proteolytic forms of osteocalcin in human urine. *Biochem Biophys Res Commun* 2003; **306**(4): 973–980.

11. Garnero P & Delmas PD. Assessment of the serum levels of bone alkaline phosphatase with a new immunoradiometric assay in patients with metabolic bone disease. *J Clin Endocrinol Metab* 1993; **77**(4): 1046–1053.

12. Prockop DJ, Kivirikko KI, Tuderman L et al. The biosynthesis of collagen and its disorders. *N Engl J Med* 1979; **310**: 13–23.

13. Melkko J, Niemi S, Risteli L et al. Radioimmunoassay of the carboxy-terminal propeptide of human type I procollagen. *Clin Chem* 1990; **36**(7): 1328–1332.

14. Charles P, Mosekilde L, Risteli L et al. Assessment of bone remodeling using biochemical indicators of type I collagen synthesis and degradation: relation to calcium kinetics. *Bone Miner* 1994; **24**(2): 81–94.

15. Ebeling PR, Peterson JM & Riggs BL. Utility of type I procollagen propeptide assays for assessing abnormalities in metabolic bone diseases. *J Bone Miner Res* 1992; **7**(11): 1243–1250.

16. Melkko J, Kauppila S, Niemi S et al. Immunoassay for intact amino-terminal propeptide of human type I procollagen. *Clin Chem* 1996; **42**(6, Pt 1): 947–954.

17. Chen P, Satterwhite JH, Licata AA et al. Early changes in biochemical markers of bone formation predict BMD response to teriparatide in postmenopausal women with osteoporosis. *J Bone Miner Res* 2005; **20**(6): 962–970.

18. Atley LM, Mort JS, Lalumiere M et al. Proteolysis of human bone collagen by cathepsin K: characterization of the cleavage sites generating by cross-linked N-telopeptide neoepitope. *Bone* 2000; **26**(3): 241–247.

19. Nishi Y, Atley L, Eyre DE et al. Determination of bone markers in pycnodysostosis: effects of cathepsin K deficiency on bone matrix degradation. *J Bone Miner Res* 1999; **14**(11): 1902–1908.

20. Garnero P, Ferreras M, Karsdal MA et al. The type I collagen fragments ICTP and CTX reveal distinct enzymatic pathways of bone collagen degradation. *J Bone Miner Res* 2003; **18**(5): 859–867.

21. Garnero P, Gineyts E, Arbault P et al. Different effects of bisphosphonate and estrogen therapy on free and peptide-bound bone cross-links excretion. *J Bone Miner Res* 1995; **10**(4): 641–649.

22. Eyre DR. The specificity of collagen cross-links as markers of bone and connective tissue degradation. *Acta Orthop Scand Suppl* 1995; **266**: 166–170.

23. Garnero P, Sornay-Rendu E, Chapuy MC et al. Increased bone turnover in late postmenopausal women is a major determinant of osteoporosis. *J Bone Miner Res* 1996; **11**(3): 337–349.

24. Risteli J, Elomaa I, Niemi S et al. Radioimmunoassay for the pyridinoline cross-linked carboxy-terminal telopeptide of type I collagen: a new serum marker of bone collagen degradation. *Clin Chem* 1993; **39**(4): 635–640.

25. Garnero P, Gineyts E, Riou JP et al. Assessment of bone resorption with a new marker of collagen degradation in patients with metabolic bone disease. *J Clin Endocrinol Metab* 1994; **79**(3): 780–785.

26. Seibel MJ, Woitge HW, Pecherstorfer M et al. Serum immunoreactive bone sialoprotein as a new marker of bone turnover in metabolic and malignant bone disease. *J Clin Endocrinol Metab* 1996; **81**(9): 3289–3294.

27. Halleen JM, Karp M, Viloma S et al. Two-site immunoassays for osteoclastic tartrate-resistant acid phosphatase based on characterization of six monoclonal antibodies. *J Bone Miner Res* 1999; **14**(3): 464–469.

28. Akesson K, Kakonen SM, Josefsson PO et al. Fracture-induced changes in bone turnover: a potential confounder in the use of biochemical markers in osteoporosis. *J Bone Miner Metab* 2005; **23**(1): 30–35.

29. Akesson K, Vergnaud P, Delmas PD et al. Serum osteocalcin increases during fracture healing in elderly women with hip fracture. *Bone* 1995; **16**(4): 427–430.

30. Ingle BM, Hay SM, Bottjer HM et al. Changes in bone mass and bone turnover following distal forearm fracture. *Osteoporosis Int* 1999; **10**(5): 399–407.

31. Zerwekh JE, Ruml LA, Gottschalk F et al. The effects of twelve weeks of bed rest on bone histology, biochemical markers of bone turnover, and calcium homeostasis in eleven normal subjects. *J Bone Miner Res* 1998; **13**(10): 1594–1601.

32. Brahm H, Strom H, Piehl-Aulin K et al. Bone metabolism in endurance trained athletes: a comparison to population-based controls based on DXA, SXA, quantitative ultrasound, and biochemical markers. *Calcif Tissue Int* 1997; **61**(6): 448–454.

33. Brahm H, Piehl-Aulin K & Ljunghall S. Biochemical markers of bone metabolism during distance running in healthy, regularly exercising men and women. *Scand J Med Sci Sports* 1996; **6**(1): 26–30.

34. Woitge HW, Friedmann B, Suttner S et al. Changes in bone turnover induced by aerobic and anaerobic exercise in young males. *J Bone Miner Res* 1998; **13**(12): 1797–1804.

35. Schlemmer A, Hassager C, Jensen SB et al. Marked diurnal variation in urinary excretion of pyridinium cross-links in premenopausal women. *J Clin Endocrinol Metab* 1992; **74**(3): 476–480.

36. Woitge HW, Scheidt-Nave C, Kissling C et al. Seasonal variation of biochemical indexes of bone turnover: results of a population-based study. *J Clin Endocrinol Metab* 1998; **83**(1): 68–75.

37. Woitge HW, Knothe A, Witte K et al. Circa-annual rhythms and interactions of vitamin D metabolites, parathyroid hormone, and biochemical markers of skeletal homeostasis: a prospective study. *J Bone Miner Res* 2000; **15**(12): 2443–2450.

38. Chapurlat RD, Garnero P, Breart G et al. Serum type I collagen breakdown product (serum CTX) predicts hip fracture risk in elderly women: the EPIDOS study. *Bone* 2000; **27**(2): 283–286.

39. Clowes JA, Allen HC, Prentis DM et al. Octreotide abolishes the acute decrease in bone turnover in response to oral glucose. *J Clin Endocrinol Metab* 2003; **88**(10): 4867–4873.

40. Uebelhart D, Schlemmer A, Johansen JS et al. Effect of menopause and hormone replacement therapy on the urinary excretion of pyridinium cross-links. *J Clin Endocrinol Metab* 1991; **72**(2): 367–373.

41. Cummings SR & Black D. Bone mass measurements and risk of fracture in Caucasian women: a review of findings from prospective studies. *Am J Med* 1995; **98**(2A): 24S–28S.

42. Johansen JS, Riis BJ, Delmas PD et al. Plasma BGP: an indicator of spontaneous bone loss and of the effect of oestrogen treatment in postmenopausal women. *Eur J Clin Invest* 1988; **18**(2): 191–195.

43. Bonde M, Qvist P, Fledelius C et al. Applications of an enzyme immunoassay for a new marker of bone resorption (CrossLaps): follow-up on hormone replacement therapy and osteoporosis risk assessment. *J Clin Endocrinol Metab* 1995; **80**(3): 864–868.

44. Slemenda C, Hui SL, Longcope C et al. Sex steroids and bone mass. A study of changes about the time of menopause. *J Clin Invest* 1987; **80**(5): 1261–1269.

45. Cosman F, Nieves J, Wilkinson C et al. Bone density change and biochemical indices of skeletal turnover. *Calcif Tissue Int* 1996; **58**(4): 236–243.

46. Chesnut CH III, Bell NH, Clark GS et al. Hormone replacement therapy in postmenopausal women: urinary N-telopeptide of type I collagen monitors therapeutic effect and predicts response of bone mineral density. *Am J Med* 1997; **102**(1): 29–37.

47. Hansen MA, Overgaard K, Riis BJ et al. Role of peak bone mass and bone loss in postmenopausal osteoporosis: 12 year study. *BMJ* 1991; **303**(6808): 961–964.

48. Ravn P, Fledelius C, Rosenquist C et al. High bone turnover is associated with low bone mass in both pre- and postmenopausal women. *Bone* 1996; **19**(3): 291–298.

49. Bauer DC, Sklarin PM, Stone KL et al. Biochemical markers of bone turnover and prediction of hip bone loss in older women: the study of osteoporotic fractures. *J Bone Miner Res* 1999; **14**(8): 1404–1410.

50. Garnero P, Sornay-Rendu E, Duboeuf F et al. Markers of bone turnover predict postmenopausal forearm bone loss over 4 years: the OFELY study. *J Bone Miner Res* 1999; **14**(9): 1614–1621.

51. Keen RW, Nguyen T, Sobnack R et al. Can biochemical markers predict bone loss at the hip and spine? A 4-year prospective study of 141 early postmenopausal women. *Osteoporosis Int* 1996; **6**(5): 399–406.

52. Akesson K, Vergnaud P, Gineyts E et al. Impairment of bone turnover in elderly women with hip fracture. *Calcif Tissue Int* 1993; **53**(3): 162–169.

53. Garnero P, Hausherr E, Chapuy MC et al. Markers of bone resorption predict hip fracture in elderly women: the EPIDOS Prospective Study. *J Bone Miner Res* 1996; **11**(10): 1531–1538.

54. Van Daele PL, Seibel MJ, Burger H et al. Case–control analysis of bone resorption markers, disability, and hip fracture risk: the Rotterdam study. *BMJ* 1996; **312**(7029): 482–483.

55. Riis BJ, Overgaard K & Christiansen C. Biochemical markers of bone turnover to monitor the bone response to postmenopausal hormone replacement therapy. *Osteoporosis Int* 1995; **5**(4): 276–280.

56. Gerdhem P, Ivaska KK, Alatalo SL et al. Biochemical markers of bone metabolism and prediction of fracture in elderly women. *J Bone Miner Res* 2004; **19**(3): 386–393.

57. Meier C, Nguyen TV, Center JR et al. Bone resorption and osteoporotic fractures in elderly men: the Dubbo Osteoporosis Epidemiology Study. *J Bone Miner Res* 2005; **20**(4): 579–587.

58. Plantalech L, Guillaumont M, Vergnaud P et al. Impairment of gamma carboxylation of circulating osteocalcin (bone gla protein) in elderly women. *J Bone Miner Res* 1991; **6**(11): 1211–1216.

59. Szulc P, Chapuy MC, Meunier PJ et al. Serum undercarboxylated osteocalcin is a marker of the risk of hip fracture in elderly women. *J Clin Invest* 1993; **91**(4): 1769–1774.

60. Vergnaud P, Garnero P, Meunier PJ et al. Undercarboxylated osteocalcin measured with a specific immunoassay predicts hip fracture in elderly women: the EPIDOS Study. *J Clin Endocrinol Metab* 1997; **82**(3): 719–724.

61. Luukinen H, Kakonen SM, Pettersson K et al. Strong prediction of fractures among older adults by the ratio of carboxylated to total serum osteocalcin. *J Bone Miner Res* 2000; **15**(12): 2473–2478.

62. Greenspan SL, Parker RA, Ferguson L et al. Early changes in biochemical markers of bone turnover predict the long-term response to alendronate therapy in representative elderly women: a randomized clinical trial. *J Bone Miner Res* 1998; **13**(9): 1431–1438.

63. Civitelli R, Gonnelli S, Zacchei F et al. Bone turnover in postmenopausal osteoporosis. Effect of calcitonin treatment. *J Clin Invest* 1988; **82**(4): 1268–1274.

64. Braga de Castro Machado A, Hannon R & Eastell R. Monitoring alendronate therapy for osteoporosis. *J Bone Miner Res* 1999; **14**(4): 602–608.

65. Rosen CJ, Hochberg MC, Bonnick SL et al. Treatment with once-weekly alendronate 70 mg compared with once-weekly risedronate 35 mg in women with postmenopausal osteoporosis: a randomized double-blind study. *J Bone Miner Res* 2005; **20**(1): 141–151.

66. Nenonen A, Cheng S, Ivaska KK et al. Serum TRACP 5b is a useful marker for monitoring alendronate treatment: comparison with other markers of bone turnover. *J Bone Miner Res* 2005; **20**(8): 1804–1812.

67. Ravn P, Hosking D, Thompson D et al. Monitoring of alendronate treatment and prediction of effect on bone mass by biochemical markers in the early postmenopausal intervention cohort study. *J Clin Endocrinol Metab* 1999; **84**(7): 2363–2368.

68. Ravn P, Clemmesen B & Christiansen C. Biochemical markers can predict the response in bone mass during alendronate treatment in early postmenopausal women. Alendronate Osteoporosis Prevention Study Group. *Bone* 1999; **24**(3): 237–244.

69. Rizzoli R, Greenspan SL, Bone G III et al. Two-year results of once-weekly administration of alendronate 70 mg for the treatment of postmenopausal osteoporosis. *J Bone Miner Res* 2002; **17**(11): 1988–1996.

70. Delmas PD, Recker RR, Chesnut CH III et al. Daily and intermittent oral ibandronate normalize bone turnover and provide significant reduction in vertebral fracture risk: results from the BONE study. *Osteoporosis Int* 2004; **15**(10): 792–798.

71. Christiansen C, Tanko LB, Warming L et al. Dose dependent effects on bone resorption and formation of intermittently administered intravenous ibandronate. *Osteoporosis Int* 2003; **14**(7): 609–613.

72. Delmas PD, Bjarnason NH, Mitlak BH et al. Effects of raloxifene on bone mineral density, serum cholesterol concentrations, and uterine endometrium in postmenopausal women. *N Engl J Med* 1997; **337**(23): 1641–1647.

73. Meunier PJ, Roux C, Seeman E et al. The effects of strontium ranelate on the risk of vertebral fracture in women with postmenopausal osteoporosis. *N Engl J Med* 2004; **350**(5): 459–468.

74. Reginster JY, Seeman E, De Vernejoul MC et al. Strontium ranelate reduces the risk of nonvertebral fractures in postmenopausal women with osteoporosis: Treatment of Peripheral Osteoporosis (TROPOS) study. *J Clin Endocrinol Metab* 2005; **90**(5): 2816–2822.

75. Hochberg MC, Greenspan S, Wasnich RD et al. Changes in bone density and turnover explain the reductions in incidence of nonvertebral fractures that occur during treatment with antiresorptive agents. *J Clin Endocrinol Metab* 2002; **87**(4): 1586–1592.

76. Eastell R, Barton I, Hannon RA et al. Relationship of early changes in bone resorption to the reduction in fracture risk with risedronate. *J Bone Miner Res* 2003; **18**(6): 1051–1056.

77. Seibel MJ, Naganathan V, Barton I et al. Relationship between pretreatment bone resorption and vertebral fracture incidence in postmenopausal osteoporotic women treated with risedronate. *J Bone Miner Res* 2004; **19**(2): 323–329.

78. Bauer DC, Black DM, Garnero P et al. Change in bone turnover and hip, non-spine, and vertebral fracture in alendronate-treated women: the fracture intervention trial. *J Bone Miner Res* 2004; **19**(8): 1250–1258.

79. Sarkar S, Reginster JY, Crans GG et al. Relationship between changes in biochemical markers of bone turnover and BMD to predict vertebral fracture risk. *J Bone Miner Res* 2004; **19**(3): 394–401.

80. Marcus R, Holloway L, Wells B et al. The relationship of biochemical markers of bone turnover to bone density changes in postmenopausal women: results from the Postmenopausal Estrogen/Progestin Interventions (PEPI) trial. *J Bone Miner Res* 1999; **14**(9): 1583–1595.

81. Cummings SR, Karpf DB, Harris F et al. Improvement in spine bone density and reduction in risk of vertebral fractures during treatment with antiresorptive drugs. *Am J Med* 2002; **112**(4): 281–289.

82. Clowes JA, Peel NF & Eastell R. The impact of monitoring on adherence and persistence with antiresorptive treatment for postmenopausal osteoporosis: a randomized controlled trial. *J Clin Endocrinol Metab* 2004; **89**(3): 1117–1123.

Chapter 10
Osteoporosis in men

Ira Pande and Roger M. Francis

EPIDEMIOLOGY OF FRACTURES IN MEN

There is a bimodal distribution of fracture incidence with age, with peaks in youth and old age. Fracture incidence rises rapidly in women above the age of 45 years, whereas the increase occurs at a later age in men, such that the fracture rate in elderly women is twice that of men of the same age. The major osteoporotic fractures are those of the vertebral body and hip, but fractures of the forearm, humerus, tibia, pelvis and ribs are also common. The lifetime risk of symptomatic fracture for a 50-year-old white man in the UK has been estimated to be 2% for the vertebra and 3% for the hip, whereas the corresponding figures for a 50-year-old woman are 11% and 14% respectively.[1]

The number of men presenting with osteoporotic fractures is rising, because of the demographic trend towards an ageing population and a doubling of the age-specific incidence of fractures over the past three decades. This makes a rise in the number of men presenting with osteoporotic fractures inevitable, in both the developed and developing world.[1] The number of men with osteoporotic fractures needing admission to hospital is similar to the number with prostate cancer, but fractures are associated with substantially more hospital-bed days. Osteoporotic fractures account for 84% of all hospital-bed days due to fracture in men and 93% in women.[2]

Hip fractures

The incidence of hip fractures increases with age in all geographical areas and ethnic groups, in both men and women. The Dubbo Osteoporosis Epidemiology Study has shown that one in four of all hip fractures occur in men. The absolute numbers peak between the ages of 80 and 84 years, with 48% occurring before the age of 80.[3] There is a greater difference in hip fracture incidence between ethnic groups and countries than between sexes, highlighting the potential importance of environmental, genetic and lifestyle factors in the aetiology of hip fractures. The lifetime risk of hip fracture is 5–6% in white men and 2.8% in black men in the USA, compared with 16–18% in white women and 6% in black women.[4]

A number of studies have shown a higher mortality after hip fracture in men than women. The Cornwall Hip Fracture Study showed that men who fractured their hip were three times more likely to die in the year following their fracture and women over

two times more than would be expected on the basis of their age.[5] Using a case–control study, the same researcher demonstrated that hip fracture in men was associated with a six- to seven-fold excess mortality compared to controls,[6] with continued increased mortality over 2 years of follow-up (Figure 10.1). Factors associated with this increased mortality included older age, pre-fracture residence in nursing or residential home, presence of co-morbid diseases and poor pre-fracture functional activity.[7]

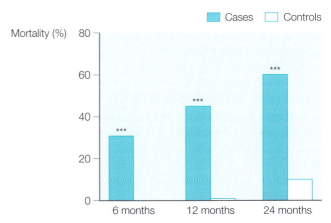

Figure 10.1. Mortality in men with hip fractures, compared with age-matched male control subjects. Data from the case–control study of Pande et al.[21] The statistical significance of differences between fracture cases and control subjects is indicated (***$P <$ 0.001).

There is also substantial morbidity after hip fracture in men.[7] Men are twice as likely as women to require nursing home care after hip fracture.[8] Most fracture survivors have reduced function, increased dependency and poor quality of life, with mean SF 36 physical component scores more than 1.7 SD below the normal 2 years following fracture.[7] Two longitudinal studies have recently shown that hip fracture is associated with a 2.5-fold increased risk of subsequent fracture in men and women, which is not entirely explained by other pre-existing risk factors.[9] The risk of subsequent fracture is highest immediately after the hip fracture and is irrespective of age.[10] This provides a rationale for early intervention after fractures to avoid subsequent fractures.

Vertebral fractures

The prevalence of vertebral deformity is higher in younger men than women, possibly due to trauma earlier in life. The European Vertebral Osteoporosis Study (EVOS) demonstrated an overall prevalence of radiological vertebral deformity of 12% in both men and women, but the relationship between prevalence and age is less steep in men.[11] The European Prospective Osteoporosis Study (EPOS) showed an overall age standardized incidence of morphometric vertebral fractures of 10.7/1000 person-years in women and 5.7/1000 person-years in men.[12] The incidence increased from 0.9/1000 in men aged 50–54 years to 6.3/1000 between the ages of 65 and 69 years and 13.6/1000 at ages 75–79 years. A further study from EPOS explored the determinants of incident vertebral fractures in men and women.[13] None of the lifestyle factors studied, including smoking, alcohol intake, physical activity or milk consumption, showed a consistent association with incident vertebral fractures in either sex. Although there was a trend for lower risk of incident vertebral fractures with higher weight and body mass index (BMI) in both sexes, this was only significant for BMI in men using qualitative assessment of vertebral fracture.[13]

Men with symptomatic vertebral fractures commonly complain of back pain, loss of height and kyphosis, but also have significantly less energy, poorer sleep, more emotional problems and impaired mobility compared with age-matched control subjects.[14] There is also excess mortality associated with vertebral fractures of about 18% at 5 years, but this appears to be due mainly to co-existing conditions rather than the fracture itself.

Recent work from the UK General Practice Research Database shows that men with a symptomatic vertebral fracture are at increased risk of a hip fracture, such that men aged 65–74 years with a clinical vertebral fracture have a 5-year risk of hip fracture of 5.7%.[15]

Cost of osteoporotic fractures in men

Most of the work on the socio-economic cost of osteoporotic fractures has concentrated on women. Nevertheless, it has been estimated that up to 20% of symptomatic vertebral fractures and 30% of hip fractures occur in men.[1] The annual cost of osteoporotic fractures in the UK has been calculated to be £1.7 billion, of which almost 25% is due to fractures in men. The cost of all osteoporotic fractures is higher than those for myocardial infarction, breast cancer and prostate cancer combined, but lower than those for stroke.[2]

PATHOGENESIS OF OSTEOPOROSIS AND FRACTURES IN MEN

The risk of fracture is influenced by a number of factors, including bone mineral density (BMD), bone turnover, skeletal size and geometry, trabecular architecture, and the frequency and severity of trauma applied to the skeleton. BMD at any age is determined by the peak bone mass, the age at which bone loss starts and the rate at which it progresses. Between 95% and 99% of the ultimate peak bone mass is attained by the age of 18 years. Although peak bone mass is higher in men than women, BMD at maturity is similar in both sexes. The adolescent rise in bone mass occurs at a younger age in females, because of their earlier onset of puberty.[16]

Genetic factors account for between 60% and 80% of the variance in peak bone mass in both sexes. Men with a family history of osteoporosis have a lower than expected BMD, but the major genetic factors determining bone density and fracture risk in men remain uncertain. Other determinants of peak bone mass in men include dietary calcium intake and exercise during childhood and adolescence, each of which may modify bone mass at maturity by about 5%.[16]

Bone loss starts between the ages of 35 and 50 years in men and women, and continues into old age in both sexes. Trabecular bone loss is less in men than women when expressed as a percentage of their higher peak bone mass, but is accompanied by trabecular thinning, rather than the reduction in trabecular number seen in women. Cortical bone loss is also lower in men, because endocortical resorption is less and periosteal bone formation is greater than in women. Biochemical and histological studies suggest that bone formation decreases with advancing age in men, but there is some evidence of increased bone resorption in elderly men.[1]

Although heredity is an important determinant of peak bone mass in men, it has much less effect on age-related bone loss. The decrease in circulating free testosterone, adrenal androgens, growth hormone and insulin-like growth factor-1 (IGF-1) with advancing age may contribute to the observed reduction in bone formation and continuing bone loss in men. It is now apparent that the actions of testosterone on the male skeleton are mediated in part by aromatization to oestradiol, such that oestrogen deficiency may contribute to age-related bone loss in men. Case reports have described osteoporosis in men with mutations in the oestrogen receptor or aromatase genes. There is also a positive correlation between serum oestradiol and BMD in healthy older men, with an inverse relationship between oestradiol and the incidence of vertebral fractures.[17,18] Other factors have been implicated in bone loss in men, including physical inactivity, tobacco and alcohol consumption, poor dietary calcium intake, vitamin D insufficiency and secondary hyperparathyroidism.[16] The development of osteoporosis in men may be accelerated by underlying causes of secondary osteoporosis, such as hypogonadism, oral corticosteroid therapy and alcohol abuse.

Hip fractures

BMD is lower in men with hip fracture than in those without proximal femur fractures[19–21] (Figure 10.2). There is a three-fold increased risk of hip fracture for each standard deviation reduction in femoral neck BMD in men, which is comparable to that seen in women.[20,21] Although skeletal geometry of the proximal femur may be an additional determinant of hip fracture risk in

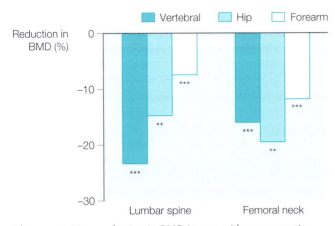

Figure 10.2. Mean reduction in BMD in men with symptomatic vertebral, hip and forearm fractures, compared with age-matched male control subjects. Data from the case–control studies of Scane et al.,[14] Pande et al.[21] and Tuck et al.[33] The statistical significance of differences from the mean values for male control subjects is indicated (**$P < 0.01$; ***$P < 0.001$).

women, the only study examining this in men found no effect of hip axis length.[21]

A number of studies have examined the effect of anthropometric measurements, lifestyle factors and underlying conditions on the risk of hip fractures in men. These studies suggest that increased height[22,23] and low body weight[19,24] are independent risk factors for hip fracture in men.

A recent meta-analysis concluded that a history of smoking results in fracture risk that is substantially greater than that explained by BMD alone.[25] Studies of the effect of alcohol consumption on BMD and fracture risk are inconsistent.[6,19,22,24] Several studies have shown a positive correlation between dietary calcium intake and BMD in men,[26] with the suggestion of a lower risk of hip fracture in men with a higher calcium intake.[24,27] Physical activity has also been shown to protect against hip fracture risk in men.[6,19,24,27]

The results of studies of the effect of medication on the risk of hip fracture are inconsistent. No association has been reported between diuretic use and hip fracture incidence in men,[23,24] but psychotropic drugs appear to double the risk of fracture.[23] A study from the Mayo Clinic did not demonstrate a deleterious effect of corticosteroids and anticonvulsants on hip fracture incidence in men,[22] in contrast to their effect on vertebral fracture risk in men.[14]

Almost all studies confirm the presence of co-morbid diseases (stroke, Parkinson's disease, dementia and poor vision) as risk factors for hip fracture in men.[6,22,23] These conditions may be associated with reduced BMD and/or an increased risk of falling. Biochemical evidence of hypogonadism has been reported in up to 50% of men with hip fractures.[28,29] A case–control study from the UK shows consistently lower androgen levels in men with hip fracture, compared with control subjects from the

time of fracture until 1 year later, confirming that hypogonadism is a risk factor for low trauma hip fracture in men.[6] The only published study evaluating oestradiol concentrations in men with hip fracture showed no difference from healthy controls.[29] Studies suggest that vitamin D deficiency is a risk factor for hip fracture in elderly men,[6,29] but it is unclear if vitamin D deficiency is a marker of physical frailty rather than a direct cause of increased fracture risk.

Vertebral fractures

Recent work from the Rotterdam Study shows a similar relationship between BMD and the incidence of vertebral fractures in men and women.[30] Men with symptomatic vertebral fractures have a mean lumbar spine BMD over 20% lower than age-matched control subjects (Figure 10.2), but also have a significant reduction in BMD in the proximal femur.[14] Although the high incidence and prevalence of vertebral deformation in young men compared with women in the EVOS and EPOS[11,12] suggest that vertebral deformities in men may be due to antecedent trauma, these data indicate that this is relatively uncommon in men presenting clinically with vertebral fractures.

Men with symptomatic vertebral fractures are significantly shorter than control subjects, but the mean difference in stature is accounted for by the reported loss of height.[14] Body weight and body mass index are significantly lower in men with vertebral fractures than control subjects. There is also significant reduction in mid-arm circumference and lean body mass in men with vertebral fractures, suggesting that they have a lower muscle mass than control subjects.[14] It has also been suggested that bone size is an important determinant of fracture risk in men.[31] A study of men with idiopathic osteoporosis and vertebral fractures showed reduced BMD and vertebral dimensions compared with aged-matched control subjects.[31] This suggests that the achievement of a reduced bone size at the end of the growth period or failure of periosteal increase during adulthood may contribute to the pathogenesis of vertebral fractures in older men.

Previous studies have shown underlying causes of secondary osteoporosis in over 50% of men presenting with vertebral fractures, of which oral steroid therapy and hypogonadism are the most common.[14,32] A case–control study from the Mayo Clinic showed an increased risk of vertebral fractures in men with smoking, alcohol consumption and underlying causes of secondary osteoporosis, whereas the risk was reduced in the presence of obesity.[32] A subsequent case–control study from the UK demonstrated an increased risk of symptomatic vertebral fractures with oral corticosteroid therapy, anticonvulsant treatment, family history of bone disease, current smoking and high alcohol consumption.[14] This study also showed a higher sex hormone-binding globulin (SHBG) and lower free testosterone index in men with symptomatic vertebral fractures compared with age-matched control subjects.[14] Further analysis showed a lower free oestradiol index in men with vertebral fractures, indicating the importance of sex steroids for the maintenance of bone density in men.

Forearm fractures

A recent case–control study of distal forearm fractures in men[33] showed a lower BMD in the lumbar spine (7.5%), total hip (7.3%) and femoral neck (11.8%) in the men with fractures compared with male control subjects (Figure 10.2). This is consistent with the results of previous studies showing an increased risk of fractures at other sites after forearm fracture in men.[15,34]

Hypogonadism

Hypogonadism is a well-established cause of osteoporosis in men, occurring in up to 20% of men with vertebral fractures and 50% of elderly men with hip fractures. Causes of hypogonadal osteoporosis in men include Klinefelter's syndrome, idiopathic hypogonadotrophic hypogonadism, hyperprolactinaemia, haemochromatosis and primary testicular failure. It has recently become apparent that androgen therapy for prostate cancer in men causes rapid bone loss and an increase in fracture incidence.[35]

DIAGNOSIS OF OSTEOPOROSIS IN MEN

The commonest clinical presentation of osteoporosis is a low trauma fracture in the absence of a focal pathological process such as malignancy or Paget's disease. Other clinical situations that raise the possibility of osteoporosis are loss of height, radiological evidence of osteopaenia or vertebral deformity and the presence of medical disorders known to be associated with an increased risk of bone loss. The World Health Organization (WHO) has defined osteoporosis as a BMD that is 2.5 standard deviations or more below the mean value for young adults (T-score <−2.5), whereas osteopoenia is defined as a BMD that is between 1 and 2.5 standard deviations below the young adult mean. Debate on how this definition should be used in men is well summarized in a review article.[36] Population-based studies have shown a similar relationship between BMD and fracture risk in both sexes.[20,30,37] However, one must remember that, in men, only as little as 39% hip fractures, 21% of all non-vertebral fractures and 50% of low trauma vertebral fractures are associated with densitometric evidence of osteoporosis.[14,37] This suggests that although low BMD is a risk factor for fractures, using only T-scores of BMD as treatment thresholds may not sufficiently relieve the total burden of fractures in the whole population. We therefore suggest that treatment for osteoporosis should be considered in men with low trauma vertebral fractures and evidence of osteoporosis or osteopoenia at the lumbar spine or femoral neck, whereas the possibility of unrecognized antecedent trauma should be explored in those with normal bone density measurements.

INVESTIGATION OF OSTEOPOROSIS IN MEN

The clinical assessment of a man with low trauma fractures and/or low bone density should be directed towards confirming the diagnosis of osteoporosis, excluding other pathology such as osteomalacia and identifying causes of osteoporosis and bone loss. Underlying causes of secondary osteoporosis should be sought by careful history, physical examination and appropriate investigation, as treatment of underlying conditions such as hyperthyroidism, hypogonadism and hyperparathyroidism may increase bone density by 10–20%. Investigations should include full blood count, erythrocyte sedimentation rate, biochemical profile, thyroid function tests, serum testosterone, SHBG and gonadotrophins. Serum and urine electrophoresis should be performed in men with vertebral fractures, to exclude the diagnosis of myeloma. Prostate-specific antigen should also be measured in men with vertebral fractures and symptoms of prostatism or evidence of sclerosis on X-rays. In elderly men with osteoporosis, serum 25-hydroxyvitamin D and intact parathyroid hormone measurements may exclude vitamin D insufficiency and secondary hyperparathyroidism.

These investigations are usually normal in men with idiopathic osteoporosis, apart from a transient rise in serum alkaline phosphatase after fracture. The most frequently encountered causes of secondary osteoporosis in men are oral steroid therapy, hypogonadism, alcohol abuse, myeloma and skeletal metastases. In men with severe unexplained osteoporosis, it may be worthwhile considering 24-h urine calcium estimation to identify hypercalciuria, 24-h urine cortisol to exclude Cushing's syndrome and anti-endomysial antibodies to look for coeliac disease.

Iliac crest bone biopsy has also been advocated for the investigation of men with idiopathic osteoporosis, to exclude conditions such as osteomalacia and mastocytosis. Although histomorphometry can be used to assess bone turnover, which may help in decisions about further investigation and treatment, the biochemical markers of bone formation and resorption provide comparable information.

TREATMENT OF OSTEOPOROSIS IN MEN

Although the number of trials of osteoporosis treatment in men is increasing, there are no anti-fracture studies performed solely in men. Given the similar relationship between BMD and fracture risk in both sexes and the comparable increases in BMD observed with treatment in men and women, it appears likely that agents which decrease fractures in women will also be effective in men. As mentioned earlier, underlying causes of secondary osteoporosis should be treated where possible, as this may increase bone density by 10–20%. In men with idiopathic osteoporosis, bisphosphonates are now the treatment of choice, but other options include teriparatide and calcitonin.

Bisphosphonates

Observational studies in men with idiopathic and secondary osteoporosis suggest that intermittent cyclical etidronate therapy increases bone density at the lumbar spine by 5–10%, with smaller increases at the hip, but the effect on fracture incidence in men remains unclear. An observational study compared the effect of alendronate with no treatment in men and women with primary and secondary osteoporosis.[38] This showed comparable increases of 5–7% in spine lumbar BMD over 1 year in all treatment groups compared with the control group, suggesting that alendronate has similar effects on bone density in men and women with primary and secondary osteoporosis. Alendronate has since been used to treat eugonadal and hypogonadal men with osteoporosis and those with corticosteroid-induced osteoporosis.[39,40] All have shown comparable results with respect to BMD changes and reduction in vertebral fracture incidence. Although there are no published data on the use of risedronate and intermittent bisphosphonates (ibandronate and zoledronate) in men, studies using other agents suggest that bisphosphonates are equally effective in the management of men and women with osteoporosis.

Teriparatide

Teriparatide (synthetic parathyroid hormone 1–34) has been licensed in the USA for the treatment of osteoporosis in men and women, but it is not licensed for men in the UK or elsewhere in Europe. In a study of 437 men with low BMD (T-score < −2.0), 11-month treatment with subcutaneous teriparatide increased spine BMD by 5.9% (20 μg) and 9.0% (40 μg), whereas femoral neck BMD increased by 1.5% and 2.9% respectively.[41] There are no data to confirm that teriparatide decreases fracture incidence in men, but this appears likely given the magnitude of the increases in BMD and the reduction in fracture risk observed in women. As teriparatide is much more expensive than the bisphophonates, its use in men is likely to be restricted to those with marked reduction in BMD and those who fail to respond to bisphosphonates. The concomitant use of alendronate in men receiving synthetic parathyroid hormone 1–34 leads to an attenuation of the anabolic effect on BMD, which may have implications for the use of teriparatide in men previously treated with a bisphosphonate.[42]

Vitamin D and vitamin D metabolites

There is little evidence that vitamin D used with or without calcium supplementation will reduce fracture risk in community-dwelling men with osteoporosis. The MRC RECORD showed no reduction in the risk of further fractures with calcium and vitamin D, either used alone or in combination.[43] Nevertheless, calcium and vitamin D may be beneficial in elderly men living in residential or nursing homes, where vitamin D deficiency and secondary hyperparathyroidism are common. Calcium and vitamin D should also be considered as an adjunct to other osteoporosis treatments, unless the clinician is confident that the patient has an adequate calcium intake and is vitamin D replete. Calcitriol has also been studied in men with osteoporosis, but no benefit on BMD or fracture incidence was found.[44]

Calcitonin

In a small study in 28 men with idiopathic osteoporosis, 12-month treatment with intranasal calcitonin (200 units daily) increased spine BMD by 7.1% compared with 2.4% in the control group receiving calcium alone.[45] Calcitonin may also be useful in the management of pain associated with vertebral fractures, as demonstrated by a double-blind, placebo-controlled trial in 32 men and 68 women.[46]

Testosterone

An observational study examined the long-term effects of testosterone replacement on bone density in 72 hypogonadal men.[47] In men who had received no previous treatment, testosterone replacement led to an increase in spine BMD of 25%, but even in those who had received treatment previously, there was a further increase of 15%.[47] Although testosterone replacement should be considered in osteoporotic men with hypogonadism, uncertainty about the long-term impact on the risk of prostatic and cardiovascular disease may restrict its use in older men, particularly as alendronate increases bone density in this situation.[39]

Fluoride salts

Initial studies with fluoride demonstrated large increases in BMD, but there was no reduction in fracture incidence. A German study showed that low-dose intermittent monofluorophosphate and calcium increased bone density and decreased the risk of vertebral fractures in men with osteoporosis.[48] Nevertheless, the narrow therapeutic window, side-effect profile and the development of more effective treatments have limited the use of fluoride in men and women with osteoporosis.

SUMMARY

Up to 20% of symptomatic vertebral fractures and 30% of hip fractures occur in men, causing substantial morbidity and greater excess mortality than the corresponding fractures in women. Almost 25% of the cost of osteoporotic fractures in the UK is due to fractures in men. The number of men with osteoporotic fractures needing admission to hospital is similar to the number with prostate cancer, but fractures are associated with substantially more hospital-bed days.

There is an inverse relationship between bone density and fracture risk in men, which is as strong as that seen in women. Peak bone mass in men is influenced by genetic factors, age at puberty, and exercise and calcium intake during childhood, whereas causes of bone loss include declining sex steroid concentrations, physical inactivity, smoking, alcohol consumption and vitamin D deficiency. Over 50% of men presenting with symptomatic vertebral crush fractures have an underlying secondary cause of osteoporosis, such as hypogonadism, oral steroid therapy and alcohol abuse. The risk of hip fractures in men is also increased by disorders associated with secondary osteoporosis and by conditions related to an increased risk of falling. Men with a forearm fracture have lower BMD and are at increased risk of future fracture at other sites.

Criteria for the diagnosis of osteoporosis in men are less well established than in women, but there is a growing consensus to use the WHO definition of a T-score <−2.5. Although the number of trials of osteoporosis treatment in men is increasing, fracture reduction is not the primary end-point of any published study so far. Given comparable increases in BMD with treatment, it appears agents that decrease fractures in women will also be effective in men.

Therapeutic options include testosterone replacement in men with hypogonadism and bisphosphonates in men with idiopathic and corticosteroid-induced osteoporosis. Calcium and vitamin D supplementation may be useful in frail, elderly men and as adjunct to other osteoporosis treatment, unless the patient is calcium and vitamin D replete. More clinical trials are needed using newer agents, such as intermittent bisphosphonates and strontium, to establish the most effective treatments for osteoporosis in men.

PRACTICE POINTS

- Up to 20% of symptomatic vertebral fractures and 30% of hip fractures occur in men, where they are associated with excess mortality, substantial morbidity and health and social service expenditure.

- Underlying causes of secondary osteoporosis should be sought in men with vertebral and hip fractures, as treatment of conditions such as hyperthyroidism and hypogonadism increases bone density by 10–20%.

- There is a comparable relationship between bone density and fracture risk in both sexes, but the optimal criteria for the diagnosis of osteoporosis in men remain uncertain.

- Bisphosphonates are currently the treatment of choice for men with osteoporosis, but other options include teriparatide and calcitonin.

RESEARCH AGENDA

- Further research is needed to investigate the pathogenesis and sequelae of osteoporosis and fractures in men.

- The criteria for the diagnosis of osteoporosis in men require further evaluation.

- More clinical trials are needed of newer agents, such as intermittent bisphosphonates and strontium, to establish the most effective treatments of osteoporosis in men.

REFERENCES

1. Eastell R, Boyle IT, Compston J et al. Management of male osteoporosis: report of the UK Consensus Group. *QJ Med* 1998; **91**: 71–92.

2. Johnell O, Kanis JA, Jonsson B et al. The burden of hospitalised fractures in Sweden. *Osteoporosis Int* 2005; **16**: 222–228.

3. Chang KP, Center JR, Nguyen TV et al. Incidence of hip and other osteoporotic fractures in elderly men and women: Dubbo Osteoporosis Epidemiology Study. *J Bone Miner Res* 2004; **19**: 532–536.

4. Cummings SR, Black DM & Rubin SM. Lifetime risks of hip, Colles', or vertebral fracture and coronary heart disease among white postmenopausal women. *Arch Intern Med* 1989; **149**: 2445–2448.

5. Pande I & Pritchard C. Osteoporotic fractures in Cornwall. *Lancet* 1999; **353**: 1707.

6. Pande I. Causes and consequences of hip fracture in men. Ph.D. thesis, University of London, 2000.

7. Pande I, Scott DL, O'Neill TW et al. Quality of life, morbidity and mortality after low trauma hip fracture in men. *Ann Rheum Dis* 2006; **65**: 87–92.

8. Osnes EK, Lofthus CM, Meyer HE et al. Consequences of hip fracture on activities of daily life and residential needs. *Osteoporosis Int* 2004; **15**: 567–574.

9. Colon-Emeric C, Kuchibhatla M, Pieper C et al. The contribution of hip fracture to risk of subsequent fractures: data from two longitudinal studies. *Osteoporosis Int* 2003; **14**: 879–883.

10. Johnell O, Kanis JA, Oden A et al. Fracture risk following an osteoporotic fracture. *Osteoporosis Int* 2004; **15**: 175–179.

11. O'Neill TW, Felsenberg D, Varlow J et al. The prevalence of vertebral deformity in European men and women. The European Vertebral Osteoporosis Study. *J Bone Miner Res* 1996; **11**: 1010–1018.

12. The European Prospective Osteoporosis Study Group. Incidence of vertebral fracture in Europe: results from the European Prospective Osteoporosis Study (EPOS). *J Bone Miner Res* 2002; **17**: 716–724.

13. Roy DK, O'Neill TW, Finn JD et al. Determinants of incident vertebral fracture in men and women: results for the European Prospective Osteoporosis Study (EPOS). *Osteoporosis Int* 2003; **14**: 19–26.

14. Scane AC, Francis RM, Sutcliffe AM et al. Case–control study of the pathogenesis and sequelae of symptomatic vertebral fractures in men. *Osteoporosis Int* 1999; **9**: 91–97.

15. Van Staa TP, Leufkens HGM & Cooper C. Does a fracture at one site predict later fractures at other sites? A British cohort study. *Osteoporosis Int* 2002; **13**: 624–629.

16. Scane AC & Francis RM. Risk factors for osteoporosis in men. *Clin Endocrinol* 1993; **38**: 15–16.

17. Amin S, Zhang Y, Sawin CT et al. Association of hypogonadism and oestradiol levels with bone mineral density in elderly men from the Framingham Study. *Ann Intern Med* 2000; **133**: 951–963.

18. Barrett-Connor E, Mueller JE, von Muhlen DG et al. Low levels of oestradiol are associated with vertebral fractures in older men, but not women: the Rancho Bernardo Study. *J Clin Endocrinol Metab* 2000; **85**: 219–223.

19. Nguyen TV, Eisman JA, Kelly PJ et al. Risk factors for osteoporotic fractures in elderly men. *Am J Epidemiol* 1996; **144**: 255–263.

20. De Laet CED, Van Hout BA, Burger H et al. Bone density and risk of hip fracture in men and women: cross-sectional analysis. *BMJ* 1997; **315**: 221–225.

21. Pande I, O'Neill TW, Pritchard C et al. Bone mineral density, hip axis length and risk of hip fracture in men: results from the Cornwall Hip Fracture Study. *Osteoporosis Int* 2000; **11**: 866–870.

22. Poor G, Atkinson EJ, O'Fallon WM et al. Predictors of hip fractures in elderly men. *J Bone Miner Res* 1995; **10**: 1900–1907.

23. Grisso JA, Kelsey JL, O'Brien LA et al. Risk factors for hip fracture in men. Hip Fracture Study Group. *Am J Epidemiol* 1997; **145**: 786–793.

24. Mussolino ME, Looker AC, Madans JH et al. Risk factors for hip fracture in white men: the NHANES I Epidemiologic Follow-up Study. *J Bone Miner Res* 1998; **13**: 918–924.

25. Kanis JA, Johnell O, Oden A et al. Smoking and fracture risk: a meta-analysis. *Osteoporosis Int* 2005; **16**: 155–162.

26. Huuskonen J, Vaisanen SB, Kroger H et al. Determinants of bone mineral density in middle aged men: a population-based study. *Osteoporosis Int* 2000; **11**: 702–708.

27. Cooper C, Barker DJ & Wickham C. Physical activity, muscle strength, and calcium intake in fracture of the proximal femur in Britain. *BMJ* 1988; **297**: 1443–1446.

28. Stanley HL, Schmitt BP, Poses RM et al. Does hypogonadism contribute to the occurrence of a minimal trauma hip fracture in elderly men? *J Am Geriatr Soc* 1991; **39**: 766–771.

29. Boonen S, Vanderschueren D, Cheng XG et al. Age-related (type II) femoral neck osteoporosis in men: biochemical evidence for both hypovitaminosis D- and androgen deficiency-induced bone resorption. *J Bone Miner Res* 1997; **12**: 2119–2126.

30. Van der Klift M, De Laet CE, McCloskey EV et al. The incidence of vertebral fractures in men and women: the Rotterdam Study. *J Bone Miner Res* 2002; **17**: 1051–1056.

31. Vega E, Ghiringelli G, Mautalen C et al. Bone mineral density and bone size in men with vertebral fractures. *Calcif Tissue Int* 1998; **62**: 465–469.

32. Seeman E, Melton LJ III, O'Fallon WM et al. Risk factors for spinal osteoporosis in men. *Am J Med* 1983; **75**: 977–983.

33. Tuck SP, Raj N & Summers GD. Is distal forearm fracture in men due to osteoporosis? *Osteoporosis Int* 2002; **13**: 630–636.

34. Cuddihy MT, Gabriel SE, Crowson CS et al. Forearm fractures as predictors of subsequent osteoporotic fracture. *Osteoporosis Int* 1999; **9**: 469–475.

35. Shahinian VB, Kuo YF, Freeman JL et al. Risk of fracture after androgen deprivation for prostate cancer. *N Engl J Med* 2005; **352**: 154–164.

36. Orwoll E. Assessing bone density in men. *J Bone Miner Res* 2000; **15**: 1867–1870.

37. Schuit SC, van der Klift M, Weel AE et al. Fracture incidence and association with bone mineral density in elderly men and women: the Rotterdam Study. *Bone* 2004; **34**: 195–202.

38. Ho YV, Frauman AG, Thomson W et al. Effects of alendronate on bone density in men with primary and secondary osteoporosis. *Osteoporosis Int* 2000; **11**: 98–101.

39. Orwoll E, Ettinger M, Weiss S et al. Alendronate for the treatment of osteoporosis in men. *N Engl J Med* 2000; **343**: 604–610.

40. Saag KG, Emkey R, Schnitzer TJ S et al. Alendronate for the prevention and treatment of glucocorticoid-induced osteoporosis. *N Engl J Med* 1998; **339**: 292–299.

41. Orwoll ES, Scheele WH, Paul S et al. The effect of teriparatide [human parathyroid hormone (1–34)] therapy on bone density in men with osteoporosis. *J Bone Miner Res* 2003; **18**: 9–17.

42. Finkelstein JS, Hayes A, Hunzelman JL et al. The effects of parathyroid hormone, alendronate, or both in men with osteoporosis. *N Engl J Med* 2003; **349**: 1216–1226.

43. The RECORD Trial Group. Oral vitamin D_3 and calcium for the secondary prevention of low-trauma fractures in elderly PEOPLE (Randomised Evaluation of Calcium Or vitamin D, RECORD): a randomised placebo-controlled trial. *Lancet* 2005; **365**: 1621–1628.

44. Ebeling PR, Wark JD, Yeung S et al. Effects of calcitriol or calcium on bone mineral density, bone turnover and fractures in men with primary osteoporosis: a two year randomised, double blind, double placebo study. *J Clin Endocrinol Metab* 2001; **86**: 4098–4103.

45. Trovas GP, Lyritis GP, Galanos A et al. A randomized trial of nasal spray calcitonin in men with idiopathic osteoporosis: effects on bone mineral density and bone markers. *J Bone Miner Res* 2002; **17**: 521–527.

46. Lyritis GP, Paspati I, Karachalios T et al. Pain relief from nasal salmon calcitonin in osteoporotic vertebral crush fractures. A double blind, placebo-controlled clinical study. *Acta Orthop Scand* 1997; **275**(Suppl.): 112–114.

47. Behre HM, von Eckardstein S, Kliesch S et al. Long-term substitution therapy of hypogonadal men with transscrotal testosterone over 7–10 years. *Clin Endocrinol* 1999; **50**: 629–635.

48. Ringe JD, Dorst A, Kipshoven C et al. Avoidance of vertebral fractures in men with idiopathic osteoporosis by a three year therapy with calcium and low-dose intermittent monofluorophosphate. *Osteoporosis Int* 1998; **8**: 47–52.

Chapter 11

Osteoporosis in paediatric rheumatic diseases: an update

Rolando Cimaz

Osteoporosis is commonly thought to be a geriatric disorder, but it is becoming of interest to paediatricians as well.[1] Bone mass is accumulated during infancy and childhood, and probably reaches its peak by the late twenties. There is rapid skeletal accretion during intrauterine growth and early infancy, followed by a linear trend during childhood. Puberty is characterized by rapid bone maturation, and this increase in bone accounts for a large proportion of the total skeletal adult mass. Peak bone mass, the highest level of bone mass achieved as a result of normal growth, is the result of an interaction between endogenous and exogenous factors. It is thought that peak bone mass represents the 'bone bank' for the future because, after it is reached, there is a slow but continuous decrease. Small gains or losses during attainment of peak bone mass can therefore have a profound effect on the prevention of osteoporotic fractures in later life. Many diseases that occur during childhood and adolescence are associated with a loss of bone mass. If the predetermined peak bone mass is not established during skeletal maturation an individual may enter adulthood with suboptimal bone mass, and therefore be at higher risk for developing osteoporosis throughout adult life.

Genetic factors play an important role in the pathogenesis of osteoporosis, because it is estimated that at least 75% of the variance in bone mineral density (BMD) is under genetic control;[2] however, chronic inflammatory diseases also have a detrimental effect.

Current diagnostic techniques such as dual X-ray absorptiometry (DXA) are not able to measure true bone density, because this method measures only a cross-sectional area of the scan and not a true volume. To measure the true density the depth of the bone would have to be known and taken into account. Volumetric BMD (i.e. three-dimensional estimates) has seldom been described in the published literature.

Osteoporosis and osteopoenia in adults are defined at a level relative to a 'normal' young adult population. The World Health Organization (WHO) criteria for the diagnosis of osteoporosis use peak bone mass and assess risk of osteoporosis by the number of standard deviations between the measured BMD and peak bone mass (T-score), measured with DXA at any skeletal site.[3] There are currently no accepted definitions for osteoporosis and osteopoenia in childhood because, in their definitions, the WHO criteria refer to the T-score (obtained by comparison with young adults) and not to the Z-score (obtained with age- and sex-matched controls). In children and adolescents who have not yet achieved peak bone mass, BMD is usually and more appropriately referred to as Z-score, which is calculated by the formula: BMD of the patient – mean BMD of the control group/SD of the control group. However, unlike in adults, no studies identify threshold Z-scores in relation to fracture risk in children. Indeed, a recent statement by the International Society for Clinical Densitometry suggests avoiding the use of the terms osteopoenia and osteoporosis when referring to children, but rather using 'low bone mass' when BMD is less than 2 SD below age- and sex-matched controls.[4]

In recent years much attention has been paid to the metabolic disorders of bone encountered in children and adolescents affected by many chronic diseases,[5] because of the improved long-term outcome. In particular, it is now known that the systemic and focal inflammation that characterizes rheumatic diseases is often accompanied by adverse effects on the skeleton also in childhood.[6,7]

LOW BONE MASS IN CHILDHOOD ARTHRITIS (JUVENILE IDIOPATHIC/RHEUMATOID/ CHRONIC ARTHRITIS)

In juvenile idiopathic arthritis (JIA) there are multiple risk factors known to be associated with decreased bone mass (Table 11.1), and many studies have been published on this subject.[8–26] Active arthritis has an osteopoenic effect, both around affected joints and systemically, by means of a complex and still partly unknown network of proinflammatory cytokines. In particular, interleukin-6 (IL-6) is known to have a profound effect on bone metabolism.[27,28] IL-6 knockout mice do not develop osteoporosis after ovariectomy, and the same effect can be obtained in experimental models after IL-6 neutralization by specific antibodies.[29] The balance between bone formation and resorption is

Table 11.1. Risk factors for osteoporosis in children with juvenile idiopathic arthritis.

Active inflammatory disease

Decreased mobility

Glucocorticoid medication

Protein/caloric malnutrition

Poor calcium/vitamin D intake

Decreased sun exposure

Decreased height and weight

Pubertal delay

controlled by a variety of factors, and studies on this subject have yielded conflicting results.[30,31]

Moreover, the discovery of the receptor activator of NF-κB (RANK) signalling pathway has provided insight into the mechanisms of osteoclastogenesis and activation of bone resorption. In JIA this might be an important mechanism of secondary bone loss, and our group has provided preliminary data on osteoprotogerin (OPG) and RANK ligand (RANKL) in children with JIA. A higher OPG/RANKL ratio was found in patients with JIA, likely as a result of a compensatory production of OPG. Moreover, the presence of the T allele of the OPG gene appeared to be associated with low BMD in our study.[32] Among other genetic characteristics that may play a role in the osteopoenia secondary to JIA, we have also studied the polymorphisms in the calcitonin receptor (CTR) and vitamin D receptor (VDR) genes. In a group of 50 patients with JIA, patients with the TT genotype had lumbar BMD (L-BMD) that was lower in comparison to those with the CC genotype. For VDR gene polymorphism, we observed that patients with the ff genotype had lower L-BMD in comparison with the FF genotype. Patients with heterozygosity for the two genotypes showed intermediate L-BMD.[33]

Effects of childhood arthritis on bone mass in adulthood

Zak et al.[34] have assessed BMD of the hip and spine in 65 young adults with a history of juvenile chronic arthritis (JCA). They found that BMD was significantly lower (and the frequency of osteopoenia and osteoporosis was higher) in patients than in age-, sex-, height- and weight-matched healthy controls. Factors associated with a lower BMD included active disease at the time of the study, baseline erosions, higher Steinbrocker functional class, polyarticular course and chronic corticosteroid treatment. The presence of JCA by itself explained about 20% of BMD variation. In another recent study[35] the impact of disease activity on peak bone mass was assessed in 229 young adults in their mid-twenties with juvenile arthritis, at a mean of period of 15 years after disease onset. Patients with persistent disease had a significantly lower BMD than did healthy subjects, while patients whose disease was in remission had a normal bone mass overall.

However, even in women with only a history of arthritis, BMD was significantly lower in the total body, but not in the lumbar spine or the radius. Moreover, almost half of the patients who were in remission had a history of pauciarticular arthritis. This type of disease is more frequent and more benign than the other childhood arthritides and could partly explain the discrepancies between the results of this study and those of Zak et al.,[34] where the percentage of patients with pauciarticular disease was lower. However, French et al.[36] observed that although many adults with a history of juvenile rheumatoid arthritis (JRA) have normal bone density, a substantial subset are osteopoenic, placing them at increased risk of fractures later in life. This observation is particularly striking given the predominance of patients with pauciarticular JRA in their population-based group.

Effect of drug treatment on BMD

One of the more serious side-effects of glucocorticoid therapy is the detrimental effect on bone mass, leading to osteoporosis.[37]

Glucocorticoids reduce bone formation and increase its resorption. The reduction in bone formation is thought to be due to a direct inhibitory effect on osteoblasts, while several mechanisms may account for the increased resorption. Corticosteroids directly increase osteoclast activity, decrease levels of sex steroids, and may decrease intestinal calcium absorption and increase its excretion, causing secondary hyperparathyroidism. The American College of Rheumatology revised guidelines for the prevention and treatment of glucocorticoid-induced osteoporosis in adult patients are also relevant to children and adolescents.[38] Recommendations include modification of lifestyle factors, weight-bearing physical exercise, calcium and vitamin D supplementation, avoidance/reduction of alcohol and tobacco consumption, and periodic measurement of BMD. A baseline measurement of BMD at the lumbar spine is therefore recommended when initiating long-term (>6 months) glucocorticoid therapy, and longitudinal measurements may be repeated periodically (as often as every 12 months) during treatment in order to monitor bone status.

The threshold for adverse skeletal effects of oral corticosteroids still remains to be defined in children. In a recent large study, Van Staa et al.[39] estimated the incidence rates of fractures of children taking oral corticosteroids. The medical records of general practitioners in the UK were used, and 37,562 children taking oral corticosteroids were compared to 345,748 control children taking non-systemic corticosteroids. Also, each child with a fracture ($n = 22,846$) was matched to one child without a fracture. The risk of fractures was increased in children with a history of frequent use of oral corticosteroids, with an odds ratio of 1.32 (95% CI: 1.03–1.69) for those who took four or more courses. Children who had discontinued oral corticosteroid treatment had fracture risks that were comparable with non-users. However, it has to be noted that this study refers mostly to patients who took short courses of steroids, unlike those used in rheumatic disorders; in fact, the most common indication for prescription of steroids was respiratory disease such as asthma.

The osteopoenic effect of methotrexate (MTX) has been described in children with malignancy treated with high-dose

MTX, and confirmed by in vitro studies.[40–44] Lower-dose MTX, now widely used in the treatment of JIA, was not associated with an osteopoenic effect in the studies of Henderson et al.[25,26] Moreover, our group has performed a study with the specific aim of evaluating possible effects of MTX on BMD of patients with JIA.[45] We studied 32 children with JIA for an average period of 18 months with serial BMD measurements during MTX treatment. BMD was measured by DXA on lumbar spine and total body. During MTX therapy the increase in BMD (4–5% per year) was smaller than in healthy controls, and increases in axial and appendicular BMD were similar. BMD, either as an absolute value or as the percentage variation from baseline, did not correlate with MTX dose or duration of therapy. Therefore, long-term, low-dose MTX does not seem to induce osteopoenia in children with JIA. Most likely, the significant beneficial effect on arthritis may counterbalance in vivo the demonstrated inhibitory effect on osteoblasts. This was further confirmed by Minaur et al.,[46,47] in both in vitro and in vivo studies.

Cyclosporin, a drug widely used in rheumatology for its immunosuppressive effects, can cause a high turnover osteopoenia.[48] The use of new drugs, such as mycophenolate mofetil and etanercept, and new therapeutical approaches, such as stem cell transplantation, will require specific studies to evaluate their impact on bone mass and bone metabolism, which is not yet fully understood. Stem cell transplantation seems to induce bone loss.[49]

OTHER CONNECTIVE TISSUE DISEASES

Children and adolescents with systemic lupus erythematosus (SLE), juvenile dermatomyositis (JDM) and the vasculitides are at risk for osteopoenia and/or osteoporosis – from the disease itself and from medical treatment. Corticosteroid therapy, often in high doses for prolonged periods of time, is the basis of treatment for all of these diseases, unlike JIA, where it is used in more selective situations. Moreover, the need to avoid sun exposure in SLE and limited mobility in JDM contribute to decreased

bone mineralization. Bone loss is a well-known complication of adult-onset SLE, while data on paediatric SLE are scarce in this regard. In a small study on juvenile SLE, Castro et al.[50] observed a non-significant decrease of spine BMD in 16 girls aged 6–17 years versus controls. On the contrary, Trapani et al.[51] observed a significant decrease of BMD in 20 young patients affected by juvenile SLE versus controls, both at baseline and after 1 year. Moreover, they found a significant inverse correlation between the cumulative dose of steroids and BMD. Both these studies are small, and more data are certainly needed.

Ellis et al.,[52] evaluating total body bone mineral content (BMC) in children with a novel Z-score prediction model, also included 29 children affected by JDM, and observed a reduced Z-score (<–1.5) in 27.6% of JDM cases. A recent study was performed on a cohort of patients with JDM.[53] Ten patients had active disease, while five had inactive disease and had not taken steroids for an average of 6 years. Osteopoenia or frank osteoporosis were observed in the majority of patients, and persisted or worsened in patients with ongoing active disease, but was still present also after a remission. Three patients with vertebral compression fractures were treated with bisphosphonates with a significant increase in bone mass. The number of JDM patients studied until now is, however, quite small, and further studies are required to better define bone damage in this disease and to identify the best treatment for the prevention of osteoporosis.

DIAGNOSTIC TOOLS

For effective prevention and treatment of osteoporosis, a correct measurement of bone mass or BMD is fundamental (Table 11.2). Today the gold standard is considered to be dual X-ray absorptiometry (DXA). It is preferable to other methods such as single- or dual-photon absorptiometry because of its increased precision and accuracy, low radiation dose and increased speed of scans. However, equipment costs limit its use to referral centres. With BMD measurement in paediatric patients there are some general problems and problems specific to the measure-

Table 11.2. Comparison of different methods for bone density measurement.

Method	Site	Precision (%)	Accuracy (%)	Dose (mRem)	Time (min)	Comments
SPA	Radius	1–3	4–5	5–18	15	Rarely used
DPA	Spine, femur	2–4	3–10	1–15	20–30	Rarely used
DXA	Spine, hip, radius, total body	1	3–9	1–3 (0.1 if pDXA)	10–20	Gold standard (best method available today); machinery is expensive
QCT	Spine	1–3	5–20	100–1000	10–20	Promising (true volumetric density measured), but still a research tool
US	Finger, heel	3		0	1	Ease of scan; fast, no radiations; cheap; portable

SPA, single-photon absorptiometry; DPA, dual-photon absorptiometry; DXA, dual X-ray absorptiometry; pDXA, peripheral DXA (at distal radius); QCT, quantitative computed tomography; US, ultrasound. Spine, lumbar spine. Time, time for scanning.

ment technique. In a recent study,[54] it was found that the diagnosis of osteoporosis in children is often due to misinterpretation of DXA scans. Thirty (88%) of the scans revised had at least one error in interpretation. The most frequent error was the use of a T-score (SD score compared with young adults) to diagnose osteoporosis, which is inappropriate for children. Other errors included use of a reference database that does not consider gender or ethnic differences, incorrect bone map, inattention to short stature and other measurement or statistical errors.

When interpreting the results of DXA scans, one has also to consider that, in children, even a stable BMD value, i.e. a lack of BMD increase during a period of skeletal growth, represents an abnormality of bone metabolism. Moreover, it is important to recognize that DXA gives a two-dimensional (areal) view of the bones, measuring areas and not true (i.e. three-dimensional) density. Therefore, comparison of bones of the same true density but of different sizes might artificially give different results. Also, 'areal' BMD should be interpreted in relation not only to age-matched controls, but also to height and weight. Unfortunately, published paediatric standards for BMD are limited; the lack of normal control values often makes the interpretation of data difficult. Finally, growth and pubertal status, frequently delayed in children with rheumatic diseases, are fundamental in the process of bone acquisition and should always be taken into account when comparing patients and controls.

Very few of the diagnostic tools currently in use are able to measure the true bone density (content divided by volume, and not by area). Quantitative computerized tomography (QCT) is one of these; however, this technique delivers a larger radiation dose than DXA and is limited in availability. In a recent cross-sectional study, Roth et al.[55] analysed bone density and bone geometry in 57 children with JIA using peripheral QCT. They found that trabecular density was affected only in polyarticular JIA and cortical density was normal in all subgroups, and concluded that an abnormal bone geometry was present. The thinned bony cortices might predispose to fractures even though cortical bone density itself is normal.

The quantitative high-frequency sound (ultrasound) technique is a radiation-free procedure that measures the transmission of ultrasound waves through bones such as the heel. With this technique the speed of sound and the broadband ultrasound attenuation (BUA) can be determined. Paediatric studies are in an early development stage; we showed a good correlation between contact ultrasound bone analyser (CUBA) and DXA in 53 children with rheumatic diseases.[56] The study group included 29 patients with JIA, 13 with SLE and 11 with JDM, with a mean age of 13 years. Calcaneal BUA was significantly correlated with lumbar DXA ($P < 0.001$), with a significant correlation also between the mean percentages of variation in 22 patients who were evaluated prospectively with both methods. We have also used this technique in a prospective follow-up study, and believe that contact ultrasound bone analysis at the calcaneus is a useful tool in the assessment and monitoring of bone status in children with chronic rheumatic disorders.[57,58] Low cost, portability, ease of use and absence of radiation are all potential

advantages of CUBA over DXA. Moreover, ultrasound may give information on bone structure as well, and further studies in this regard are warranted. However, this technique is largely operator-dependent, and the presence of arthritis or intra-articular drug injection in adjacent joints must be taken into account when interpreting the results.

PREVENTION

Prevention of osteopoenia and osteoporosis during the critical developmental stages of skeletal maturation contributes to decrease fracture risk later in life. It is now known that prevention of osteoporosis in children with arthritis is closely linked to the control of disease activity, and hopefully with the newer therapeutic options the frequency of this complication will decrease.

Optimal calcium intake is also very important, because it accounts for 5–10% of the variance in peak bone mass. Adequate dietary calcium intake is therefore recommended in all children, according to the published guidelines (800 mg/day from 1 to 5 years, 1200 mg/day from 6 to 10 years, and 1500 mg/day from 11 to 24 years); doses might be higher during corticosteroid treatment. Likewise, vitamin D intake should be maximized to at least 400 U per day and, when not contraindicated, sun exposure should be recommended in order to facilitate vitamin D synthesis. Control of chronic illness, adequate nutrition and appropriate weight-bearing activity are other determinants of bone accretion. Finally, smoking and excessive alcohol consumption in adolescents should be avoided because they are likely to be risk factors for a decreased peak bone mass.

THERAPY

Studies on drug treatment of osteoporosis in childhood are relatively new. It is always difficult to perform controlled trials in uncommon diseases, and there should be additional caution when interpreting the results of published studies. For example, bone loss tends to taper or plateau after 6–12 months of corticosteroid treatment, and during this time period any given therapy might show benefit. Moreover, there are methodological problems, some of which are specific to childhood (described earlier when discussing the limitations of diagnostic tools and interpretation of results). Calcium and vitamin D supplementation might have some benefit in mild disease, but severely affected patients need more potent intervention.[59] There is a paucity of intervention studies of calcium/vitamin D supplementation in paediatric rheumatic diseases, and pharmacological interventions with vitamin D in children with arthritis have yielded conflicting results. In a pilot study, we administered calcifediol (0.5 mg/kg/day) to 15 children with JIA and low levels of 25-hydroxyvitamin D.[60] Their BMD was markedly reduced, and their yearly increase of bone density was <2%, in comparison to about 11% in age-matched healthy controls. The administration of calcifediol for 1 year induced a significant rise in 25-hydroxyvitamin D and was followed by an increase in bone mass ($8.9 \pm 2.4\%$/year), similar to that of normal controls.

There was a significant correlation between the increase in 25-hydroxyvitamin D levels and the increase in BMD values ($P < 0.02$). Other investigators have used this approach. Reed et al.[61] supplemented 13 children with JIA with 25-hydroxyvitamin D for 1 year, but no significant BMD increase was obtained. Warady et al.[20] administered calcium and vitamin D for 6 months to 10 children with rheumatic diseases who were taking corticosteroids. In this crossover study patients were subsequently followed for 6 months without added supplements and acted as their own controls. The results were inconsistent, only some patients having an increase in BMD. The small size of these studies, and differences in the selection of patients and in the methods used, may all account for these discrepancies.

Among promising candidates for treatment of juvenile osteoporosis, growth hormone (GH) has been shown to be effective in improving the bone mass of patients with chronic arthritis. Rooney et al.[62] measured bone mineral content in 20 children with severe JCA (17 of whom were treated with corticosteroids) before and after a 1-year trial with recombinant human GH. BMC increased during the treatment period and correlated with increasing height. In an uncontrolled study, Simon et al.[63] observed that in 14 children treated for 1 year with GH and followed for 2 more years after stopping it, height velocity and height as well as lean mass increased significantly during the year on GH, but fell to pretreatment values after withdrawal. The authors also observed an increase in both formation and resorption bone markers during the treatment with GH. The same group showed[64] that a significant increase in bone turnover was present in 14 children with systemic JRA on long-term steroid therapy, treated with GH for 1 year. Bone turnover returned to the pre-GH velocity after discontinuation of the growth hormone. Finally, they also showed[65] that lumbar bone mineral density increased by 36.6% in 13 JIA patients treated with GH for 3 years. Bechtold et al.[66] followed 11 children with JIA treated with GH over 4 years, and it is worth noting that in this study BMD was converted to volumetric BMD (vBMD) after adjustment for vertebral size. Despite biochemical changes, there was no statistically significant improvement of vBMD, with a percentage increase comparable to healthy children. Long-term controlled studies are therefore needed to determine the risks and benefits of GH therapy in JIA and the real impact on bone mass and bone turnover.[67] Moreover, GH must be given almost every day by injection, is expensive, is not free of potential side-effects, and there are legal limitations to its prescription in several countries. Therefore, it is the author's opinion that its therapeutic use for osteoporosis should be restricted to patients with severe growth retardation as well.

Calcitonin inhibits bone resorption by osteoclasts and is useful treatment for osteoporosis, reducing vertebral and hip fractures in adult patients. Its main side-effects are gastrointestinal (nausea and vomiting). It can be administered by injection, orally or intranasally. It has been used only rarely in paediatric rheumatic diseases, but two Japanese groups have reported a good efficacy and safety profile in steroid-induced osteoporosis in children with nephrotic syndrome, and in osteogenesis imperfecta.[68,69] Moreover, a recent open study[70] of intranasal salmon calcitonin in 10 children with JIA showed a decrease in bone resorption markers and an increase in BMD (7.2–9.5%/year) measured with dual-photon absorptiometry. However, despite the fact that it can rapidly improve symptoms of vertebral fractures, calcitonin treatment for osteoporosis in paediatric patients is still considered to be experimental. A therapeutic rationale for the use of fluoride in osteoporosis is based on its ability to stimulate osteoblasts to make new bone. However, at high concentrations fluoride may cause the formation of abnormally mineralized bone of impaired quality.[71] Indeed, some studies in adults have shown that there was an increase in the number of fractures, especially at higher doses.[72,73]

Bisphosphonates

Of all the new agents in clinical use, bisphosphonates (BPs) seem to be the most promising. BPs are analogues of pyrophosphate, and several chemical features contribute to their biological action: the P–C–P moiety gives these compounds the ability to adsorb to hydroxyapatite and target bone, while variations in the side-chains determine the potency and spectrum of action of each compound. BPs are selectively concentrated in bone and they inhibit bone resorption by interfering with the action of osteoclasts. Some of the biochemical mechanisms that account for these effects have recently been elucidated.[74–78] BPs have been extensively used in adults; until recently their use in paediatric patients has been limited by fear of adverse effects on a growing skeleton, because of the potential risks to a foetus if administered to a girl approaching child-bearing age, and because the drug is not appreciably eliminated in the short to medium term. More recently, BPs have been shown to be quite safe, at least in the short term, even in paediatric patients, and their use has been expanding.[79–83]

The conditions for which BPs have been used in children are different from those for which BPs have been used in adults, and can be divided into four categories: primary defects in bone mineralization (juvenile idiopathic osteoporosis); bone matrix abnormalities (osteogenesis imperfecta);[84] bone abnormalities secondary to systemic diseases or treatments; and soft-tissue calcifications. Adverse effects in children have not been reported in greater frequency than in adults (Table 11.3). With the newer, nitrogen-containing BPs, osteomalacia does not seem to be a problem, although it has been reported in adults treated with etidronate.[85] Hypocalcaemia and fever are infrequent and transient, and mild abdominal discomfort or dyspepsia are also occasional complaints. Radiological alterations described in prepubertal patients include band-like metaphyseal sclerosis and concentric epi- and apophyseal sclerosis.[86] However, no adverse effects on growth have been noted, even after a long follow-up, and after drug discontinuation the radiographic abnormalities tend to disappear. Bone biopsies of treated patients showed normal bone structure and no mineralization defects.[87]

An open multicentre prospective study evaluated the safety and efficacy of alendronate in children with rheumatic diseases who were either on chronic corticosteroid treatment or had a low

Table 11.3. Adverse effects of bisphosphonates.

Observed

Increase in body temperature following intravenous infusion, flu-like symptoms

Nausea, dyspepsia, oesophagitis, abdominal pain, diarrhoea, constipation

Hypocalcaemia, hypophosphataemia, hypomagnesaemia

Transient lymphopoenia

Iritis, conjunctivitis, uveitis, scleritis

Mineralization defects (with etidronate), transient skeletal pain, reversible epiphyseal and metaphyseal sclerosis in growing skeleton

Feared but not observed

Irreversible and permanent effect on bone remodelling

Damage to growth plates and impairment in linear growth

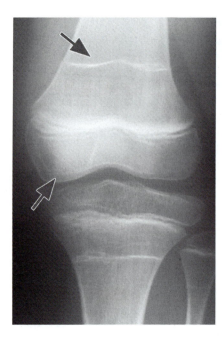

Figure 11.1. Radiological alterations (metaphyseal lines) following treatment with alendronate in a pre-pubertal child.

bone mineral density determined by DXA.[88] Forty-three patients (30 females and 13 males), with JIA (17 patients), SLE (12), JDM (7) or other connective tissue diseases (7) were studied. Mean age at study entrance was 12.9 ± 3.7 years; 14 patients were post-pubertal. Alendronate was administered orally at the daily dosage of 5 or 10 mg according to body weight (less or greater than 20 kg). Baseline Z-scores ranged from −1.3 to −5.3. Each patient underwent serial clinical and laboratory evaluations. Lumbar spine bone mineral density (BMD) was measured at baseline and after 6 and 12 months using a standardized protocol, and Z-scores were calculated by comparing results with age- and sex-matched controls from a reference population of healthy subjects. There was a substantial increase of bone mass in all children, with an average BMD increase of 14.2 ± 10% after 1 year. One-third of patients attained normal BMD. In comparison, BMD had increased by only 1% in the 16 study patients followed during the year immediately preceding onset of alendronate therapy. Height increased by an average of 4.3 ± 3.7 cm during the study period. Knee radiographs performed in pre-pubertal children showed absence of rickets and presence of metaphyseal lines (Figure 11.1). The drug was well tolerated, except for occasional abdominal pain and one episode of oesophagitis. Variations in parameters of bone metabolism and disease activity were also evaluated.[89] Relevant variables entered into a database included demographic and anthropometric data, biochemical parameters of bone metabolism (serum levels of Ca, P, bone-specific alkaline phosphatase, deoxypyridinolines, osteocalcin, parathyroid hormone and urinary procollagen telopeptide), serological markers of inflammation, and BMD values. Over the first 12-month treatment period, both bone resorption and bone formation parameters significantly decreased, while over the same time period none of the disease activity indices changed significantly. BMD Z-score variations did not correlate with variations of inflammatory parameters (erythrocyte sedimentation rate, matrix metalloproteinase-3, IL-6, C-reactive protein). It was concluded that the observed BMD increase was not secondary to a change in disease activity, but was most likely an effect of the biological activity of alendronate. After the first year, 10 patients continued treatment for another year, while 20 stopped treatment. During the second year the treated group showed an additional BMD increase of 9.6 ± 3.8%, while in the untreated group BMD increase was only 3.6 ± 4.9%. Seven patients of this latter group had an actual BMD decrease.

We concluded that alendronate significantly improves bone mass in children or adolescents with rheumatic diseases and secondary osteoporosis. However, many questions still remain unanswered. Will the positive effects last over time? For how long can this treatment be given? Will bone be more resistant to fracture? Are there any potential risks for young women in their child-bearing years with respect to foetal toxicity? Will there be any unexpected medium- to long-term adverse effects? Will newer bisphosphonates be safer and/or more effective? At present, BPs should be considered as valuable tools, even in paediatric patients, but only for treating severe osteoporotic disease or in the setting of experimental protocols.

PRACTICE POINTS

- There are multiple risk factors involved in increasing the risk of osteoporosis in patients with paediatric rheumatic diseases.

- Optimal achievement of peak bone mass during childhood and adolescence is essential in order to minimize the future risk of fracture.

- New treatments such as bisphosphonates are now available, although their use for paediatric patients has been limited.

RESEARCH AGENDA

- Further studies aimed at delineating other important risk factors in the prediction of fracture and bone mineral density.

- Studies on new diagnostic tools, such as computed tomography.

- Longer follow-up for patients treated with bisphosphonates, in order to better understand the long-term safety of these compounds when administered during the paediatric age.

REFERENCES

1. Cassidy JT. Osteopenia and osteoporosis in children. *Clin Exp Rheumatol* 1999; **17**: 245–250.
2. Ralston SH. The genetics of osteoporosis. *Bone* 1999; **25**: 85–86.
3. Kanis JA, Melton LJ, Christiansen C et al. The diagnosis of osteoporosis. *J Bone Miner Res* 1994; **9**: 1137–1140.
4. Lewiecki EM, Watts NB, McClung MR et al. Official positions of the International Society for Clinical Densitometry *J Clin Endocrinol Metab* 2004; **89**: 3651 3655.
5. Ward LM & Glorieux FH. The spectrum of pediatric osteoporosis. In: Glorieux FH, Pettifor JM & Jüppner H, eds. *Pediatric Bone: Biology and Diseases.* Amsterdam: Academic Press, 2003; 401–442.
6. Rabinovich CE. Osteoporosis: a pediatric perspective. *Arthritis Rheum* 2004; **50**: 1023–1025.
7. McDonagh JE. Osteoporosis in juvenile idiopathic arthritis. *Curr Opin Rheumatol* 2001; **13**: 399–404.
8. Cetin A, Celiker R, Dincer F et al. Bone mineral density in children with juvenile chronic arthritis. *Clin Rheumatol* 1998; **17**: 551–553.
9. Falcini F, Ermini M, Bagnoli F et al. Bone turnover is reduced in children with juvenile rheumatoid arthritis. *J Endocrinol Invest* 1998; **21**: 31–36.
10. Havelka S, Vavrincova P & Stepan J. Metabolic bone status in young women with juvenile chronic arthritis. *J Rheumatol* 1993; **37**: 14–16.
11. Henderson CJ & Lovell DJ. Bone mineral content in juvenile rheumatoid arthritis – pilot project results. *J Rheumatol* 1991; **18**: 1–22.
12. Hillman L, Cassidy JT, Johnson L et al. Vitamin D metabolism and bone mineralization in children with juvenile rheumatoid arthritis. *J Pediatr* 1994; **121**: 910–916.
13. Hopp R, Degan J, Gallagher JC et al. Estimation of bone mineral density in children with juvenile rheumatoid arthritis. *J Rheumatol* 1991; **18**: 1235–1239.
14. Kotaniemi A, Savolainen A, Kontiainen H et al. Estimation of central osteopenia in children with chronic polyarthritis treated with glucocorticoids. *Pediatrics* 1993; **91**: 1127–1130.
15. Kotaniemi A. Growth retardation and bone loss as determinants of axial osteopenia in juvenile chronic arthritis. *Scand J Rheumatol* 1997; **26**: 14–18.
16. Pereira RMR, Corrente JE, Chahade WH et al. Evaluation by dual X-ray absorptiometry (DXA) of bone mineral density in children with juvenile chronic arthritis. *Clin Exp Rheumatol* 1998; **16**: 495–501.
17. Polito C, Strano CG, Rea L et al. Reduced bone mineral content and normal serum osteocalcin in non steroid-treated patients with juvenile rheumatoid arthritis. *Ann Rheum Dis* 1995; **54**: 193–196.
18. Rabinovich EC. Bone mineral status in juvenile rheumatoid arthritis. *J Rheumatol* 2000; **27**: 34–37.
19. Varamos S, Ansell BM & Reeve J. Vertebral collapse in juvenile chronic arthritis: its relationships with glucocorticoid therapy. *Calcif Tissue Int* 1987; **41**: 75–78.
20. Warady BD, Lindsley CB, Robinson RG et al. Effects of nutritional supplementation on bone mineral status of children with rheumatic diseases receiving corticosteroid therapy. *J Rheumatol* 1994; **21**: 530–535.
21. Pepmueller PH, Cassidy JT, Allen SH et al. Bone mineralization and bone mineral metabolism in children with juvenile rheumatoid arthritis. *Arthritis Rheum* 1996; **39**: 746–757.
22. Brik R, Keidar Z, Schapira D et al. Bone mineral density and turnover in children with systemic juvenile chronic arthritis. *J Rheumatol* 1998; **25**: 990–992.
23. Kotaniemi A, Savolainen A, Kroger H et al. Development of bone mineral density at the lumbar spine and femoral neck in juvenile chronic arthritis. A prospective one year follow-up study *J Rheumatol* 1998; **25**: 2450–2455.
24. Kotaniemi A, Savolainen A, Kroger H et al. Weight-bearing physical activity, calcium intake, systemic glucocorticoids, chronic inflammation, and body constitution as determinants of lumbar and femoral bone in juvenile chronic arthritis. *Scand J Rheumatol* 1999; **28**: 19–26.
25. Henderson CJ, Cawkwell GD, Specker BL et al. Predictors of total body bone mineral density in non-corticosteroid-treated prepubertal children with juvenile rheumatoid arthritis. *Arthritis Rheum* 1997; **40**: 1967–1975.
26. Henderson CJ, Specker BL, Sierra RI et al. Total-body bone mineral content in non-corticosteroid-treated postpubertal females with juvenile rheumatoid arthritis. Frequency of osteopenia and contributing factors. *Arthritis Rheum* 2000; **43**: 531–540.
27. Manolagas SC & Jilka RL. Bone marrow, cytokines, and bone remodeling. Emerging insights into the pathophysiology of osteoporosis. *N Engl J Med* 1995; **332**: 305–311.
28. Jilka RL, Hangoc G, Girasole G et al. Increased osteoclast development after estrogen loss: mediation by interleukin-6. *Science* 1992; **257**: 88–91.
29. Poli V, Balena R, Fattori E et al. Interleukin-6 deficient mice are protected from bone loss caused by estrogen depletion. *EMBO J* 1994; **13**: 1189–1196.
30. Pereira RMR, Falco V, Corrente JE et al. Abnormalities in the biochemical markers of bone turnover in children with juvenile chronic arthritis. *Clin Exp Rheumatol* 1999; **17**: 251–255.
31. Rabinovich CE. Bone metabolism in childhood rheumatic disease. *Rheum Dis Clin North Am* 2002; **28**: 655–667.
32. Masi L, Simonini G, Piscitelli E et al. Osteoprotegerin (OPG)/RANK-L system in juvenile idiopathic arthritis: is there a potential modulating role for OPG/RANK-L in bone injury? *J Rheumatol* 2004; **31**: 986–991.
33. Masi L, Cimaz R, Simonini G et al. Association of low bone mass with vitamin D receptor gene and calcitonin receptor gene polymorphism in juvenile idiopathic arthritis. *J Rheumatol* 2002; **29**: 2225–2231.
34. Zak M, Hassager C, Lovell DJ et al. Assessment of bone mineral density in adults with a history of juvenile chronic arthritis: a cross-sectional long-term follow-up study. *Arthritis Rheum* 1999; **42**: 790–798.
35. Haugen M, Lien G, Flato B et al. Young adults with juvenile arthritis in remission attain normal peak bone mass at the lumbar spine and forearm. *Arthritis Rheum* 2000; **43**: 1504–1510.
36. French AR, Mason T, Nelson AM et al. Osteopenia in adults with a history of juvenile rheumatoid arthritis. A population based study. *J Rheumatol* 2002; **29**: 1065–1070.
37. Mul D, van Suijlekom-Smit LW, ten Cate R et al. Bone mineral density and body composition and influencing factors in children with rheumatic diseases treated with corticosteroids. *J Pediatr Endocrinol Metab* 2002; **15**: 187–192.
38. American College of Rheumatology ad hoc Committee on glucocorticoid-induced osteoporosis. Recommendations for the prevention and treatment of glucocorticoid-induced osteoporosis. 2001 Update. *Arthritis Rheum* 2001; **44**: 1496–1503.

39. Van Staa TP, Cooper C, Leufkens HGM et al. Children and the risk of fractures caused by oral corticosteroids. *J Bone Miner Res* 2003; **18**: 913–918.

40. Bologna C, Edno L, Anaya JM et al. Methotrexate concentrations in synovial membrane and trabecular and cortical bone in rheumatoid arthritis patients. *Arthritis Rheum* 1994; **37**: 1770–1773.

41. May KP, Mercill D, McDermott MT et al. The effect of methotrexate on mouse bone cells in culture. *Arthritis Rheum* 1996; **39**: 489–494.

42. May KP, West SG, McDermott MT et al. The effect of low-dose methotrexate on bone metabolism and histomorphometry in rats. *Arthritis Rheum* 1994; **37**: 201–206.

43. Scheven BA, van der Veen MJ, Damen CA et al. Effects of methotrexate on human osteoblasts in vitro: modulation by 1,25-dihydroxyvitamin D₃. *J Bone Miner Res* 1995; **10**: 874–880.

44. Uehara R, Suzuki Y, Ichikawa Y. Methotrexate (MTX) inhibits osteoblastic differentiation in vitro: possible mechanism of MTX osteopathy. *J Rheumatol* 2001; **28**: 251–256.

45. Bianchi ML, Cimaz R, Galbiati E et al. Bone mass change during methotrexate treatment in patients with juvenile rheumatoid arthritis. *Osteoporosis Int* 1999; **10**: 20–25.

46. Minaur NJ, Kounali D, Vedi S et al. Methotrexate in the treatment of rheumatoid arthritis. II: In vivo effects on bone mineral density. *Rheumatology (Oxford)* 2002; **41**: 741–749.

47. Minaur NJ, Jefferiss C, Bhalla AK et al. Methotrexate in the treatment of rheumatoid arthritis. I: In vitro effects on cells of the osteoblast lineage. *Rheumatology (Oxford)* 2002; **41**: 735–740.

48. Abdelhadi M, Ericzon BG, Hultenby K et al. Structural skeletal impairment induced by immunosuppressive therapy in rats: cyclosporine A vs tacrolimus. *Transplant Int* 2002; **15**: 180–187.

49. Tauchmanova L, Serio B, Del Puente A et al. Long-lasting bone damage detected by dual-energy X-ray absorptiometry, phalangeal osteosonogrammetry, and in vitro growth of marrow stromal cells after allogeneic stem cell transplantation. *J Clin Endocrinol Metab* 2002; **87**: 5058–5065.

50. Castro TC, Terreri MT, Szejnfeld VL et al. Bone mineral density in juvenile systemic lupus erythematosus. *Braz J Med Biol Res* 2002; **35**: 1159–1163.

51. Trapani S, Civinini R, Ermini M et al. Osteoporosis in juvenile systemic lupus erythematosus: a longitudinal study on the effects of steroids on bone mineral density. *Rheumatol Int* 1998; **18**: 45–49.

52. Ellis KJ, Shypailo RJ, Hardin DS et al. Z score prediction model for assessment of bone mineral content in pediatric diseases. *J Bone Miner Res* 2001; **16**: 1658–1664.

53. Stewart WA, Acott PD, Salisbury SR et al. Bone mineral density in juvenile dermatomyositis: assessment using dual X-ray absorptiometry. *Arthritis Rheum* 2003; **48**: 2294–2298.

54. Gafni RI & Baron J. Overdiagnosis of osteoporosis in children due to misinterpretation of dual-energy X-ray absorptiometry (DEXA). *J Pediatr* 2004; **144**: 253–257.

55. Roth J, Palm C, Scheunemann I et al. Musculoskeletal abnormalities of the forearm in patients with juvenile idiopathic arthritis relate mainly to bone geometry. *Arthritis Rheum* 2004; **50**: 1277–1285.

56. Falcini F, Bindi G, Ermini M et al. Comparison of quantitative calcaneal ultrasound and dual energy X-ray absorptiometry in the evaluation of osteoporotic risk in children with chronic rheumatic diseases. *Calcif Tissue Int* 2000; **67**: 19–23.

57. Falcini F, Bindi G, Simonini G et al. Bone status evaluation with calcaneal ultrasound in children with chronic rheumatic diseases. A one year followup study. *J Rheumatol* 2003; **30**: 179–184.

58. Simonini G, Cimaz R & Falcini F. Usefulness of bone ultrasound techniques in pediatric rheumatic diseases. *J Rheumatol* 2005; **32**: 198–199.

59. Adachi JD & Ioannidis G. Calcium and vitamin D therapy in corticosteroid-induced bone loss: what is the evidence? *Calcif Tissue Int* 1999; **65**: 332–336.

60. Bianchi ML, Bardare M, Galbiati E et al. Bone development in juvenile rheumatoid arthritis. In: Schonau E & Matkovic V, eds. *Paediatric Osteology. Prevention of Osteoporosis – A Paediatric Task?* Singapore: Elsevier Science, 1998; 173–181.

61. Reed A, Haugen M, Pachman L et al. 25-Hydroxyvitamin D therapy in children with active juvenile rheumatoid arthritis. Short-term effects on serum osteocalcin levels and bone mineral density. *J Pediatr* 1991; **119**: 657–660.

62. Rooney M, Davies UM, Reeve J et al. Bone mineral content and bone mineral metabolism: changes after growth hormone treatment in juvenile chronic arthritis. *J Rheumatol* 2000; **27**: 1073–1081.

63. Simon D, Prewar A & Czernichow P. Treatment of juvenile rheumatoid arthritis with growth hormone. *Horm Res* 2000; **53**: 82–86.

64. Touati G, Ruiz JC, Porquet D et al. Effects on bone metabolism of one year recombinant human growth hormone administration to children with juvenile chronic arthritis undergoing chronic steroid therapy. *J Rheumatol* 2000; **27**: 1287–1293.

65. Simon D, Lucidarme N, Prieur AM et al. Effects on growth and body composition of growth hormone treatment in children with juvenile idiopathic arthritis requiring steroid therapy. *J Rheumatol* 2003; **30**: 2492–2499.

66. Bechtold S, Ripperger P, Bonfig W et al. Bone mass development and bone metabolism in juvenile idiopathic arthritis: treatment with growth hormone for 4 years. *J Rheumatol* 2004; **31**: 1407–1412.

67. Bechtold S, Ripperger P, Muhlbayer D et al. GH therapy in juvenile chronic arthritis: results of a two-year controlled study on growth and bone. *J Clin Endocrinol Metab* 2001; **86**: 5737–5744.

68. Nishioka T, Kurayama H, Yasuda T et al. Nasal administration of salmon calcitonin for prevention of glucocorticoid-induced osteoporosis in children with nephrosis. *J Pediatr* 1991; **118**: 703–707.

69. Nishi Y, Hamamoto K, Kajiyama M et al. Effect of long-term calcitonin therapy by injection and nasal spray on the incidence of fractures in osteogenesis imperfecta. *J Pediatr* 1992; **121**: 477–480.

70. Siamopoulou A, Challa A, Kapoglou P et al. Effects of intranasal salmon calcitonin in juvenile idiopathic arthritis: an observational study. *Calcif Tissue Int* 2001; **69**: 25–30.

71. Pak CY, Zerwekh JE & Antich P. Anabolic effects of fluoride on bone. *Trends Endocrinol Metab* 1995; **7**: 229–234.

72. Lane N. Osteoporosis and metabolic bone diseases. In: Klippel JH, ed. *Primer on the Rheumatic Diseases*. Atlanta: Arthritis Foundation, 1997; 385–390.

73. Lems WF, Jacobs WG, Bijlsma JW et al. Is the addition of sodium fluoride to cyclical etidronate beneficial in the treatment of corticosteroid-induced osteoporosis? *Ann Rheum Dis* 1997; **56**: 357–363.

74. Russell RGG & Rogers MJ. Bisphosphonates: from the laboratory to the clinic and back again. *Bone* 1999; **25**: 97–106.

75. Breuil V, Cosman F, Stein L et al. Osteoclast formation and activity in vitro: effects of alendronate. *J Bone Miner Res* 1998; **13**: 1721–1729.

76. Fisher GE, Rogers MJ, Halasy JM et al. Alendronate mechanism of action: geranylgeraniol, an intermediate in the mevalonate pathway, prevents inhibition of osteoclast formation, bone resorption, and kinase activation in vitro. *Proc Natl Acad Sci USA* 1999; **96**: 133–138.

77. Van Beek E, Lowik C, Van Der Pluijm G et al. The role of geranylgeranylation in bone resorption and its suppression by bisphosphonates in fetal bone explants in vitro: a clue to the mechanism of action of nitrogen-containing bisphosphonates. *J Bone Miner Res* 1999; **14**: 722–729.

78. Grove JE, Brown RJ & Watts DJ. The intracellular target for the antiresorptive aminobisphosphonate drugs in *Dictyostelium discoideum* is the enzyme farnesyl diphosphate synthase. *J Bone Miner Res* 2000; **15**: 971–981.

79. Falcini F, Trapani S, Ermini M et al. Intravenous administration of alendronate counteracts the in vivo effects of glucocorticoids on bone remodelling. *Calcif Tissue Int* 1996; **58**: 166–169.

80. Shaw NJ, Boivin CM & Crabtree NJ. Intravenous pamidronate in juvenile osteoporosis. *Arch Dis Child* 2000; **83**: 143–145.

81. Shoemaker LR. Expanding role of bisphosphonate therapy in children. *J Pediatr* 1999; **134**: 264–267.

82. Srivastava T & Alon US. Bisphosphonates: from grandparents to grandchildren. *Clin Pediatr* 1999; **38**: 687–702.

83. Noguera A, Ros JB, Pavia C et al. Bisphosphonates, a new treatment for glucocorticoid-induced osteoporosis in children. *J Pediatr Endocrinol Metab* 2003; **16**: 529–536.

84. Glorieux FH, Bishop NJ, Plotkin H et al. Cyclic administration of pamidronate in children with severe osteogenesis imperfecta. *N Engl J Med* 1998; **339**: 947–952.

85. Boyce BF, Fogelman I, Ralston S et al. Focal osteomalacia due to low-dose diphosphonate therapy in Paget's disease. *Lancet* 1984; **1**: 821–824.

86. Van Persijn van Meerten EL, Kroon HM et al. Epi- and metaphyseal changes in children causes by administration of bisphosphonates. *Radiology* 1992; **184**: 249–254.

87. Brumsen C, Hamdy NA & Papopoulos SE. Long-term effects of bisphosphonates on the growing skeleton: studies of young patients with severe osteoporosis. *Medicine (Baltimore)* 1997; **76**: 266–283.

88. Bianchi ML, Cimaz R, Bardare M et al. Efficacy and safety of alendronate for the treatment of osteoporosis in diffuse connective tissue diseases in children. *Arthritis Rheum* 2000; **43**: 1960–1966.

89. Cimaz R, Gattorno M, Sormani MP et al. Changes in markers of bone turnover and inflammatory parameters during alendronate therapy in pediatric patients with rheumatic disease. *J Rheumatol* 2002; **29**: 1786–1792.

Chapter 12

How to prevent fractures in the individual with osteoporosis

M. Kassim Javaid and Cyrus Cooper

FRACTURE IMPACT

At the age of 50 years, the remaining lifetime risk of at least one fracture of the hip, vertebral body or distal forearm approaches 40% among white women and 13% among white men (Table 12.1).[1] The most frequent site of fracture is the thoracolumbar spine, with prevalence rates of morphometric vertebral deformities being around 25% among white women in the USA aged 50 years and over.[2,3] Around two-thirds of these morphometric vertebral deformities are subclinical. Other skeletal sites linked with osteoporosis include the hand, rib, foot and toe.

Whilst fragility fractures of the proximal femur occur less frequently (lifetime risk = 18% among women aged 50 years), the mortality and morbidity associated with fractures at this site is considerably greater than that associated with vertebral deformity. Hip fractures invariably require hospitalization; 1 year following fracture, 27% of patients enter a nursing home for the first time, 40% are unable to walk independently, 60% have difficulty with at least one essential activity of daily living, and 80% are restricted in other activities such as driving and shopping. Mortality rates are increased among subjects with both hip and vertebral fractures; reductions in survival of around 15% are reported during the 5 years following fracture at both of these sites. The excess mortality in the case of vertebral deformities is apparent among patients with clinically diagnosed vertebral fracture, as well as those with asymptomatic, morphometric deformities. Figure 12.1 shows the age- and sex-specific incidence rates for fractures of the hip, distal forearm and vertebral body.

The economic burden of fragility fractures is considerable. In the USA, the care of these fractures costs around US $20 billion each year. In the UK, this figure totals UK £1.5 billion. The most expensive fracture is hip fracture, and around half of hip fracture costs arise from care required after departure from hospital. In the UK, 20% of all orthopaedic beds are occupied by patients with a hip fracture, and 19% of patients require long-term nursing care.

PATHOPHYSIOLOGY OF FRACTURE

Fracture incidence depends on two factors: bone strength and trauma. During the first three decades of life, fractures typically arise from high-energy trauma, such as road traffic accidents. Above the age of 65 years, around 90% of fractures result from a fall from standing height or less.[4] Reduced bone strength is therefore an important, modifiable, determinant of fracture risk in the elderly. Bone mineral density (BMD) is a major determinant of bone strength; dual-energy X-ray absorptiometric (DXA) measurements of BMD account for 75–90% of the variance in bone strength observed during in vitro and in vivo studies.[5] However, bone strength is determined by other aspects of bone structure, including size, geometry, microarchitecture and turnover.

Bone density in adult life is a function of the peak bone mass attained during early adulthood and the subsequent rate of bone loss. The two major causes of involutional bone loss are secondary hyperparathyroidism (consequent upon reduced calcium intake and hypovitaminosis D) and reduced physical activity. In addition, oestrogen deficiency predisposes to bone loss among women. Other important causes of bone loss include thinness, cigarette smoking, heavy alcohol

Table 12.1. The impact of osteoporotic fracture.

	Hip	Spine	Wrist
Lifetime risk (%)			
Women	14	11	13
Men	3	2	2
Cases/year	400,000	270,000	330,000
Hospitalization	100	2–10	22
Relative survival	0.83	0.82	1.00

Costs: All sites combined approx. UK £1.5 billion.
Reprinted with permission from: Cooper C. *Osteoporosis Int* 1999; **9**(Suppl. 2): S2–S8.[79]

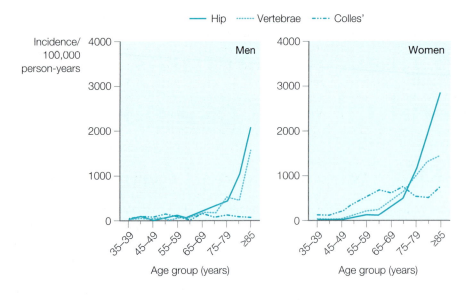

Figure 12.1. Epidemiology of fracture: age-specific incidence rates for men and women derived from the population of Rochester, MN, USA. Reproduced with permission from: Cooper C & Melton MJ. *Trends Endocrinol Metab* 1992; **3**: 224–229.[81]

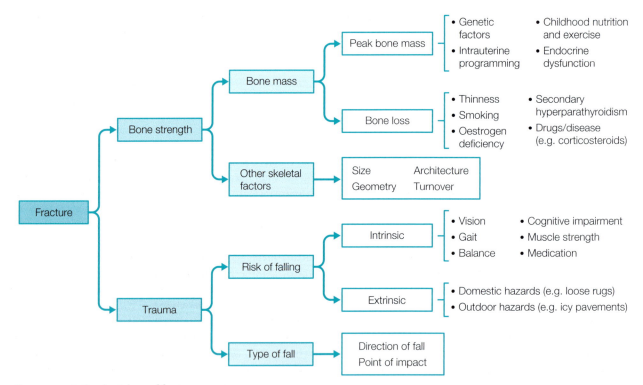

Figure 12.2. Pathophysiology of fracture.

consumption and drugs/diseases that secondarily predispose to osteoporosis (most importantly glucocorticoids). The multifactorial aetiology of fracture is illustrated in Figure 12.2.

PREVENTIVE STRATEGIES

For regulatory purposes, specific definitions of prevention and treatment are used in the context of osteoporosis. The term 'pre-

vention' is used to denote the prevention of bone loss in post-menopausal women with osteopoenia, whereas 'treatment' is defined as a reduction in fracture risk in post-menopausal women with osteoporosis. In clinical practice, this distinction between prevention and treatment is less appropriate, since many agents currently in use act fundamentally in the same manner, i.e. by inhibition of bone resorption. Furthermore, with the increasing evidence for a relatively rapid rate of treatment onset and offset for these interventions, there has been a move away from long-term preventive strategies towards the use of shorter-term therapy in high-risk individuals. The latter approach is supported by the demonstration of a significant reduction in vertebral and non-vertebral fracture rate among post-menopausal women with established osteoporosis after only 1 year of treatment with anti-resorptive agents.

A variety of bone mass measurement techniques is predictive of fracture, including DXA and quantitative ultrasound (QUS). Site-specific measurements are more predictive (relative risk (RR): 2.0–2.8 for 1 SD reduction in BMD) than assessments at more distant sites (RR: 1.5–2.2 for 1 SD reduction in BMD). The definition of osteoporosis, according to WHO guidelines,[6,7] is a T-score of <–2.5 for Caucasian post-menopausal women. Diagnostic thresholds for those patients using glucocorticoids tend to be lower, ranging from a T-score of –1 to –1.5.[8] Since different approaches to bone mineral measurement result in a variable classification of individuals as having osteoporosis, it has recently been proposed that the gold standard for diagnostic purposes is total hip BMD measured by DXA. However, the most rational utility of these measurements is in fracture risk prediction, and measures are already under way in order that bone mineral measurements be expressed as absolute fracture risk related to a relative time interval – for example, 10 years.

The aim of preventive strategies is to reduce the number of subsequent fractures in someone who has been diagnosed with low bone mass or who may already have fragility fractures. The first line in such preventive approaches is to correct the underlying cause of osteoporosis (hypogonadism in men, hyperthyroidism, hyperparathyroidism or glucocorticoid exposure).

LIFESTYLE MEASURES

The main lifestyle changes which may impact on the occurrence of fracture in patients with osteoporosis are smoking, exercise and diet. Smoking affects the skeleton in many ways; there is a direct toxic effect on new bone growth. Smoking may also reduce calcium absorption as well as increasing the risk of falling in elderly patients. The smoking-related increase in the risk of hip fracture is age related, with greater deleterious effects in the post-menopausal age group.[9] The effect of smoking cessation on bone mass and fracture rate has been studied in a 5-year Norwegian cohort. Despite adjustment for confounding variables such as body mass index, physical inactivity and self-reported poor health, ex-smokers still had an increased risk of hip fracture compared with non-smokers, but a lower risk than current smokers.[10,11] This would suggest that the effect of smoking is partially reversible, but perhaps a portion of the damage to the skeleton is irreversible. However, these findings have not been supported by a study of younger women, where there was no effect of smoking status on wrist fracture,[12] or by the Framingham Study, which found a reduction in the benefit from oestrogen replacement therapy (ERT) in smokers but no independent effect of smoking on BMD.[13]

The level of physical activity has been shown to be associated with increased bone mass[14] and also reduced fracture rate[15] in observational studies. Exercise therapy can be used to prevent fracture in those at risk or form part of a rehabilitation programme after a fracture. A study of patients with vertebral osteoporosis having twice-weekly exercise classes showed a significant reduction in back pain and a non-significant trend in reduced further vertebral fractures.[16]

A small study has assessed a simple home exercise programme after hip fracture and found an increase in quadriceps strength, walking speed and subjective measures.[17] However, there was no effect on postural stability nor any comment possible on fall prevention. Another study has examined the role of early mobilization following Colles' fracture and confirmed previous evidence that there is quicker regain of wrist movement and that this is not at the expense of increased analgesic use nor worsening bony deformity.[18]

Although most non-vertebral fractures occur following a fall, no study has shown an intervention that has reduced fracture.[19] Protecting the hip with hip protectors has been shown to reduce hip fracture.[20] However, in view of their cumbersome design, compliance is poor.

DIETARY MODIFICATION (NUTRITIONAL OR PHARMACOLOGICAL SUPPLEMENTATION WITH CALCIUM AND VITAMIN D)

Both calcium and vitamin D act to reduce parathyroid hormone (PTH) levels and so may preserve bone mass. Some epidemiological studies of calcium intake comparing different populations have shown a protective effect against fracture in men,[21] whilst others have not.[22] After the menopause, calcium has been shown to reduce bone loss by reducing bone turnover and increasing bone density.[23] Calcium alone in pharmacological doses (1.2 g) has been shown to reduce the risk of further vertebral fracture in patients who have a prevalent vertebral fracture.[24] The evidence for hip fracture reduction has only been shown by epidemiological studies (Figure 12.3).[25,26]

Vitamin D is biologically inert from dietary sources or from the skin. It is metabolized by the liver and then the kidney to the active moiety 1,25-dihydroxyvitamin D. Its main action is to increase the absorption of calcium and to a lesser extent phosphorus from the small bowel. In the calcium-deficient state, it also acts on bone via osteoblasts to increase osteoclast numbers and mobilize calcium from the skeleton. Importantly, active vitamin D inhibits the synthesis and secretion of PTH. In this way, vitamin D may act to inhibit PTH-mediated, age-related bone loss.

The effects of calcitriol on bone mass have been inconsistent, reflecting the different calcium intakes in each of the studies.[27,28] Calcitriol, compared with calcium, has been shown to reduce vertebral fracture rates in post-menopausal women with prevalent vertebral deformity,[28] but other studies have found no benefit. A side-effect of calcitriol therapy includes hypercalcaemia, causing nephrocalcinosis and renal failure.

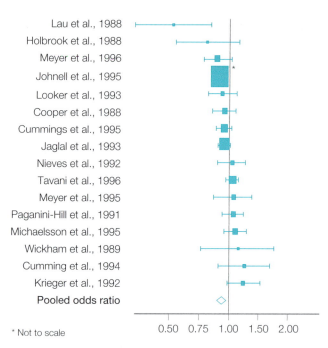

* Not to scale

Figure 12.3. Calcium treatment and risk of hip fracture. The odds ratios and 95% confidence intervals are shown for an increase of 300 mg/day of calcium and the risk of hip fracture in post-menopausal women. Reproduced with permission from: Cumming RG & Nevitt MC. *J Bone Miner Res* 1997; **12**: 1321–1329.[26]

One of the main mechanisms of age-related bone loss involves increased resorptive activity of PTH on the bone, secondary to hypovitaminosis D. In ambulatory elderly women resident in nursing homes, the combination of 1.2 g of calcium and 800 IU of vitamin D$_3$ (cholecalciferol) daily was given for 3 years. After 18 months the treatment group had significant increases of 2.7% in total femur BMD compared with a decline in the placebo group of 4.6%.[29] By the end of the 3-year period, there was a significant reduction in fracture rates at non-vertebral sites (OR: 0.70; 95% confidence interval (CI): 0.51–0.91) including the hip (OR: 0.70; 95% CI: 0.51–0.91).[30] Another study has shown that an annual intramuscular injection of 150,000–200,000 units of vitamin D to those over 75 years resulted in a significant reduction in all fractures.[31] Although participants in these studies were not diagnosed as osteoporotic before entry, the benefit would seem to be greatest in those at greatest risk.[32] However, more recent work has not demonstrated a benefit for either calcium and/or vitamin D oral supplementation[33] or annual vitamin D depot injection.[34]

OESTROGEN REPLACEMENT THERAPY AND SELECTIVE OESTROGEN RECEPTOR MODULATORS

Oestrogen deficiency is the major cause of bone loss leading to osteoporosis in women. Oestrogen inhibits osteoclast activity and, in the post-menopausal state, there is an imbalance between osteoclast resorption and osteoblast formation of bone, resulting in a net loss of bone density. The risk of fracture is increased in women who have early menopause. Treatment is aimed at restoring oestrogenic control of bone metabolism. There are three treatments available: oestrogen replacement therapy (ERT), selective oestrogen receptor modulators (SERMs) and gonadomimetic agents.

Epidemiological studies have shown that ERT increases bone density and reduces fracture by up to 50%.[35] In a small 1-year trial transdermal oestrogen increased lumbar spine BMD by 5.3% and radius BMD by 1%.[36] There was no significant benefit at the femoral neck. The incidence of vertebral fracture was reduced in the treatment group (RR: 0.39). Contrary to epidemiological evidence, the HERS investigation,[37] a large prospective study of ERT use in patients with established coronary artery disease, failed to observe a reduction in fracture incidence. However, fracture was not a primary outcome of this trial. It has also been suggested that differences between ERT users and non-users may have biased results from epidemiological studies of ERT use.[38]

Although there is evidence that oestrogen deficiency is important in early post-menopausal-related bone loss, osteoporotic fracture occurs in the later post-menopausal period. It has been shown that, during this time, ERT is less effective in reducing bone loss,[39] suggesting that the more important mechanism of bone loss for women at this time is age related.[40] The duration of ERT needed to protect against fracture is also unclear. The benefit in bone density, however, seems to be present only whilst the woman takes ERT. It has been shown that there is a little benefit in women who took ERT more than 5 years ago, suggesting a catch-up bone loss in the large group of women who stop ERT. Hence, the duration of therapy necessary to protect women against a fragility fracture may well be indefinite.

The benefits of ERT extend beyond the skeletal system. ERT is a good treatment for vasomotor instability, evidenced by flushing, in the peri-menopausal period. The effect of ERT on cardiovascular disease is complex. Although ERT improves the lipid profile by reducing total cholesterol and low density lipid (LDL$_c$) and causes vasodilation by a calcium antagonism, both the WHI and the HERS study have questioned the beneficial effect of ERT in reducing cardiovascular events by showing an increase in events in the first year with only a trend for reduction in years 4–5. The major risks associated with ERT are venous thrombo-embolism (VTE), endometrial cancer and breast cancer.[41] The occurence of VTE is associated with an increase in deep venous thrombosis (relative hazard: 2.8) and pulmonary embolism (relative hazard: 2.8), both fatal and non-fatal.[40] Overall, the excess event rate was 3.9/1000 woman-years. For this reason, ERT is contraindicated in women who have a previous history of VTE.

The unopposed oestrogenic effect on the uterus by ERT leads to an increase in endometrial cancer. To prevent this, progesterone needs to be given to those post-menopausal women who still have their uterus. This causes the resumption of menses, which is an important cause of non-compliance, and also symptoms similar to the pre-menstrual tension syndrome.

The other major concern is of excess cases of breast cancer after long-term use. This effect may be dose related and it may be that using lower doses of oestrogen in ERT preparations may limit this adverse effect. Other effects include breast tenderness and nipple sensitivity.

SERMs have oestrogenic and anti-oestrogenic effects, which are tissue dependent. The effect reflects the different concentration of oestrogen receptor subtype a or b. In bone, SERMs increase osteoblast production as well as reducing osteoclast activity and life span. There are two SERMs in current wide use, raloxifene and tamoxifen. The latter is used in breast cancer chemotherapy but is not in wider use due to endometrial adverse effects.

The Multiple Outcomes of Raloxifene Evaluation (MORE) randomized trial evaluated raloxifene (at 60 and 120 mg daily) with placebo in 7705 osteoporotic post-menopausal women over a median of 40 months.[42,43] Raloxifene increased bone density at the femoral neck and lumbar spine by 2.4% and 2.7% respectively. There was a peak in bone density, which was reached after 24 months and sustained thereafter. Although there was no reduction in non-vertebral fracture, there was a significant reduction in incident vertebral fracture. The greatest benefit was in women with pre-existing vertebral fracture on the 120 mg dose of raloxifene. In this group the number needed to treat (NNT) was 10.

The cardiovascular effects of raloxifene are unclear to date; the agent increases high-density lipid$_2$ (HDL$_2$) levels, suggesting the drug may have a cardioprotective role.[44]

The risk of long-term treatment with SERMs is similar to that of ERT with two important exceptions: SERMs are probably neutral at the endometrium and protective against carcinoma at the breast. In the large multicentre, randomized, controlled trial of raloxifene, there was a reduction in cases of endometrial cancer (RR: 0.8; 95% CI: 0.2–2.7), with a mean increase in endometrial thickness over 3 years of 0.01 mm, compared with a thinning of 0.27 mm in the placebo group. There was also a reduction in the incidence of invasive breast cancer (RR: 0.24) with an NNT over 40 months of 126. The apparently protective effect on breast cancer was most pronounced among oestrogen receptor-positive cases.

After 3 years of treatment with raloxifene, the prevalence of VTE was 1% in the raloxifene-treated group and 0.3% in the placebo group (RR: 3 1; 95% CI: 1.5–6.2). Other adverse effects included leg cramps and hot flushing, which precludes the use of SERMs in women during the peri-menopausal period.

Tibolone is a synthetic steroid with oestrogenic effects as well as effects on the androgen and progesterone receptors. Due to combined oestrogenic and progesterone effects, the effect on the endometrium is perceived to be neutral. Over a period of 2 years of treatment, it has been shown to increase bone mass at the hip and spine by 4.5% (95% CI: 2.3–6.6) and 6.9% (95% CI: 5.2–11.0) respectively.[45] There are no fracture data available at present. Side-effects of tibolone include breast tenderness, weight gain, hirsutism, disturbances in liver enzymes and irregular vaginal bleeding.

BISPHOSPHONATES

Bisphosphonates represent a group of potent anti-resorptive drugs related to naturally occurring pyrophosphate. Bisphosphonates are selectively distributed to bone, where they are taken up by osteoclasts. They inhibit osteoclast activity and shorten their lifespan. In addition, the amino-bisphosphonates also appear to interfere with the metabolism of mevalonic acid, leading to a loss of geranylated proteins, which are essential for osteoclast function.[46]

Etidronate was the first bisphosphonate to be used to prevent fracture in patients with osteoporosis. More recently, alendronate and risedronate have also become available.

Cyclical etidronate is licensed for the prevention and treatment of osteoporosis in post-menopausal women and for the prevention and treatment of glucocorticoid-induced osteoporosis. Etidronate in a dose of 400 mg daily is given for 14 days followed by 500 mg calcium daily for 76 days. The cycle is then repeated for the duration of treatment. The agent has been shown to increase bone density at the lumbar spine, but the effect at the hip is less clear.[47] Randomized controlled trials have demonstrated that cyclic etidronate reduces vertebral fracture rate in post-menopausal women with established osteoporosis,[46] but there is no significant reduction in non-vertebral fracture. Etidronate is also beneficial in corticosteroid-induced osteoporosis.[48]

Alendronate is licensed for the prevention and treatment of post-menopausal osteoporosis and for the prevention and treatment of glucocorticoid-induced osteoporosis.[49–52] For the latter indication, the recommended daily dose is 5 mg for all categories of patients except post-menopausal women not receiving hormone replacement therapy (HRT), in whom the recommended daily dose is 10 mg. Subsequent to the demonstration of anti-fracture efficacy in the Fracture Intervention Trial among post-menopausal women with established osteoporosis, the results of the second arm of this study have also been published. This included 4432 post-menopausal women with a low femoral neck BMD, but no vertebral fracture at baseline, who were randomized to placebo or alendronate. Significant treatment benefits in BMD were seen in the alendronate-treated women at the femoral neck when compared to the placebo group. There was a non-significant reduction in all clinical fractures (relative hazard: 0.86; 95% CI: 0.73–1.01). In the subgroup of women who had a baseline femoral neck BMD T-score below −2.5, the reduction in clinical fractures was statistically significant (RR: 0.64; 95% CI: 0.50–0.82).

Risedronate is a peridynal bisphosphonate that has recently been licensed for the treatment and prevention of osteoporosis in post-menopausal women, and for prevention and treatment of glucocorticoid-induced osteoporosis in post-menopausal women. Two randomized controlled trials of the effects of risedronate on vertebral and non-vertebral fracture rates in postmenopausal women with established osteoporosis (at least one vertebral fracture at baseline) have recently been published. In the North American study, 2458 women with established osteoporosis were treated with risedronate (2.5 or 5 mg daily) versus placebo.[53] Treatment was associated with an RR of new vertebral fracture of 0.35 (95% CI: 0.19–0.62) after 1 year and 0.59 (95% CI: 0.43–0.82) after 3 years. At 3 years, there was also a significant reduction in non-vertebral fracture (RR: 0.6; 95% CI: 0.39–0.94). Significant increases in BMD compared with placebo were seen at the lumbar spine (mean: 4.3%), femoral neck (mean: 2.8%) and trochanter (mean: 4.0%).

In a second randomized controlled trial performed in Europe and Australia,[54] the effects of risedronate were studied in 1226 post-menopausal women with established osteoporosis. A significant reduction in vertebral fractures was seen in the treatment arm at 1 year (RR: 0.39; 95% CI: 0.22–0.68), as well as at 3 years (RR: 0.51; 95% CI: 0.36–0.73) (Figure 12.4).[55] The overall incidence of adverse events was similar in treatment and placebo groups in both these trials. In particular, the incidence of upper gastrointestinal tract adverse events was similar across groups. The place of intermittent bisphosphonate therapy with ibandronate and zolendronate within the context of existing anti-resorptive therapies has yet to be clarified.

The optimal duration of bisphosphonate therapy is unknown. There are theoretical risks of long-term inhibition of bone turnover and mineralization abnormality. Seven-year follow-up of patients using alendronate has shown progressive gains in lumbar spine BMD of 11.4% compared with baseline. Change at the hip has been less marked (4.9% after a similar duration of use).[56] Ten-year follow-up data show no gross effect on bone architecture and mineralizaion. Data are also scarce on the pattern of bone loss after cessation of bisphosphonate therapy. It appears that skeletal benefits may be preserved for at least the first year after cessation, but data are urgently required for more protracted follow-up periods.

Two studies have examined the role of combination therapy with a bisphosphonate and ERT.[57,58] In women already taking a combined preparation of ERT, the addition of alendronate increased bone density both at the lumbar spine and femoral trochanter, and there was a non-significant trend in higher bone density at the hip after 12 months of treatment. Despite this there was a non-significant increase in fracture prevalence in the alendronate group. A longer study over 4 years, with smaller patient numbers, demonstrated similar gains in bone mass at total hip and that there was a non-significant reduction in the number of incident vertebral fractures per group (1 versus 5).[57] Alendronate has also been shown to be superior to calcitonin therapy in a comparative study.[59]

CALCITONIN

Calcitonin is a naturally occurring polypeptide hormone, usually secreted by the parafollicular cells of the thyroid. Its physiological action is to reduce calcium content in the blood by inhibiting osteoclast adsorption in the short term and reducing

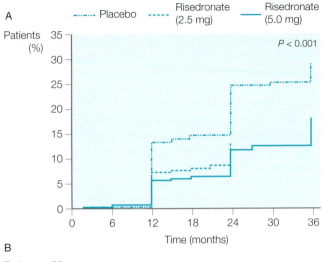

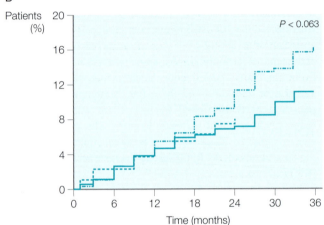

Figure 12.4. Risedronate and the incidence of fracture. The incidence of new vertebral (A) and non-vertebral (B) osteoporotic-related fractures in osteoporotic post-menopausal women taking either risedronate (2.5 or 5 mg) or placebo. Reproduced with permission from: Reginster J et al. *Osteoporosis Int* 2000; **11**: 83–91.[55]

osteoclast formation in the longer term. A major hurdle to successful pharmacological benefit is the development of down-regulation of the osteoclast receptor to calcitonin. Thus, in the long term, this enables bone resorption to escape the suppressive effects of calcitonin.

Calcitonin has minor effects on renal reabsorption and gut absorption of calcium, which oppose the greater physiological effect of PTH. The overall activity of calcitonin on calcium is faster acting and of shorter duration than that of the more potent PTH. In the animal kingdom, calcitonin has a much more prominent role in calcium homeostasis, especially in species that change from freshwater to sea water when there are large calcium losses. The source of pharmaceutical calcitonin is from salmon or human sources.

Calcitonin can be given either subcutaneously or intranasally. The dosing and frequency of calcitonin administration varies.

A 5-year multi-dosage regime of calcitonin in post-menopausal women has shown an increase in lumbar spine BMD after 1 year, which was sustained over the next 4 years for the 200 IU dose.[60] There was no appreciable benefit at the femur. After 3 years there was a reduction in new vertebral fracture (RR: 0.67), giving an NNT of 11 to be treated for 3 years to prevent a single new vertebral fracture.[59] A major limitation of this study was the substantial 59% of patients who were lost to follow-up.[61]

Other studies of calcitonin use have shown increases in spinal and arm BMD in post-menopausal women with osteoporosis with a similar reduction in vertebral fracture by 60%.[59,62,63] On stopping calcitonin treatment, bone loss restarts, indicating that an intermittent therapeutic regimen with 1 year on and 1 year off may be required. There are no serious side-effects with calcitonin use. The side-effects are not dose related and tend to be inconvenient but nevertheless are important in terms of non-compliance. They include flushing, vomiting, diarrhoea and local irritation when injected, or nasal crusting or secretion when it is taken by the nasal route.

ANABOLIC AGENTS

While there are many different pharmacological methods to prevent bone resorption, agents that directly increase bone formation are less well developed. The two most widely studied anabolic agents that may play a role in the management of osteoporosis are PTH and sodium fluoride.

Parathyroid hormone

Parathyroid hormone (PTH) is a single-chain peptide hormone that is secreted by the chief cells in the parathyroid glands located posteriorly to the thyroid gland. Its major physiological effects are to increase plasma calcium and reduce plasma phosphate. PTH acts physiologically on the bone in two separate phases. In the short term it stimulates osteolysis of the bone matrix by promoting calcium phosphate removal from the matrix using an osteocyte/osteoblast membrane system. In the longer term, PTH, via osteoblasts, stimulates osteoclast activity and formation. This increase in osteoclast activity after a few weeks leads to a secondary stimulation of osteoblast activity and thereby enhances bone formation. PTH has multiple actions on the renal system. It is a potent stimulator of phosphate excretion by the kidneys; this outweighs the effect of increased phosphate released by the bone, causing a reduction in plasma phosphate. PTH increases renal calcium reabsorption and also stimulates the renal metabolism of vitamin D to its active form. In this way, PTH indirectly stimulates gut calcium absorption. In the case of hyperparathyroidism, the constant high levels of PTH cause substantial bone loss and fracture.

However, when given once daily, studies have shown that this intermittent PTH use conversely increases bone mass. The effect on bone is mediated by both increasing the amount of calcium available to the skeleton from the plasma and also by directly stimulating osteoblast function and number, either by increased recruitment[64] or by preventing apoptosis.[65,66]

A 21-month study of daily subcutaneous teriparatide, a recombinant human PTH (1–34) fragment, in post-menopausal women demonstrated a significant reduction in both vertebral (4% versus 14%) and non-vertebral (3% versus 5%) fracture rates.[67] The study was stopped prematurely because animal studies suggested an increase in osteosarcoma risk in rats given high dose PTH from infancy to old age. However, the relevance to humans treated with teriparatide for short durations may be minimal and the approved labelling suggests therapy for no more than 2 years. While serum calcium increases with teriparatide therapy, the increase is transient and less than 5% of treated patients required dose reductions. However, the optimal timing and agent for co-therapy, especially anti-resorptive therapy after PTH, has not yet been resolved.

In a small study of post-menopausal women with osteoporosis, a daily injection of PTH increased BMD at the spine progressively by 13% over 3 years. The benefit at the femur was less impressive. There was no loss at cortical sites, such as the radius, which is a concern with PTH use. There was a significant reduction in vertebral fracture rates.[68] Similar findings have been found in osteoporotic men. However, in this study there was a small but significant decline in radial BMD as compared with the placebo group.[69]

Adverse effects of PTH administration include hypercalcaemia and local injection site reactions.

Sodium fluoride

Sodium fluoride has been used to treat established osteoporosis for at least three decades. There is an enormous geographical variation in the use of this agent, but two large prospective randomized controlled trials of high-dose sodium fluoride[70–75] suggested that, despite a marked improvement in lumbar spine BMD, fluoride-treated individuals showed no reduction in spine fracture incidence over a 4-year period, and had a worrying loss of bone mineral from the appendicular skeleton. The results of these studies have led to the large-scale abandonment of high-dose sodium fluoride in the treatment of established osteoporosis.

Data on the use of lower doses (25–50 mg daily) have been more encouraging, but despite gains of bone density observed in some of these studies, the incidence of vertebral fractures has again not been observed. Side-effects of fluoride therapy, which are common but mainly transient, include gastrointestinal irritation, arthralgia and bone pain. These tend to reverse when treatment is stopped and recur less frequently when treatment is restarted at a lower dose. At present, fluoride cannot be widely recommended for the prevention and treatment of osteoporosis. It retains a role in the management of difficult cases, under hospital supervision.

Strontium ranelate

Strontium ranelate is a novel agent for the prevention of osteoporotic fractures. The mechanism of action is unclear and may involve enhancing osteoblast replication while reducing osteo-clast differentiation. Two large multicentre studies have demon-strated a 49% reduction in vertebral fracture which was maintained over 3 years[76] and 19% reduction in significant non-vertebral fracture.[77] The most commonly reported side-effect was diarrhoea, with transient rises in both creatine kinase and calci-um also observed. As strontium is denser than calcium, there is an artefactual increase in areal BMD as measured by DXA.

SUMMARY

In view of the current weight of evidence, there is an expanding range of treatment options available for preventing fracture. Despite this, the rate of utilization of these agents in those at very high risk of fracture is still low.[78] A framework for treating the osteoporotic patient would ideally operate on three tiers (Figure 12.5).

Firstly, there should be an assessment of the patient with the view to correcting or ameliorating underlying pathologies, such as hypogonadism in men or corticosteroid use. The sec-ond tier would involve lifestyle and dietary measures. Lifestyle measures include regular exercise, smoking cessation and wearing of a hip protector. Dietary intervention should be aimed at ensuring an adequate intake of calcium and vitamin D. The intervention could be aimed either at changes in the patient's diet or by adding specific food supplements. Vitamin D and calcium supplementation have been shown to reduce the rates of all fragility fractures. If such measures were instituted in a population-wide measure, a 10% increase in average bone density would result in a 50% decline in fractures. However, compliance to such lifestyle measures is poor.

Finally, the use of specific bone agents should be tailored according to a patient's individual characteristics. Prescribing HRT should involve consideration of the potential benefits with

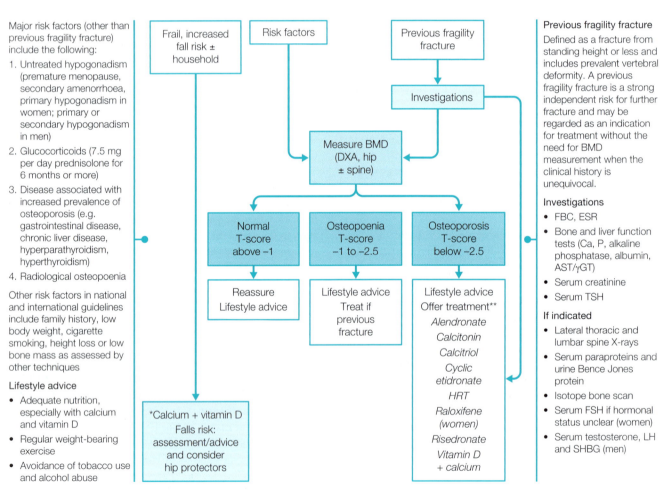

Figure 12.5. Medical management of men and women aged over 45 years who have or are at risk of osteoporosis. Reproduced with permission from: Royal College of Physicians. *Osteoporosis: Clinical Guidelines for Prevention*, 1999.[82] AST/γGT, asparate transaminase/glutamyl transpeptidase; BMD, bone mineral density; DXA, dual-energy X-ray absoptiometry; ESR, erythrocyte sedimentation rate; FBC, full blood count; HRT, hormone replacement therapy (oestrogen in women, testosterone in hypogonadal men); LH, luteinizing hormone; SHBG, sex hormone-binding globulin; TSH, thyroid-stimulating hormone.

Table 12.2. Examples of treatment groups for fracture prevention.

Treatment	Annual cost (effectiveness)	Patient group (annual fracture rate)	Treatment cost per fracture avoided (cost after accounting for savings from avoiding fractures)
Calcium with vitamin D	£55 (30%)	Women below the mean in body weight (<67 kg), mean age of 81 years living in nursing homes, sheltered accommodation (hip fracture rate = 2.5%)	£7400 per hip fracture avoided (£2361 per hip fracture avoided)
HRT (unopposed)	£23 (53%)	52-year-old women had a hysterectomy <50 years and 1+ previous fractures (all fracture rate = 3.6%)	£1204 per any fracture avoided (£736 per any fracture avoided)
Etidronate	£161 (34%)	79-year-old women <57 kg and 1+ previous fracture living in community (hip fracture rate = 2.63%)	£18,000 per hip fracture averted (£5420 per hip fracture avoided)
Alendronate	£335 (50%)	79-year-old women <57 kg and 1+ fracture and smoker living in community (hip fracture rate = 4.4%)	£15,227 per hip fracture averted (£3227 per hip fracture averted)
Etidronate	£161 (34%)	79-year-old women <57 kg and 1+ previous fracture and smoker living in community (hip fracture rate = 4.4%)	Saves 1.5 hip fractures/100 women (£1852 saving/100 patients prescribed)

Source: data extracted from National Osteoporosis Society. *A Primary Care Service Framework for Osteoporosis*, 1999.[80]
Costs are cheapest preparations in MIMS.

the risks of thrombo-embolic events, recent cardiac history, breast and endometrial cancer. The benefit of ERT on fracture prevention is dose dependent, with 5 years of continuous use needed to show a reduction in fracture and little effect after treatment is stopped. Whilst tibolone does increase BMD there is, at present, no evidence of fracture prevention.

SERMs represent a useful alternative to ERT to post-menopausal women. Raloxifene has been shown to reduce vertebral fracture but also to be protective against breast cancer. This may further influence prescribing in those osteoporotic women with risk factors for breast cancer.

Bisphosphonates are appropriate for those intolerant of hormone therapy or those at higher risk of fracture. Both of the amino bisphosphonates used, alendronate and risedronate, reduce vertebral and non-vertebral fractures. Their use is limited by upper gastrointestinal tolerance. This necessitates following guidelines for administration that may be poorly complied with by some in the community. The cost-effectiveness of such treatments is outlined in Table 12.2.

The use of nasal calcitonin is effective in preventing fracture; however, its cost and need for intermittent therapy limit its use except in certain patients. Calcitonin is suitable in those patients with acute pain following a vertebral fracture, taking advantage of calcitonin's analgesic properties. Whilst fluoride therapy may reduce vertebral fracture, potential increases in hip fracture preclude the recommendation of fluoride for the treatment of osteoporosis except by specialist centres. For those with more

aggressive bone loss and fracture despite bisphosphonate therapy, teriparatide may be considered. The placing of strontium within this framework is not yet clear.

PRACTICE POINTS

- There is under-utilization of treatments to prevent fracture in osteoporotic patients.

- Supplemental vitamin D with calcium has been shown to reduce fracture in the immobile elderly.

- While SERMs have been shown to reduce vertebral fracture, the bisphosphonates are more potent, with alendronate and risedronate also reducing fracture at non-vertebral sites.

- PTH is a promising anabolic agent and has been shown to increase bone density and reduce fracture.

- Strontium ranelate has both anabolic and anti-catabolic effects, and has also been shown to reduce fracture.

RESEARCH AGENDA

- Controlled studies to compare alternate osteoporotic strategies (the high-risk and population approaches) at the level of the general population are needed.

- Longer-term studies to confirm the optimal duration of therapy with bisphosphonates and, importantly, the effect of cessation of therapy on continued fracture prevention are needed.

- The optimal combination of anabolic and anti-catabolic agents in patients with high risk of fracture is needed.

ACKNOWLEDGEMENTS

Dr M. K. Javaid was supported by the Arthritis Research Campaign of Great Britain. The manuscript was prepared by Mrs G. Strange.

REFERENCES

1. Seeley DG, Browner WS, Nevitt MC et al. Which fractures are associated with low appendicular bone mass in elderly women? The Study of Osteoporotic Fractures Research Group. *Ann Intern Med* 1991; **115**: 837–842.

2. Melton LJ, Lane AW, Cooper C et al. Prevalence and incidence of vertebral deformities. *Osteoporosis Int* 1993; **3**: 113–119.

3. Matthis C, Weber U, O'Neill TW et al. Health impact associated with vertebral deformities: results from the European Vertebral Osteoporosis Study (EVOS). *Osteoporosis Int* 1998; **8**: 364–372.

4. Parkkari J, Kannus P, Palvanen M et al. Majority of hip fractures occur as a result of a fall and impact on the greater trochanter of the femur: a prospective controlled hip fracture study with 206 consecutive patients. *Calcif Tissue Int* 1999; **65**: 183–187.

5. Lauritzen JB. Hip fractures: incidence, risk factors, energy absorption, and prevention. *Bone* 1996; **18**: 65S–75S.

6. Meunier PJ. Evidence-based medicine and osteoporosis: a comparison of fracture risk reduction data from osteoporosis randomised clinical trials. *Int J Clin Pract* 1999; **53**: 122–129.

7. World Health Organization Study Group. *Assessment of Fracture Risk and its Application to Screening for Postmenopausal Osteoporosis*. Geneva: WHO, 1994.

8. Eastell R, Reid DM, Compston J et al. A UK consensus on management of glucocorticoid-induced osteoporosis: an update. *J Intern Med* 1998; **244**: 271–292.

9. Law MR & Hackshaw AK. A meta-analysis of cigarette smoking, bone mineral density and risk of hip fracture: recognition of a major effect. *BMJ* 1997; **315**: 841–846.

10. Forsen L, Bjartveit K, Bjorndal A et al. Ex-smokers and risk of hip fracture. *Am J Public Health* 1998; **88**: 1481–1483.

11. Cornuz J, Feskanich D, Willett WC et al. Smoking, smoking cessation, and risk of hip fracture in women. *Am J Med* 1999; **106**: 311–314.

12. Hemenway D, Colditz GA, Willett WC et al. Fractures and lifestyle: effect of cigarette smoking, alcohol intake, and relative weight on the risk of hip and forearm fractures in middle-aged women. *Am J Public Health* 1988; **78**: 1554–1558.

13. Kiel DP, Baron JA, Anderson JJ et al. Smoking eliminates the protective effect of oral estrogens on the risk for hip fracture among women. *Ann Intern Med* 1992; **116**: 716–721.

14. Chow R, Harrison JE & Notarius C. Effect of two randomised exercise programmes on bone mass of healthy postmenopausal women. *BMJ (Clin Res Ed)* 1987; **295**: 1441–1444.

15. Joakimsen RM, Magnus JH & Fonnebo V. Physical activity and predisposition for hip fractures: a review. *Osteoporosis Int* 1997; **7**: 503–513.

16. Harrison JE, Chow R, Dornan J et al. Evaluation of a program for rehabilitation of osteoporotic patients (PRO): 4-year follow-up. The Bone and Mineral Group of the University of Toronto. *Osteoporosis Int* 1993; **3**: 13–17.

17. Sherrington C & Lord SR. Home exercise to improve strength and walking velocity after hip fracture: a randomized controlled trial. *Arch Phys Med Rehab* 1997; **78**: 208–212.

18. Dias JJ, Wray CC, Jones JM et al. The value of early mobilisation in the treatment of Colles' fractures. *J Bone Joint Surg (Br)* 1987; **69**: 463–467.

19. Tinetti ME, Baker DI, McAvay G et al. A multifactorial intervention to reduce the risk of falling among elderly people living in the community. *N Engl J Med* 1994; **331**: 821–827.

20. Lauritzen JB, Petersen MM & Lund B. Effect of external hip protectors on hip fractures. *Lancet* 1993; **341**: 11–13.

21. Cooper C, Barker DJ & Wickham C. Physical activity, muscle strength, and calcium intake in fracture of the proximal femur in Britain. *BMJ* 1988; **297**: 1443–1446.

22. Smith RW & Frame B. Concurrent axial and appendicular osteoporosis: its relation to calcium consumption. *N Engl J Med* 1965; **273**: 72–78.

23. Kanis JA. Calcium nutrition and its implications for osteoporosis. Part II. After menopause. *Eur J Clin Nutr* 1994; **48**: 833–841.

24. Recker RR, Hinders S, Davies KM et al. Correcting calcium nutritional deficiency prevents spine fractures in elderly women. *J Bone Miner Res* 1996; **11**: 1961–1996.

25. Kanis JA, Johnell O, Gullberg B et al. Evidence for efficacy of drugs affecting bone metabolism in preventing hip fracture. *BMJ* 1992; **305**: 1124–1128.

26. Cumming RG & Nevitt MC. Calcium for the prevention of osteoporotic fractures in post-menopausal women. *J Bone Miner Res* 1997; **12**: 1321–1329.

27. Aloia JF, Vaswani A, Yeh JK et al. Calcitriol in the treatment of postmenopausal osteoporosis. *Am J Med* 1988; **84**: 401–408.

28. Falch JA, Odegaard OR, Finnanger AM et al. Postmenopausal osteoporosis: no effect of three years treatment with 1,25-dihydroxycholecalciferol. *Acta Med Scand* 1987; **221**: 199–204.

29. Chapuy MC, Arlot ME, Duboeuf F et al. Vitamin D3 and calcium to prevent hip fractures in the elderly women. *N Engl J Med* 1992; **327**: 1637–1642.

30. Chapuy MC, Arlot ME, Delmas PD et al. Effect of calcium and cholecalciferol treatment for three years on hip fractures in elderly women. *BMJ* 1994; **308**: 1081–1082.

31. Heikinheimo RJ, Inkovaara JA, Harju EJ et al. Annual injection of vitamin D and fractures of aged bones. *Calcif Tissue Int* 1992; **51**: 105–110.

32. Ranstam J & Kanis JA. Influence of age and body mass on the effects of vitamin D on hip fracture risk. *Osteoporosis Int* 1995; **5**: 450–454.

33. Grant AM, Avenell A, Campbell MK et al. RECORD Trial Group. Oral vitamin D3 and calcium for secondary prevention of low-trauma fractures in elderly people (Randomised Evaluation of Calcium Or vitamin D, RECORD): a randomised placebo-controlled trial. *Lancet* 2005; **365**(9471): 1621–1628.

34. Anderson FH, Smith HE, Raphael HM et al. Effect of annual intramuscular D supplementation on fracture risk in 9440 community living older people: the Wessex Fracture Prevention Trial. *J Bone Miner Res* 2004; **19**(Suppl. 1): 1220.

35. Kiel DP, Felson DT, Anderson JJ et al. Hip fracture and the use of estrogens in postmenopausal women. The Framingham Study. *N Engl J Med* 1987; **317**: 1169–1174.

36. Lufkin EG, Wahner HW, O'Fallon WM et al. Treatment of postmenopausal osteoporosis with transdermal estrogen. *Ann Intern Med* 1992; **117**: 1–9.

37. Hulley S, Grady D, Bush T et al. Randomized trial of estrogen plus progestin for secondary prevention of coronary heart disease in postmenopausal women. Heart and Estrogen/Progestin Replacement Study (HERS) Research. *JAMA* 1998; **280**: 605–613.

38. Posthuma WF, Westendorp RG & Vandenbroucke JP. Cardioprotective effect of hormone replacement therapy in postmenopausal women: is the evidence biased? *BMJ* 1994; **308**: 1268–1269.

39. Ensrud KE, Palermo L, Black DM et al. Hip and calcaneal bone loss increase with advancing age: longitudinal results from the study of osteoporotic fractures. *J Bone Miner Res* 1995; **10**: 1778–1787.

40. Orwoll ES & Nelson HD. Does estrogen adequately protect postmenopausal women against osteoporosis: an iconoclastic perspective. *J Clin Endocrinol Metab* 1999; **84**: 1872–1874.

41. Grady D, Wenger NK, Herrington D et al. Postmenopausal hormone therapy increases risk for venous thromboembolic disease. The Heart and Estrogen/progestin Replacement Study. *Ann Intern Med* 2000; **132**: 689–696.

42. Ettinger B, Black DM, Mitlak BH et al. Reduction of vertebral fracture risk in postmenopausal women with osteoporosis treated with raloxifene: results from a 3-year randomized clinical trial. Multiple Outcomes of Raloxifene Evaluation (MORE) Investigators. *JAMA* 1999; **282**: 637–645.

43. Cummings SR, Eckert S, Krueger KA et al. The effect of raloxifene on risk of breast cancer in postmenopausal women: results from the MORE randomized trial. Multiple Outcomes of Raloxifene Evaluation. *JAMA* 1999; **281**: 2189–2197.

44. Delmas PD, Bjarnason NH, Mitlak BH et al. Effects of raloxifene on bone mineral density, serum cholesterol concentrations, and uterine endometrium in postmenopausal women. *N Engl J Med* 1997; **337**: 1641–1647.

45. Studd J, Arnala I, Kicovic PM et al. A randomized study of tibolone on bone mineral density in osteoporotic postmenopausal women with previous fractures. *Obstet Gynecol* 1998; **92**: 574–579.

46. Rodan GA. Bone mass homeostasis and bisphosphonate action. *Bone* 1997; **20**: 1–4.

47. Harris ST, Watts NB, Jackson RD et al. Four-year study of intermittent cyclic etidronate treatment of postmenopausal osteoporosis: three years of blinded therapy followed by one year of open therapy. *Am J Med* 1993; **95**: 557–567.

48. Adachi JD, Roux C, Pitt PI et al. A pooled data analysis on the use of intermittent cyclical etidronate therapy for the prevention and treatment of corticosteroid induced bone loss. *J Rheumatol* 2000; **27**: 2424–2431.

49. Liberman UA, Weiss SR, Broll J et al. Effect of oral alendronate on bone mineral density and the incidence of fractures in postmenopausal osteoporosis. The Alendronate Phase III Osteoporosis Treatment Study Group. *N Engl J Med* 1995; **333**: 1437–1443.

50. Black DM, Cummings SR, Karpf DB et al. Randomised trial of effect of alendronate on risk of fracture in women with existing vertebral fractures. Fracture Intervention Trial Research Group. *Lancet* 1996; **348**: 1535–1541.

51. Pols HA, Felsenberg D, Hanley DA et al. Multinational, placebo-controlled, randomized trial of the effects of alendronate on bone density and fracture risk in postmenopausal women with low bone mass: results of the FOSIT study. Foxamax International Trial Study Group. *Osteoporosis Int* 1999; **9**: 461–468.

52. Cummings SR, Black DM, Thompson DE et al. Effect of alendronate on risk of fracture in women with low bone density but without vertebral fractures: results from the Fracture Intervention Trial. *JAMA* 1998; **280**: 2077–2082.

53. Harris ST, Watts NB, Genant HK et al. Effects of risedronate treatment on vertebral and nonvertebral fractures in women with postmenopausal osteoporosis: a randomized controlled trial. Vertebral Efficacy With Risedronate Therapy (VERT) Study Group. *JAMA* 1999; **282**: 1344–1352.

54. Reginster J, Minne HW, Sorensen OH et al. Randomized trial of the effects of risedronate on vertebral fractures in women with established postmenopausal osteoporosis. Vertebral Efficacy with Risedronate Therapy (VERT) Study Group. *Osteoporosis Int* 2000; **11**: 83–91.

55. Reginster J, Minne HW, Sorenson ON et al. Randomised trial of the effects of risedronate on vertebral fractures in women with established postmenopausal osteoporosis. *Osteoporosis Int* 2000; **11**: 83–91.

56. Tonino RP, Meunier PJ, Emkey R et al. Skeletal benefits of alendronate: 7-year treatment of postmenopausal osteoporotic women. Phase III Osteoporosis Treatment Study Group. *J Clin Endocrinol Metab* 2000; **85**: 3109–3115.

57. Wimalawansa SJ. A four-year randomized controlled trial of hormone replacement and bisphosphonate, alone or in combination, in women with postmenopausal osteoporosis. *Am J Med* 1998; **104**: 219–226.

58. Lindsay R, Cosman F, Lobo RA et al. Addition of alendronate to ongoing hormone replacement therapy in the treatment of osteoporosis: a randomized, controlled clinical trial. *J Clin Endocrinol Metab* 1999; **84**: 3076–3081.

59. Adami S, Passeri M, Ortolani S et al. Effects of oral alendronate and intranasal salmon calcitonin on bone mass and biochemical markers of bone turnover in postmenopausal women with osteoporosis. *Bone* 1995; **17**: 383–390.

60. Chesnut CH, Silverman S, Andriano K et al. A randomized trial of nasal spray salmon calcitonin in postmenopausal women with established osteoporosis: the prevent recurrence of osteoporotic fractures study. *Am J Med* 2000; **109**: 267–276.

61. Cummings SR & Chapurlat RD. What proof proves about calcitonin and clinical trials. *Am J Med* 2000; **109**: 330–331.

62. Rico H, Revilla M, Hernandez ER et al. Total and regional bone mineral content and fracture rate in postmenopausal osteoporosis treated with salmon calcitonin: a prospective study. *Calcif Tissue Int* 1995; **56**: 181–185.

63. Overgaard K, Hansen MA, Jensen SB et al. Effect of salcatonin given intranasally on bone mass and fracture rates in established osteoporosis: a dose–response study. *BMJ* 1992; **305**: 556–561.

64. MacDonald BR, Gallagher JA & Russell RG. Parathyroid hormone stimulates the proliferation of cells derived from human bone. *Endocrinology* 1986; **118**: 2445–2449.

65. Stanislaus D, Yang X, Liang JD et al. In vivo regulation of apoptosis in metaphyseal trabecular bone of young rats by synthetic human parathyroid hormone (1–34) fragment. *Bone* 2000; **27**: 209–218.

66. Jilka RL, Weinstein RS, Bellido T et al. Increased bone formation by prevention of osteoblast apoptosis with parathyroid hormone. *J Clin Invest* 1999; **104**: 439–446.

67. Neer RM, Arnaud CD, Zanchetta JR et al. Effect of parathyroid hormone (1–34) on fractures and bone mineral density in postmenopausal women with osteoporosis. *N Engl J Med* 2001; **344**: 1434–1441.

68. Lindsay R, Nieves J, Formica C et al. Randomised controlled study of effect of parathyroid hormone on vertebral-bone mass and fracture incidence among postmenopausal women on estrogen with osteoporosis. *Lancet* 1997; **350**: 550–555.

69. Kurland ES, Cosman F, McMahon DJ et al. Parathyroid hormone as a therapy for idiopathic osteoporosis in men: effects on bone mineral density and bone markers. *J Clin Endocrinol Metab* 2000; **85**: 3069–3076.

70. Jones G, Riley M, Couper D & Dwyer T. Water fluoridation, bone mass and fracture: a quantitative overview of the literature. *Aust NZ J Public Health* 1999; **3**(23): 34–40.

71. Pak CY, Sakhaee K, Piziak V et al. Slow-release sodium fluoride in the management of postmenopausal osteoporosis. A randomized controlled trial. *Ann Intern Med* 1994; **120**: 625–632.

72. Riggs BL, Hodgson SF, O'Fallon WM et al. Effect of fluoride treatment on the fracture rate in postmenopausal women with osteoporosis. *N Engl J Med* 1990; **322**: 802–809.

73. Christiansen C, Christensen MS, McNair P et al. Prevention of early postmenopausal bone loss: controlled 2-year study in 315 normal females. *Eur J Clin Invest* 1980; **10**: 273–279.

74. Meunier PJ, Sebert JL, Reginster JY et al. Fluoride salts are no better at preventing new vertebral fractures than calcium–vitamin D in postmenopausal osteoporosis: the FAVO Study. *Osteoporosis Int* 1998; **8**: 4–12.

75. Phipps KR, Orwoll ES, Mason JD et al. Community water fluoridation, bone mineral density, and fractures: prospective study of effects in older women. *BMJ* 2000; **321**: 860–864 (in process citation).

76. Meunier PJ, Roux C, Seeman E et al. The effects of strontium ranelate on the risk of vertebral fracture in women with postmenopausal osteoporosis. *N Engl J Med* 2004; **350**: 459–468.

77. Reginster JY, Seeman E, De Vernejoul MC et al. Strontium ranelate reduces the risk of nonvertebral fractures in postmenopausal women with osteoporosis: Treatment of Peripheral Osteoporosis (TROPOS) study. *J Clin Endocrinol Metab* 2005; **90**: 2816–2822.

78. Kamel HK, Hussain MS, Tariq S et al. Failure to diagnose and treat osteoporosis in elderly patients hospitalized with hip fracture. *Am J Med* 2000; **109**: 326–328 (in process citation).

79. Cooper C. Epidemiology of osteoporosis. *Osteoporosis Int* 1999; **9**(Suppl. 2): S2–S8.

80. National Osteoporosis Society. *A Primary Care Service Framework for Osteoporosis*. London: National Osteoporosis Society of Great Britain, 1999.

81. Cooper C & Melton MJ. Epidemiology of osteoporosis. *Trends Endocrinol Metab* 1992; **3**: 224–229.

82. Royal College of Physicians. *Osteoporosis: Clinical Guidelines for Prevention*. London: Royal College of Physicians, 1999.

Chapter 13

Non-pharmacological interventions

Paul Lips and Natasja M. van Schoor

THE EFFECT OF EXERCISE

Physical exercise influences bone mass, muscle strength and coordination in younger as well as in elderly people. Immobilization rapidly causes bone loss that can only be regained very slowly.[1] The prevention of immobility-induced bone loss requires a moderate amount of physical exercise.[2] The benefit of intense exercise programmes on bone mass is, however, moderate at best. Exercise is important in young people for the attainment of peak bone mass. In the elderly it may decrease bone loss, maintain or increase muscle strength and improve balance. In this section studies on exercise will be reviewed with an emphasis on its effect in the elderly.

Exercise stimulates bone formation and decreases bone resorption by inducing strain (deformation, compression). It is now widely accepted that the induced strain generates fluid streams in the bone channels (canaliculi) connecting osteocytes. The osteocytes secrete growth factors into the fluid stream and the latter stimulate the osteoblasts. In this system the osteocyte acts as a mechanosensor.[3]

Animal experiments have shown that dynamic (intermittent) loading is more effective in stimulating bone formation than static loading. The peak strain induced by loading is more important than the total duration of loading, while the number of repetitions (cycles) is only important up to a certain threshold.[4] High peak strains are generated by high-impact loading. The highest bone mineral densities were observed in weightlifters and squash players,[5] followed by other sports, whereas little gain was obtained in swimmers.

Epidemiological studies

Many epidemiological studies have shown an effect of mobility and physical exercise on bone mineral density (BMD) and fracture risk. The Study of Osteoporotic Fractures, a prospective cohort study in 9516 women, showed an increased risk ratio (RR) for hip fractures in women who could not stand from a chair without using their hands (RR: 2.1) and women who were mobile (standing or walking) for fewer than 4 h per day (RR: 1.7), whereas walking for exercise decreased the risk (RR: 0.7).[6] In the EPIDOS study, a slow gait and the inability to walk on toes were identified as risk factors for hip fracture.[7] In the Amsterdam Vitamin D Study, low mobility, measured by a walk-

ing score, was a risk factor for hip fracture (RR: 2.4).[8] Immobility (i.e. not walking for over 4 weeks in the previous year) was an important risk factor for hip fractures (RR: 3.6) and all fractures (RR: 2.6) in another prospective cohort study.[9]

Low physical activity, low hand-grip strength and a poor walking test were risk factors for falls and fractures in the Longitudinal Aging Study Amsterdam.[10–13] The Nurses' Health Study showed that walking for at least 4 h per week was associated with a 40% lower risk of hip fracture.[14] Impaired balance and walking were risk factors for falls in another prospective cohort study.[15]

Effects of exercise on bone mass

In children, weight-bearing activity (three times a week) was associated with greater increases of BMD compared to a control group.[16,17] A longitudinal cohort study in 84 men and 98 women in Amsterdam followed from 13 to 28 years demonstrated that weight-bearing activity during youth was a more important determinant for BMD than calcium intake.[18] Several randomized trials have addressed the effect of physical exercise in young, peri-menopausal and post-menopausal women. These have been recently reviewed.[19] These studies generally show a small increase or no change of BMD in the exercise groups and a small loss in the control groups. High-intensity strength training two times per week for 45 minutes was done in a randomized trial of 40 women 50–70 years of age. The bone mineral density of the lumbar spine and femoral neck increased significantly in the exercise group compared to the control group (+1 versus –2%). A significant increase of muscle mass and muscle strength and improvement of balance was also demonstrated in the exercise group.[20] Other studies have shown similar results[21,22] or non-significant changes.[23–25] High-resistance training appeared to be more effective than aerobic exercise, but the effect is site specific.[19] The effects of alendronate and weight-bearing jumping exercise were compared in a double-blind randomized trial in post-menopausal women. While alendronate increased bone mass at the lumbar spine and femoral neck, exercise increased cortical bone mass in the distal tibia.[26] Both effects disappeared after discontinuation of therapy.[27]

A meta-analysis of controlled trials concluded that exercise training programmes in pre- and post-menopausal women prevented or reversed almost 1% of bone loss per year in the lumbar spine and femoral neck.[28] The maximal study duration was 24 months, so that conclusions on long-term effects cannot be extended beyond that time period. Resistance training in combination with oestrogen therapy in women after surgical menopause was more effective in increasing BMD than oestrogen alone.[29] Similar results were obtained in frail elderly women.[30]

The separate and combined effects of weight-bearing exercise and oestrogen were investigated in 60- to 72-year-old post-menopausal women. Both oestrogen and exercise had a positive effect on BMD of the lumbar spine, femoral neck and trochanteric region. The effect of the combined treatment was additive in the lumbar spine and synergistic for total body BMD.[31]

Long-term effects of exercise (>2 years) were investigated in two studies. The Erlangen Fitness Osteoporosis Prevention Study compared endurance/strength training and jumping during 26 months with no exercise in post-menopausal women with osteopoenia. Bone density of the spine and hip, and muscle strength as well as the pain index improved.[32] The effect of impact exercise during 30 months was investigated in elderly women. Bone mineral density in the femoral neck and trochanter decreased in the control group, while no change occurred in the exercise group. Participants of the exercise group experienced less falls with fractures than the control subjects (6 versus 16, P = 0.02).[33]

Tai chi has been promoted for improving balance, and in a randomized study for 1 year, it significantly decreased bone loss in the distal tibia.[34] High-frequency loading by a vibration platform may also increase bone mass of the hip and muscle strength according to one 6-month trial, but more data are needed.[35]

Effects of exercise on balance and fall risk

Poor physical performance and impaired balance are important risk factors for falls.[12] The effect of exercise on balance and falls has been studied in the elderly in the FICSIT trials (Frailty and Injuries: Cooperative Studies of Intervention Techniques).[36] These seven randomized controlled trials were performed in nursing homes or community-dwelling elderly and included various types of exercise, such as endurance, flexibility, balance platform, tai chi and resistance for 10–36 weeks.[36] Follow-up for falls and injuries was done for up to 2–4 years. The fall incidence ratio for general exercise versus control was 0.9 (CI: 0.81–0.99) and for balance versus control 0.83 (CI: 0.70–0.98). Resistance and endurance training did not have an effect on fall incidence. The most successful intervention was multifactorial and included individual attention to postural hypotension, medication, transfer skills, environmental hazards, gait and balance impairment, and focal muscle weakness. This individual-tailored programme led to a 25% reduction of the number of subjects who fell.[37]

The Cochrane review concluded that exercise alone did not establish protection against falling. Significant protection was only achieved with a multifactorial intervention.[38] The components of successful multifactorial intervention to prevent falls have recently been reviewed.[39] Whereas it has been demonstrated that exercise can increase bone density, there is little evidence that exercise decreases the number of fractures.[40] Controlled clinical trials with exercise as intervention and fracture as end-point have not been performed. Another problem is patient adherence. Exercise studies demand professional trainers or physiotherapists. It is questionable that patients will continue exercise on their own, once the intervention programme has been discontinued. It cannot be assumed that patient compliance with exercise will be better than that with bisphosphonate or oestrogen treatment.

Risks of exercise

The most effective training to increase bone mass is high-impact exercise. This, however, carries increased risks of (stress) fracture and osteoarthritis.[41] Endurance training, such as running, may bring cardiovascular risks, but this is very low for walking and moderate strength exercise programmes. Questionnaires for risk assessment can be used to select high-risk individuals.[42]

The emphasis of physical exercise programmes in post-menopausal women, in the elderly or in patients with osteoporosis should not be on increasing bone mass, but on improving muscle strength and balance. The first aim is to decrease fracture risk by decreasing the risk of falling.[41] Such a programme may also decrease bone loss in comparison with an inactive life, but increase of bone mass should not be expected.

Practical considerations

What type of exercise should a doctor advise to his patients? The exercise should be weight-bearing, easy to complete and enjoyable, and it should fit in a daily routine. Most patients can walk and do sitting and standing exercise. An increase in muscle strength and an improvement of balance can thus be obtained without too much effort. The American College of Sports Medicine recommends weight-bearing endurance activities such as stairclimbing, jogging, jumping activities (volleyball) and resistance exercise, with moderate to high intensity at least three times per week for 30–60 minutes.[43]

The social aspect should not be forgotten. When the exercise provides pleasure and well-being, the adherence will be better. An example from a geriatrician is: 'Get a dog and the dog will walk you every day.'

MANAGEMENT OF PAIN

The main consequence of osteoporosis is fracture and fractures are accompanied by pain. An acute fracture causes pain usually lasting until repair has occurred. An acute vertebral fracture may cause pain lasting for several weeks to months, which is slowly abating. The pain may also become chronic. Longitudinal observation in patients following vertebral fracture indicated that the total disappearance of pain may take 2–3 years.[44] Pain increases with the number of prevalent vertebral fractures, and lumbar fractures cause more pain and decrease of physical function than thoracic fractures.[45,46] About one in three vertebral fractures is clinical, i.e. immediately comes to medical attention, usually because of pain. However, subclinical vertebral fractures are also associated with increased back pain and functional limitations.[47,48]

After an acute vertebral fracture, bed rest may be needed for a few days. An analgesic (e.g. paracetamol, 500–1000 mg, three times a day) can be prescribed. When pain is more severe, codeine (10 mg) can be added to each tablet of paracetamol (500 mg). However, this may cause constipation. When bedrest is needed, a laxative should be given. A muscle relaxant (diazepam, 5 mg) can be prescribed especially in cases with very severe pain when bed rest for some days is necessary. Opioids are rarely indicated and should be avoided as far as possible. Non-steroidal anti-inflammatory drugs such as ibuprofen or naproxen can also be used during the first weeks.

Other drugs that decrease pain in the acute stage include calcitonin, a hormone that inhibits osteoclastic bone resorption. Calcitonin (100 IU salmon calcitonin, i.m.) was more effective than placebo in decreasing pain in patients with acute vertebral fractures.[49,50] This applies not only to calcitonin per injection, but also when administered as nasal spray or suppository.[51,52] When prescribed, calcitonin can be administered subcutaneously or intranasally at night.[53,54]

Chronic back pain often results from postural changes inducing muscular tension and traction on ligaments. The kyphosis causes realignment of muscles and tendons, leading to chronic pain. Extension exercises increase the strength of the back musculature, reduce the deformity as far as possible and correct kyphosis. Exercise in a heated swimming pool (29–31°C) results in muscle relaxation and often decreases pain.[55] Another possibility is transcutaneous electrical nerve stimulation (TENS), which can be applied on the most painful area of the back.

Severe long-lasting pain after vertebral compression fractures has succesfully been treated for up to a year with intrathecal infusion of bupivacain with a pump.[56] Another, experimental, option for severe pain due to vertebral compression is vertebroplasty, i.e. the percutaneous injection of polymethylmethacrylate under fluoroscopic guidance.[57,58] Treatment was done in up to seven vertebrae in one patient and resulted in considerable symptomatic improvement. With kyphoplasty, a balloon is inserted transpedicularly in the collapsed vertebra and inflated to restore vertebral height. Subsequently polymethylmethacrylate or calcium phosphate is injected.[59] The procedure may result in (partly) restoration of vertebral height and reduction of pain. Complications of vertebro- and kyphoplasty include paresis or sensory loss in a leg, pulmonary embolism and new vertebral fractures in the vicinity of the treated vertebral fracture. Data on these techniques from randomized controlled trials are not available.

Practical management of pain

In cases of acute back pain, the first step is paracetamol (500 mg) up to a maximum of six tablets per day. When the reponse is not adequate, codeine (10 mg) may be added. Combined tablets (paracetamol with codeine) are available. The next step is to try a non-steroidal anti-inflammatory drug, such as ibuprofen (400 mg, three times a day) or naproxen. Alternatively, the codeine dose can be increased from 10 to 20 mg in combination with 500 mg paracetamol. In cases of very severe pain, calcitonin (50–100 IU) may be given by subcutaneous or intramuscular injection or 200 IU intranasally at night. Improvement should be observed within a week.

MOBILIZATION AND REHABILITATION FOLLOWING FRACTURE

Rehabilitation medicine is aimed at enabling patients to reach and maintain an optimal level of functional abilities. The central goal is restoration of autonomy and well-being. In established osteoporosis, this pertains to maintaining or improving posture, relieving or lessening pain, improving ambulation and preventing falls.

Mobilization and rehabilitation: hip fracture

Treatment of hip fracture may be conservative (undisplaced intracapsular fractures in younger people) or surgical. The latter method allows early mobilization and weight-bearing, and is therefore the treatment of choice in most patients. Over 90% of hip fracture patients receive internal fixation or replacement of one or more components of the hip.[60] Post-operative mobilization and weight-bearing on the affected limb within 24–48 h after surgery are recommended.[61] In acute care, isometric strengthening exercises and mobilizing exercises can start on the first post-operative day. On the fourth post-operative day, supervised full weight-bearing exercises and gait training using parallel bars can be initiated.[62,63]

Seventy-five per cent of elderly, previously independent, home-dwelling individuals who receive early post-operative mobilization and weight-bearing can return home within days or 2 weeks, if adequate after-care from physiotherapist, home help and physician is available.[61] More complex patients with comorbidity will often be discharged to an institution for rehabilitation or long-term care. Between and within countries, a wide variety of after-care is available, ranging from orthopaedic and geriatric wards, orthopaedic–geriatric units, rehabilitation institutions to nursing homes. Depending on pre-existing health and social support status of the patient, the choice will vary.[60]

Overall, the outcome of hip fracture in the elderly is poor. Between one-quarter and one-half of home-dwelling patients admitted to hospital for a hip fracture will never be able to return home.[64,65] In this regard, patients with intracapsular (transcervical) fractures have a greater chance of returning home than patients with extracapsular (pertrochanteric) fractures,[66] who are usually older and have more co-morbid conditions. Admission to a nursing home or a rehabilitation centre after fracture is associated with reduced social functioning.[67]

The success of rehabilitation, i.e. recovery of activities of daily living (ADL) functioning and discharge home, can partly be explained by internal and external patient characteristics.

A pre-morbid impairment of cognitive functioning, ADL status and nutritional status are associated with lower rehabilitation outcomes in elderly patients.[68,69] Having a close relative to provide care obviously increases the chance of discharge home.[70] Admission from acute care to specialized rehabilitation facilities has been associated with improved long-term functional outcome.[71]

Early rehabilitation with a multidisciplinary approach, whether in a specialized unit or at home, appears to influence outcome favourably.[72] Very little research has been done on the contents of the rehabilitation programme. There is some evidence that high-frequency, i.e. more than five sessions per week, physical and occupational therapy can result in earlier ambulation and more frequent discharge home.[73] An exercise programme on strength, postural control and mobility was beneficial 7 months after a hip fracture in a randomized trial among elderly patients.[71] However, evidence from randomized trials and a meta-analysis yielded conflicting results on the effects of special multidisciplinary rehabilitation programmes after hip fracture.[74]

Mobilization and rehabilitation: vertebral compression fractures

Although vertebral compression fractures often go unrecognized until discovered radiographically, they can be the cause of considerable pain, acute as well as chronic. Frost[75] has reported a programme for managing acute compression fractures. In the acute phase, 4–8 days of bed rest at home or in the hospital is followed by getting out of bed for short periods with a thoracolumbar back support and an intermittent horizontal rest regimen for 3 months. However, controlled trials on rehabilitation after vertebral compression fractures have not been performed. When the pain has become chronic, improving muscular support of the spine by exercises may be helpful.[76] In a randomized trial among patients with chronic pain from vertebral crush fractures, positive effects of physiotherapy twice a week for 10 weeks were found. The therapy consisted of balance and muscle strength training with stabilization of the lumbar spine during exercise.[77] The training resulted in a lower pain level, decreased use of analgetics, improved functional score and increased quadriceps strength in comparison with the control group. As stated above, multifactorial programmes including gait, balance and strength training can improve muscle strength and balance and lower the risk of falls.[37] In severe cases with multiple fractures, chest deformities will hamper normal respiration[78] and increased abdominal pressure may cause gastro-oesophageal reflux. Due to thoracic kyphosis and height loss, the lower ribs may touch the iliac crest, causing pain. A kypho-orthesis with additional weights or surgical removal of the 12th rib may be of help.[79] Walking aids may facilitate stretching, decrease kyphosis and lower intra-abdominal pressure.

Orthesis, back supports and walking aids

Despite the lack of formal evidence for their efficacy and safety, bracing of the spine with back ortheses is widely used to treat back pain and to prevent further complications. Most often, rigid or soft thoracolumbar and lumbosacral supports are used, but patient compliance is problematic.[80] A promising alternative is the Posture Training Support, a weighted kypho-orthesis. There is some evidence that it is more effective and has a higher compliance rate than conventional spinal ortheses.[79,80] A newer type of orthesis was reported to increase trunk–muscle strength, which may be explained by increased muscular activity while wearing the orthesis as a consequence of biofeedback.[81]

Walking aids can be of great help in improving and maintaining mobility in patients with hip fracture or multiple vertebral fractures. Following the supervised ambulation with parallel bars, hip fracture patients can slowly advance to the use of a walker or cane. A properly fitted cane should have a rubber tip and be long enough to allow 20° or 30° of flexion at the elbow. Adequate supervision and instruction is of great importance. The cane should be held in the hand opposite the affected side and should support no more than 20–25% of the body weight.

If a patient lacks upper body strength or is unstable with a cane, a walker should be prescribed. First, the walker must be advanced 20–30 cm, followed by the affected leg and finally the other leg. Carrying objects is difficult when using a walker. Adding a basket to store small items can overcome this problem.[82] In recent years, four-wheeled walkers ('rollators') are used with rapidly increasing frequency. They are easy to use, do not need to be lifted and are often outfitted with a seat to enable a rest on longer trajectories. However, a four-wheeled walker also carries some risks.[83] When sitting on a walker, it may slide away, even with properly applied brakes. The brakes may fail, or the walker may tip over. A well-designed walker and proper instructions may minimize these risks.

HIP PROTECTORS

Other factors besides bone strength determine the occurrence of hip fractures. When a fall occurs, the impact near the hip, the absence of protective reflexes and decreased local soft tissue energy absorption are important.[84] A relatively new development for the prevention of hip fractures is the hip protector. It consists of underpants with two hard shells or soft pads that cover the area over the greater trochanter of the hip. Usually, hip protectors are integrated into the undergarment. The general principle is simple: when a fall on the hip occurs, the protectors either aborb the energy of the fall or divert it to the surrounding tissue. As a consequence, the energy that is transferred to the hip is reduced to the extent that no fracture occurs. More than 90% of hip fractures are related to a direct impact on the hip.[84]

Mechanism of action

In a fall, the kinetic energy of the falling body is absorbed upon impact with the floor through deformation of the internal structures of the body, soft tissue layers and of the floor itself. In the absence of energy-absorbing padding, much of the energy must be absorbed by the skeleton. This results in high forces on the bone. A simple fall on the hip from a standing position generates sufficient energy to fracture the bone, even in young healthy individuals.[85] Studies have shown that the energy released during a fall may be several times the amount required to break the hip.[86] Soft tissue can absorb a large part of the energy, which may be one of the reasons for the observed protective effect of obesity on hip fracture risk.[87] A decreased amount of soft tissue covering the area over the trochanter will increase the risk of fracture.[88] Indeed, women who had suffered a hip fracture appeared to have less soft tissue covering the hip compared to controls.[89]

Protection of the greater trochanter to prevent a hip fracture is a logical consequence. Even the use of carpets as compared to a stone or wooden floor will significantly reduce the force that is exerted on the hip.[90] The hip protector is based on two main principles. Firstly, absorption of energy by soft pads placed over the hip and, secondly, redistribution of the point impact load into the surrounding soft tissue ('shunting'), by placing hard shells over the hip. However, absorption of energy by soft pads only seems insufficient to prevent a hip fracture. In vitro fall simulation experiments using seven different materials of practically usable thickness (20 mm) demonstrated that the amount of energy absorbed was relatively low, ranging from 22% to 38%. The impact forces on the femur remained above the fracture threshold of 5 kN. To go below this threshold, the thickness of the materials had to be at least 100–140 mm, which clearly is too thick to be acceptable for a preventive system that must be worn daily.[91] One of the reasons for the inadequate energy absorption of soft hip pads is the small surface of the impact site. The second principle of hip protectors, used in the 'energy-shunting shells', works much like a crash helmet. The curved hard shells increase the area of contact, and also absorb energy, but also lead the energy of the impact away from the trochanter to the surrounding tissues. Three biomechanical studies comparing soft (usually energy-absorbing) and hard (usually energy-shunting) hip protectors found that hard hip protectors were superior to soft hip protectors in reducing the force,[92–94] especially when increasing the force exerted on the hip.[93] However, patient compliance may be higher when using soft hip protectors, and many new hip protectors are developed each year, some of them using new mechanisms such as the airbag.[95] New biomechanical and patient studies should point out which hip protector can be prescribed best.

Preventive effects

The first clinical study on the effectiveness of hip protectors was performed by Lauritzen et al.[96] In this study, which included 701 elderly nursing home residents, 10 nursing home wards were randomized to hip protectors or no intervention (control group). The protectors were worn in special underwear. The protector consisted of two layers: the outer shield was made of polypropylene and the inner part of plastozote (Safehip®). During 11 months of follow-up, eight patients in the intervention group and 31 patients in the control group sustained hip fractures. The effect of hip protectors was significant, with a relative risk of hip fracture of 0.44. It was reported that none of the eight residents in the intervention group who had suffered a hip fracture was wearing hip protectors at the time of the fracture. Compliance to wearing the hip protectors proved to be a problem. Only 24% of the participants wore them regularly.

Since this first study, many different randomized controlled trials on the effectiveness of hip protectors have been carried out.[97–109] A systematic Cochrane review of these randomized controlled trials[110] found a statistically significant reduction in hip fractures for persons wearing hip protectors as compared to controls when pooling the data of studies performed in nursing homes or residential care settings (RR: 0.77; 95% CI: 0.62–0.97) (see Figure 13.1). As can be seen, the effect is only statistically significant in the subgroup of cluster-randomized trials. In cluster-randomized trials, complete homes or wards are randomized to the intervention or control group; in trials using individual randomization, individuals are randomized. The most likely explanations for the difference in effect are: (1) a higher compliance in cluster-randomized trials; (2) (unknown) co-interventions in cluster-randomized trials. One may expect that compliance is higher in cluster-randomized trials, because the whole home or ward is wearing hip protectors, and this is more clear to the nursing staff. However, five out of six cluster-randomized trials showed a compliance lower than 50%. Therefore, the second explanation seems more likely. It may be that when a complete home or ward is assigned to the intervention group, more effort is made and (unknown) co-interventions are performed by caregivers to reduce the incidence of hip fractures.

In Figure 13.2, it can be seen that no significant reduction in hip fracture incidence was found for community-dwelling older people (RR: 1.16; 95% CI: 0.85–1.59). The authors of this review concluded: 'Accumulating evidence casts some doubt on the effectiveness of the provision of hip protectors in reducing the incidence of hip fractures in older people. Acceptance and adherence by users of the protectors remain poor due to discomfort and impracticality.'[110]

Practical considerations

Compliance to wearing hip protectors is low to moderate in most studies. A pilot study by Villar et al.[111] evaluated reasons for non-compliance. Just over a quarter had managed to wear hip protectors for the full period of 12 weeks. Discomfort and poor fit were the main reasons for non-compliance. In a systematic review of the literature, compliance varied between 20% and 92% in the 18 studies that were identified, with a median compliance of 56%.[112] The reasons most frequently mentioned for not wearing hip protectors were: not being comfortable (too tight/poor fit); the extra effort (and time) needed to wear the device; urinary incontinence; and physical difficulties/illnesses. The ongoing development of new types of hip protectors may partly solve these problems. At this moment, hip protectors may be considered for older persons living in nursing homes or residential care settings with a high risk for hip fracture. Adequate and continuous supervision is needed to ensure proper wearing

Review: Hip protectors for preventing hip fractures in older people
Comparison: 01 Provision of hip protectors
Outcome: 01 Incidence of hip fractures: institutional residence

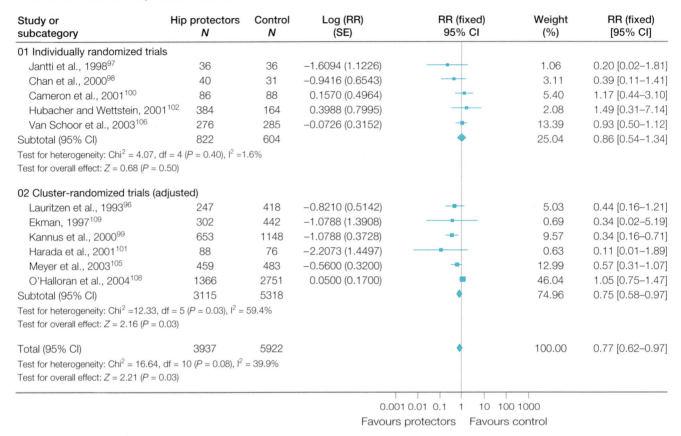

Study or subcategory	Hip protectors N	Control N	Log (RR) (SE)	RR (fixed) 95% CI	Weight (%)	RR (fixed) [95% CI]
01 Individually randomized trials						
Jantti et al., 1998[97]	36	36	−1.6094 (1.1226)		1.06	0.20 [0.02–1.81]
Chan et al., 2000[98]	40	31	−0.9416 (0.6543)		3.11	0.39 [0.11–1.41]
Cameron et al., 2001[100]	86	88	0.1570 (0.4964)		5.40	1.17 [0.44–3.10]
Hubacher and Wettstein, 2001[102]	384	164	0.3988 (0.7995)		2.08	1.49 [0.31–7.14]
Van Schoor et al., 2003[106]	276	285	−0.0726 (0.3152)		13.39	0.93 [0.50–1.12]
Subtotal (95% CI)	822	604			25.04	0.86 [0.54–1.34]
Test for heterogeneity: Chi^2 = 4.07, df = 4 (P = 0.40), I^2 = 1.6%						
Test for overall effect: Z = 0.68 (P = 0.50)						
02 Cluster-randomized trials (adjusted)						
Lauritzen et al., 1993[96]	247	418	−0.8210 (0.5142)		5.03	0.44 [0.16–1.21]
Ekman, 1997[109]	302	442	−1.0788 (1.3908)		0.69	0.34 [0.02–5.19]
Kannus et al., 2000[99]	653	1148	−1.0788 (0.3728)		9.57	0.34 [0.16–0.71]
Harada et al., 2001[101]	88	76	−2.2073 (1.4497)		0.63	0.11 [0.01–1.89]
Meyer et al., 2003[105]	459	483	−0.5600 (0.3200)		12.99	0.57 [0.31–1.07]
O'Halloran et al., 2004[108]	1366	2751	0.0500 (0.1700)		46.04	1.05 [0.75–1.47]
Subtotal (95% CI)	3115	5318			74.96	0.75 [0.58–0.97]
Test for heterogeneity: Chi^2 = 12.33, df = 5 (P = 0.03), I^2 = 59.4%						
Test for overall effect: Z = 2.16 (P = 0.03)						
Total (95% CI)	3937	5922			100.00	0.77 [0.62–0.97]
Test for heterogeneity: Chi^2 = 16.64, df = 10 (P = 0.08), I^2 = 39.9%						
Test for overall effect: Z = 2.21 (P = 0.03)						

0.001 0.01 0.1 1   10 100 1000
Favours protectors   Favours control

Figure 13.1. A systematic Cochrane review of randomized controlled trials of hip fractures in older institutionalized persons wearing hip protectors. Reproduced with permission from: Parker MJ, Gillespie WJ & Gillespie LD. *Cochrane Database Syst Rev* 2005; issue 3.[110]

Review: Hip protectors for preventing hip fractures in older people
Comparison: 01 Provision of hip protectors
Outcome: 01 Incidence of hip fractures: institutional residence

Study or subcategory	Hip protectors n/N	Control n/N	RR (fixed) 95% CI	Weight (%)	RR (fixed) [95% CI]
Birks et al., 2003[103]	6/182	2/184		2.92	3.03 [0.62–14.83]
Cameron et al., 2003[104]	21/302	22/298		32.53	0.94 [0.53–1.68]
Birks et al., 2004[107]	39/1388	66/2781		64.55	1.18 [0.80–1.75]
Total (95% CI)	1872	3263		100.00	1.16 [0.85–1.59]
Total events: 66 (Hip protectors), 90 (Control)					
Test for heterogeneity: Chi^2 = 1.92, df = 2 (P = 0.38), I^2 = 0%					
Test for overall effect: Z = 0.92 (P = 0.36)					

0.01   0.1   1   10   100
Favours protectors   Favours control

Figure 13.2. A systematic Cochrane review of randomized controlled trials of hip fractures in community-dwelling older people. Reproduced with permission from: Parker MJ, Gillespie WJ & Gillespie LD. *Cochrane Database Syst Rev* 2005; issue 3.[110]

of the protectors and to provide assistance when needed. Hip protectors may carry some risk when they are not properly applied (e.g. with the rim on the trochanter). Assistance is essential when the patient cannot put on the undergarment with the hip protectors.

SUMMARY

Non-pharmacological interventions play an important role in the prevention and treatment of osteoporosis and fractures. These interventions include exercise training, physiotherapy, pain management, rehabilitation and hip protectors.

High-resistance training can increase bone density in children and young adults. Exercise training programmes can prevent or reverse bone loss in pre- and post-menopausal women. Multifactorial programmes, including gait, balance and muscle strength training, have been shown to decrease the incidence of falls in the elderly. There is no evidence that exercise can decrease the number of fractures. Walking and moderate muscle strength training programmes should be considered for the elderly and patients with osteoporosis in order to decrease the risk of falls.

An acute vertebral fracture may cause severe pain for weeks to months. Chronic pain increases with the number of prevalent vertebral fractures. Recommended analgesics are paracetamol, paracetamol with codeine, non-steroidal anti-inflammatory drugs and, in cases of severe pain, calcitonin by injection.

The principal aims of rehabilitation are to improve posture and ambulation in order to restore autonomy and well-being. Mobilization after hip fracture surgery should start within a few days. This may contribute to discharge home within a few weeks when the pre-morbid condition was good. In more complex patients with co-morbidity, early rehabilitation with a multidisciplinary approach, whether at home or in a special unit, can favourably influence outcome. Rehabilitation for vertebral compression fracture includes intermittent bed rest, and balance and trunk muscle strength training. Although evidence for efficacy is scarce, back supports (ortheses) are also widely used. Four-wheeled walkers can increase stability. Recently, hip protectors have been introduced to absorb the energy of a fall and redistribute the load to the surrounding tissue. Hip protectors may be considered for older persons living in nursing homes or residential care settings with a high risk for hip fracture. However, adequate and continuous supervision is needed to monitor compliance, which has been identified as a problem in most studies.

PRACTICE POINTS

- Non-pharmacological interventions against osteoporotic fracture include measures to decrease pain, correct postural changes, improve mobility, enable the patient to follow a normal social life and prevent further fracture.

- Important modalities include analgesia, physiotherapy, orthotic supports, hip protectors and exercise programmes.

RESEARCH AGENDA

- Which type of exercise is most effective to prevent falls and fractures?

- The design of an effective, comfortable hip protector which ensures high compliance.

- A randomized trial to test the effect of vertebroplasty against control treatment.

REFERENCES

1. Biering F, Bohr HH & Schaadt OP. Longitudinal study on bone mineral content in the lumbar spine the forearm and the lower extremities after spinal cord injury. *Eur J Clin Invest* 1990; **20**: 330–335.
2. Van der Wiel HE, Lips P, Nauta J et al. Biochemical parameters of bone turnover during ten days of bed rest and subsequent mobilization. *Bone Miner* 1991; **13**: 123–129.
3. Burger EH & Klein-Nulend J. Mechanotransduction in bone – role of the lacuno-canalicular network. *FASEB J* 1999; **13**: S101–S112.
4. Lanyon LE & Rubin CT. Static versus dynamic loads as an influence on bone remodeling. *J Biomech* 1984; **17**(12): 897 905.
5. Heinonen A, Oja P, Kannus P et al. Bone mineral density in female athletes representing sports with different loading characteristics of the skeleton. *Bone* 1995; **17**: 197–203.
6. Cummings SR, Nevitt MC, Browner WS et al. Risk factors for hip fracture in white women. *N Engl J Med* 1995; **332**: 767–773.
7. Dargent-Molina P, Favier F, Grandjean H et al. Fall-related factors and risk of hip fracture: the EPIDOS prospective study. *Lancet* 1996; **348**: 145–149.
8. Tromp AM, Ooms ME, Popp-Snijders C et al. Predictors of fractures in elderly women. *Osteoporosis Int* 2000; **11**: 134–140.
9. Pluym SMF, Graafmans WC, Bouter LM et al. Ultrasound measurements for the prediction of osteoporotic fractures in elderly people. *Osteoporosis Int* 1999; **9**: 550–556.
10. Tromp AM, Smit JH, Deeg DJH et al. Predictors for falls and fractures in the Longitudinal Aging Study Amsterdam. *J Bone Miner Res* 1998; **13**: 1932–1939.
11. Stel VS, Pluijm SMF, Deeg DJH et al. A classification tree for predicting recurrent falling in community-dwelling older persons. *J Am Geriatr Soc* 2003; **51**: 1356–1364.
12. Stel VS, Smit JH, Pluijm SMF et al. Balance and mobility performance as treatable risk factors for recurrent falling in older persons. *J Clin Epidemiol* 2003; **56**: 659–668.
13. Stel VS, Pluijm SMF, Deeg DJ et al. Functional limitations and poor physical performance as independent risk factors for self-reported fractures in older persons. *Osteoporosis Int* 2004; **15**: 742–750.
14. Feskanich D, Willett W & Colditz G. Walking and leisure-time activity and risk of hip fracture in postmenopausal women. *JAMA* 2002; **288**: 2300–2306.
15. Tinetti ME, Speechly M & Ginter SF. Risk factors for falls among elderly persons living in the community. *N Engl J Med* 1988; **319**: 1701–1707.
16. Bradney M, Pearce G, Naughton G et al. Moderate exercise during growth in prepubertal boys: changes in bone mass, size, volumetric density and bone strength: a controlled prospective study. *J Bone Miner Res* 1998; **13**: 1814–1821.
17. Morris FL, Naughton GA, Gibbs JL et al. Prospective ten-month exercise intervention in premenarcheal girls: positive effects on bone and lean mass. *J Bone Miner Res* 1997; **12**: 1453–1462.

18. Welten DC, Kemper HC, Post GB et al. Weight-bearing activity during youth is a more important factor for peak bone mass than calcium intake. *J Bone Miner Res* 1994; **9**: 1089–1096.

19. Layne JE & Nelson ME. The effects of progressive resistance training on bone density: review. *Med Sci Sports Exerc* 1999; **31**: 25–30.

20. Nelson ME, Fiatarone MA, Morganti CM et al. Effects of high-intensity strength training on multiple risk factors for osteoporotic fractures. A randomized controlled trial. *JAMA* 1994; **272**: 1909–1914.

21. Chow R, Harrison JE & Notarius C. Effect of two randomised exercise programmes on bone mass of healthy postmenopausal women. *BMJ* 1987; **295**: 1441–1444.

22. Lohmann T, Going S, Pamenter R et al. Effects of resistance training on regional and total bone mineral density in premenopausal women: a randomized prospective study. *J Bone Miner Res* 1995; **10**: 1015–1024.

23. Nichols JF, Nelson KP, Peterson KK et al. Bone mineral density responses to high-intensity strength training in active older women. *J Aging Phys Activ* 1995; **3**: 26–38.

24. Revel M, Mayoux-Benhamou MA, Rabourdin JP et al. One-year psoas training can prevent lumbar bone loss in postmenopausal women: a randomized controlled trial. *Calcif Tissue Int* 1993; **53**: 307–311.

25. Smidt GL, Lin S, O'Dwyer KD et al. The effect of high-intensity trunk exercise on bone mineral density of postmenopausal women. *Spine* 1992; **17**: 280–285.

26. Uusi-Rasi K, Kannus P, Cheng S et al. Effect of alendronate and exercise on bone and physical performance of postmenopausal women: a randomized controlled trial. *Bone* 2003; **33**: 132–143.

27. Uusi-Rasi K, Sievanen H, Heinonen A et al. Effect of discontinuation of alendronate treatment and exercise on bone mass and physical fitness: 15-month follow-up of a randomized, controlled trial. *Bone* 2004; **35**: 799–805.

28. Wolff I, Croonenborg van JJ, Kemper HCG et al. The effect of exercise training programs on bone mass: a meta-analysis of published controlled trials in pre- and postmenopausal women. *Osteoporosis Int* 1999; **9**: 1–12.

29. Notelovitz M, Martin D, Tesar R et al. Estrogen therapy and variable-resistance weight training increases bone mineral in surgically menopausal women. *J Bone Miner Res* 1991; **6**: 583–590.

30. Villareal DT, Binder EF, Yarasheski KE et al. Effects of exercise training added to ongoing hormone replacement therapy on bone mineral density in frail elderly women. *J Am Geriatr Soc* 2003; **51**: 985–990.

31. Kohrt WM, Snead DB, Slatopolsky E et al. Additive effects of weight-bearing exercise and estrogen on bone mineral density in older women. *J Bone Miner Res* 1995; **10**: 1303–1311.

32. Kemmler W, Lauber D, Weineck J et al. Benefits of 2 years of intense exercise on bone density, physical fitness and blood lipids in early postmenopausal osteopenic women. *Arch Intern Med* 2004; **164**: 1084–1091.

33. Korperlainen R, Keinanen-Kiukaanniemi S, Heikkinen J et al. Effect of impact exercise on bone mineral density in elderly women with low BMD: a population-based randomized controlled 30-month intervention. *Osteoporosis Int* 2005; PMID 15889312.

34. Chan K, Qin L, Lau M et al. A randomized, prospective study on the effects of Tai Chi Chun exercise on bone mineral density in postmenopausal women. *Arch Psych Med Rehab* 2004; **85**: 717–722.

35. Verschueren SM, Roelants M, Delecluse C et al. Effect of 6-month whole body vibration training on hip density, muscle strength, and postural control in postmenopausal women: a randomized controlled pilot study. *J Bone Miner Res* 2004; **19**: 352–359.

36. Province MA, Hadley EC, Hornbrook MC et al. The effects of exercise on falls in elderly patients. A preplanned meta-analysis of the FICSIT Trials. Frailty and Injuries: Cooperative Studies of Intervention Techniques. *JAMA* 1995; **273**: 1341–1347.

37. Tinetti MJ, Baker DI, McAvay F et al. Multifactorial intervention to reduce the risk of falling among elderly people living in the community. *N Engl J Med* 1994; **331**: 821–827.

38. Gillespie LD, Gillespie WJ, Cumming R et al. Interventions to reduce the incidence of falling in the elderly. *Cochrane Collab* 1997; **4**: 1–34.

39. Chang JT, Morton SC, Rubenstein LZ et al. Interventions for the prevention of falls in older adults: systematic review and meta-analysis of randomised clinical trials. *BMJ* 2004; **328**: 653–654.

40. Seeman E. Getting younger and older people moving may seem sensible, but evidence is lacking. *BMJ* 1999; **318**: 1695 (letter).

41. Turner CH. Exercise as a therapy for osteoporosis: the drunk and the street lamp, revisited. *Bone* 1998; **23**: 83–85.

42. Sharkey NA, Williams NI & Guerin JB. The role of exercise in the prevention and treatment of osteoporosis and osteoarthritis. *Nurs Clin North Am* 2000; **35**: 209–221.

43. Kohrt WM, Bloomfield SA, Little KD et al. Position Stand American College of Sports Medicine. Physical activity and bone health. *Med Sci Sports Exerc* 2004; 1985–1996.

44. Ross PD, Davis JW, Epstein RS et al. Pain and disability associated with new vertebral fractures and other spinal conditions. *J Clin Epidemiol* 1994; **47**: 231–239.

45. Oleksik A, Lips P, Dawson A et al. Health-related quality of life in postmenopausal women with low BMD with or without prevalent vertebral fractures. *J Bone Miner Res* 2000; **15**: 1384–1392.

46. Lips P & van Schoor NM. Quality of life in patients with osteoporosis. *Osteoporosis Int* 2005; **16**: 447–455.

47. Nevitt MC, Ettinger B, Black DM et al. The association of radiographically detected vertebral fractures with back pain and function: a prospective study. *Ann Intern Med* 1998; **128**: 793–800.

48. Oleksik AM, Ewing S, Shen W et al. Impact of incident vertebral fractures on health related quality of life (HRQOL) in postmenopausal women with prevalent vertebral fractures. *Osteoporosis Int* 2005; **16**: 861–870.

49. Lyritis GP, Tsakalakos N, Magiasis B et al. Analgesic effect of salmon calcitonin in osteoporotic vertebral fracture: a double-blind placebo-controlled clinical study. *Calcif Tissue Int* 1991; **49**: 369–372.

50. Gennari C, Agnusdei D & Camporeale A. Use of calcitonin in the treatment of bone pain associated with osteoporosis. *Calcif Tissue Int* 1991; **49**(Suppl. 2): S9–S13.

51. Punn KK & Chan MB. Analgesic effect of intranasal salmon calcitonin in the treatment of osteoporotic vertebral fractures. *Clin Ther* 1989; **11**: 205–209.

52. Lyritis GP, Ioannidis GV, Karachalios Th. et al. Analgesic effect of salmon calcitonin suppositories in patients with acute pain due to recent osteoporotic vertebral crush fractures: a prospective double-blind randomized, placebo-controlled clinical study. *Clin J Pain* 1999; **15**: 284–289.

53. Eastell R. Practical management of the patient with osteoporotic vertebral fracture. In: Meunier PJ, ed. *Osteoporosis, Diagnosis and Management.* London: Martin Dunitz, 1999; 175–190.

54. Frances RM, Baillie SP, Chuck AJ et al. Acute and long-term management of patients with vertebral fractures. *Q J Med* 2004; **97**: 63–74.

55. Gold DT, Shipp KM & Lyles KW. Managing patients with complications of osteoporosis. *Endocrinol Metab Clin North Am* 1998; **27**: 485–496.

56. Dahm PO, Nitescu PV, Appelgren LK et al. Intrathecal infusion of bupivacaine with or without buprenorphine relieved intractable pain in three patients with vertebral compression fractures caused by osteoporosis. *Reg Anesth Pain Med* 1999; **24**: 352–357.

57. Mathis JM, Petri M & Naff N. Percutaneous vertebroplasty treatment of steroid-induced osteoporotic compression fractures. *Arthritis Rheum* 1998; **41**: 171–175.

58. Cortet B, Cotten A, Boutry N et al. Percutaneous vertebroplasty in the treatment of osteoporotic vertebral compression fractures: an open prospective study. *J Rheumatol* 1999; **26**: 2222–2228.

59. Kasperk C, Hillmeyer J, Nöldge G et al. Treatment of painful vertebral fractures by kyphoplasty in patients with primary osteoporosis: a prospective non-randomized controlled study. *J Bone Miner Res* 2005; **20**: 604–612.

60. Eldar R & Isakov E. Rehabilitation of hip fractures: a review. *Crit Rev Phys Rehab Med* 1998; **10**: 1–13.

61. Thorngren KF. Fractures in older persons. *Disabil Rehab* 1994; **16**: 119–126.

62. Cheng CL, Lan S, Hui PW et al. Prognostic factors and progress for ambulation in elderly patients after hip fracture. *Am J Phys Med Rehab* 1989; **68**: 230–234.

63. Kyo T, Takaoaka K & Ono F. Femoral neck fractures – factors related to ambulation and progress. *Clin Orthop* 1993; **45**: M101–M104.

64. Melton LJ. Epidemiology of fractures. In: Riggs BL & Melton LJ, eds. *Osteoporosis: Etiology, Diagnosis and Management.* New York: Raven Press, 1995.

65. Borgqvist L, Ceder L & Thorngren KG. Function and social status 10 years after fracture. Prospective follow up of 103 patients. *Acta Orthop Scand* 1990; **61**: 404–410.

66. Keene GS, Parker MJ & Pryor GA. Mortality and morbidity after hip fractures. *BMJ* 1993; **307**: 1248–1250.

67. Jensen JS & Bagger J. Long term social prognosis after hip fracture. *Acta Orthop Scand* 1982; **53**: 97–101.

68. Delmi M, Rapin CH, Bengoa JM et al. Dietary supplementation in elderly patients with fractured neck of the femur. *Lancet* 1990; **335**: 1013–1016.

69. Heruti RJ, Lusjy A, Barell V et al. Cognitive status at admission: does it affect the rehabilitation outcome of elderly patients with hip fracture? *Arch Phys Med Rehab* 1999; **80**: 432–436.

70. Parker MJ & Palmer CR. Prediction of rehabilitation after hip fracture. *Age Ageing* 1995; **24**: 96–98.

71. Kane RJ, Chen Q, Finch M et al. Functional outcome of posthospital care for stroke and hip fracture patients under medicare. *J Am Geriatr Soc* 1998; **12**: 1525–1533.

72. Lyons AR. Clinical outcomes and treatment of hip fractures. *Am J Med* 1997; **103**: S51–S64.

73. Hoenig H, Rubenstein LV, Sloane R et al. What is the role of timing in the surgical and rehabilitative care of community-dwelling persons with acute hip fracture? *Arch Intern Med* 1997; **157**: 513–520.

74. Pfeifer M, Sinaki M, Geusens P et al. Musculoskeletal rehabilitation in osteoporosis: a review. *J Bone Miner Res* 2004; **19**: 1208–1214.

75. Frost HM. Personal experience in managing acute compression fractures, their aftermath, and the bone pain syndrome, in osteoporosis. *Osteoporosis Int* 1998; **8**: 13–15.

76. Sinaki M & Grubbs NC. Back strengthening exercises: a quantative evaluation of their efficacy for women aged 40 to 65 years. *Arch Phys Med Rehab* 1989; **70**: 16–20.

77. Malmros B, Mortensen L, Jensen MB et al. Positive effects of physiotherapy on chronic pain and performance in osteoporosis. *Osteoporosis Int* 1998; **8**: 215–221.

78. Schlaich C, Minne HW, Bruckner T et al. Reduced pulmonary function in patients with spinal osteoporotic fractures. *Osteoporosis Int* 1998; **8**: 261–267.

79. Sinaki M. Musculoskeletal rehabilitation. In: Riggs BL & Melton LJ, eds. *Osteoporosis: Etiology, Diagnosis and Management*. New York: Raven Press, 1995.

80. Kaplan RS, Sinaki M & Hameister MD. Effect of back supports on back strength in patients with osteoporosis: a pilot study. *Mayo Clin Proc* 1996; **71**: 235–241.

81. Pfeifer M, Begerow B & Minne HW. Effects of a new spinal orthosis on posture, trunk strength and quality of life in women with postmenopausal osteoporosis: a randomized trial. *Am J Phys Med Rehab* 2004; **83**: 177–186.

82. Brummel Smith K. Rehabilitation. In: Cassel CK, Reisenberg DE, Sorensen LB & Walsh JR, eds. *Geriatric Medicine*, 2nd edn. New York: Springer-Verlag, 1990.

83. Finkel J, Fernie G & Cleghorn W. A guideline for the design of a four-wheeled walker. *Assist Technol* 1997; **9**: 116–129.

84. Cummings SR & Nevitt MC. A hypothesis: the causes of hip fractures. *J Gerontol* 1989; **44**: M107–M111.

85. Robinovich SN, Hayes WC & McMahon TA. Prediction of femoral impact forces in falls on the hip. *J Biochem Eng* 1991; **113**: 366–374.

86. Lotz JC & Hayes WC. The use of quantitative computed tomography to estimate risk of fracture of the hip from falls. *J Bone Joint Surg (Am)* 1990; **72**: 689–700.

87. Lauritzen JB & Askegaard V. Protection against hip fractures by energy absorption. *Dan Med Bull* 1992; **39**: 91–93.

88. Maitland LA, Myers ER, Hipp JA et al. Read my hips: measuring trochanteric soft tissue thickness. *Calcif Tissue Int* 1993; **52**: 85–89.

89. Lauritzen JB, Petersen MM, Jensen PK et al. Body fat distribution and hip fracture. *Acta Orthop Scand* 1992; **63**(Suppl. 248): 89.

90. Maki BE & Fernie GR. Impact attenuation of floor coverings in simulated falling accidents. *Appl Ergonom* 1990; **21**: 107–114.

91. Parkkari J, Kannus P, Poutala J et al. Force attenuation properties of various trochanteric padding materials under typical falling conditions of the elderly. *J Bone Miner Res* 1994; **9**: 1391–1396.

92. Robinovitch SN, Hayes WC & McMahon TA. Energy-shunting hip padding system attenuates femoral impact force in a simulated fall. *J Biomech Eng* 1995; **117**: 409–413.

93. Kannus P, Parkkari J & Poutala J. Comparison of force attenuation properties of four different hip protectors under simulated falling conditions in the elderly: an in vitro biomechanical study. *Bone* 1999; **25**: 229–235.

94. Schmitt K-U, Spierings AB & Derler S. A finite element approach and experiments to assess the effectiveness of hip protectors. *Technol Health Care* 2004; **12**: 43–49.

95. Charpentier PJ. A hip protector based on airbag technology. *Bone* 1996; **18**(Suppl. 1): 117S.

96. Lauritzen JB, Petersen MM & Lund B. Effect of external hip protectors on hip fractures. *Lancet* 1993; **341**: 11–13.

97. Jantti PO, Aho HJ, Maki-Jokela PL et al. Hip protectors and hip fractures. *Age Ageing* 1998; **27**: 758–759.

98. Chan DK, Hillier G, Coore M et al. Effectiveness and acceptability of a newly designed hip protector: a pilot study. *Arch Gerontol Geriatr* 2000; **30**: 25–34.

99. Kannus P, Parkkari J, Niemi S et al. Prevention of hip fracture in elderly people with use of a hip protector. *N Engl J Med* 2000; **343**: 1506–1513.

100. Cameron ID, Venman J, Kurrle SE et al. Hip protectors in aged-care facilities: a randomized trial of use by individual higher-risk residents. *Age Ageing* 2001; **30**: 477–481.

101. Harada A, Mizuno M, Takemura M et al. Hip fracture prevention trial using hip protectors in Japanese nursing homes. *Osteoporosis Int* 2001; **12**: 215–221.

102. Hubacher M & Wettstein A. Acceptance of hip protectors for hip fracture prevention in nursing homes. *Osteoporosis Int* 2001; **12**: 794–799.

103. Birks YF, Hildreth R, Campbell P et al. Randomised controlled trial of hip protectors for the prevention of second hip fractures. *Age Ageing* 2003; **32**: 442–444.

104. Cameron ID, Cumming RG, Kurrle SE et al. A randomised trial of hip protector use by frail older women living in their own homes. *Injury Prev* 2003; **9**: 138–141.

105. Meyer G, Warnke A, Bender R et al. Effect on hip fractures of increased use of hip protectors in nursing homes: cluster randomised controlled trial. *BMJ* 2003; **326**: 76–78.

106. Van Schoor NM, Smit JH, Twisk JW et al. Prevention of hip fractures by external hip protectors: a randomized controlled trial. *JAMA* 2003; **289**: 1957–1962.

107. Birks YF, Porthouse J, Addie C et al. Randomized controlled trial of hip protectors among women living in the community. *Osteoporosis Int* 2004; **15**: 701–706.

108. O'Halloran PD, Cran GW, Beringer TR et al. A cluster randomised controlled trial to evaluate a policy of making hip protectors available to residents of nursing homes. *Age Ageing* 2004; **33**(6): 582–588.

109. Ekman A, Mallmin H, Michaelsson K et al. External hip protectors to prevent osteoporotic hip fractures. *Lancet* 1997; **350**(9077): 563–564.

110. Parker MJ, Gillespie WJ & Gillespie LD. Hip protectors for preventing hip fractures in older people. *Cochrane Database Syst Rev* 2005; issue 3.

111. Villar MTA, Hill P, Inskip H et al. Will elderly rest home residents wear hip protectors? *Age Ageing* 1998; **27**: 195–198.

112. Van Schoor NM, Devillé WL, Bouter LM et al. Acceptance and compliance with external hip protectors: a systematic review of the literature. *Osteoporosis Int* 2002; **13**: 917–924.

Alison M. Duncan, William R. Phipps and Mindy S. Kurzer

INTRODUCTION

Phyto-oestrogens are naturally occurring compounds found in plants to varying degrees. The classic definition of a phyto-oestrogen is a non-steroidal plant compound that is able to exert oestrogenic effects.[1] Phyto-oestrogens consist of numerous classes including isoflavones, lignans and coumestans.[1] A fourth class of compounds referred to as resorcylic acid lactones might better be classified as myco- or fungal-oestrogens due to their production by moulds found on cereal crops.[1] This review will focus on the isoflavones and lignans, which have received the most attention regarding their classification, food sources, absorption, metabolism and human health effects.

CLASSIFICATION AND FOOD SOURCES

Although isoflavones and lignans are non-steroidal compounds, they are structurally similar to naturally occurring oestrogens, synthetic oestrogens and anti-oestrogens (Figure 14.1). Isoflavones are found in highest amounts in soybeans and soy foods, although they are also present in other beans and legumes.[2] Soy foods generally contain 1.2–3.3 mg isoflavones/g dry weight, with the precise amount depending on numerous factors including the type of soy food,[3] as well as soybean variety, harvest year and geographical location.[4] Studies have estimated typical isoflavone intakes to be 25–40 mg/day for Asians[5,6] and less than 1 mg/day for post-menopausal women living in the USA.[7] The major isoflavones present in soy foods include genistein and daidzein, and to a lesser extent glycitein.[2] They occur in soy conjugated to sugar moieties as glycosides, termed genistin, daidzin and glycitin.[3,4] Clover is another dietary source of isoflavones as it contains high concentrations of formononetin, which is a precursor of daidzein, and biochanin A, which is a precursor of genistein.[2]

Lignans are more widely distributed in plants, found in oilseeds, seaweed, legumes, seeds, fruits, vegetables, whole grains and are particularly concentrated in flaxseed.[8] Flaxseed generally contains 0.96–3.15 μmol lignans/g, with the precise amount depending on factors such as variety, growing location and harvest year.[9] The median daily intake of lignans has been estimated at 578 μg in American post-menopausal women.[7]

Lignans present in flaxseed and other plant foods are termed plant lignans, and include secoisolariciresinol-diglucoside (SECO-DG) and matairesinol (MAT).[9] These compounds serve as precursors to the mammalian lignans, enterodiol and enterolactone.[9]

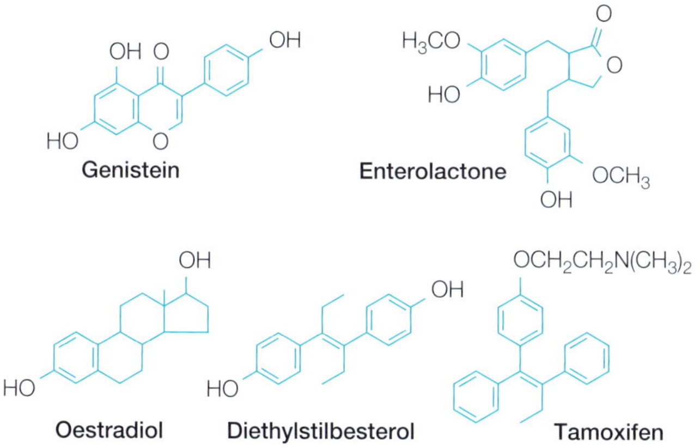

Figure 14.1. Structures of phyto-oestrogens including an isoflavone (genistein) and a mammalian lignan (enterolactone), relative to structures of an endogenous oestrogen (oestradiol), a synthetic oestrogen (diethylstilbesterol, DES) and a synthetic anti-oestrogen (tamoxifen).

PRACTICE POINTS

- Soybeans are the richest food source of isoflavones.
- Isoflavones are present in foods bound to glycosidic linkages.
- Lignans are more widespread in the plant kingdom, with particularly high concentrations in flaxseed.
- Lignans are present in food as plant lignans, which are precursors to mammalian lignans.

ABSORPTION AND METABOLISM

Intestinal bacteria are central to the absorption and metabolism of both isoflavones and lignans.[10–12] Steps involved in the absorption and metabolism of isoflavones are illustrated in Figure 14.2. Following oral ingestion, glucosidases, which are produced by intestinal bacteria, metabolize the glycosidic isoflavones to their corresponding aglycones, which are termed genistein, daidzein and glycitein.[10,11] Before absorption occurs, however, intestinal bacteria may further metabolize the isoflavone aglycones to isoflavone metabolites, specifically genistein to p-ethyl phenol, and daidzein to equol and/or O-desmethylangolensin (O-DMA), all of which may also be absorbed.[10,11] Following absorption, isoflavones undergo hepatic conjugation to glucuronic acid or sulphate,[10,11] to produce forms that are measured in biological fluids.[13,14] Similar to endogenous steroids, they undergo enterohepatic circulation, whereby they are deconjugated in the intestine and reabsorbed or excreted in the faeces.[10,11] Human studies demonstrate that serum and urinary concentrations of isoflavones increase in accordance with the amount consumed, indicating absorption in a dose-dependent manner.[15]

The absorption and metabolism of lignans are similar to that of isoflavones, as illustrated in Figure 14.3. Following oral consumption, the plant lignans, SECO-DG and MAT, are metabolized by intestinal bacteria at various steps.[12] SECO-DG is first metabolized to SECO through hydrolysis of the sugar moieties by intestinal bacteria,[12] followed by dehydroxylation and demethylation to enterodiol, reactions which are also catalysed by bacterial enzymes.[12] Enterodiol may then be absorbed or further oxidized irreversibly to enterolactone, which is then absorbed.[12] Intestinal bacterial enzymes also catalyse dehydroxylation and demethylation reactions to convert MAT to enterolactone, which can then be absorbed.[12] The conversion of plant lignans to mammalian lignans is thought to be efficient; however, the detection of SECO and MAT in the urine[12] suggests it is not a necessary process. It is also possible that there may be other unidentified plant precursors of enterodiol and enterolactone.[12]

Once the mammalian lignans are absorbed, they are conjugated to glucuronic acid or sulphate, enter the circulation and may then be excreted in the urine[14] or undergo enterohepatic circulation.[12] Urinary and plasma concentrations of the mammalian lignans have been shown to increase significantly in a dose-dependent manner following consumption of lignan-rich flaxseed.[16,17] Dietary studies focusing on the effect of specific foods on lignan metabolism have shown significant increases in serum and urinary concentrations of enterolactone following consumption of numerous grains and fruits, including whole grains[18] and strawberries,[19] in healthy adults. In addition, a cross-sectional study reported that plasma enterolactone was positively associated with vegetable and fibre intake as expected; however, there were also positive associations observed with alcohol and caffeine intake, raising concern regarding the specificity of plasma enterolactone as a biomarker for exposure to lignan-containing foods.[20]

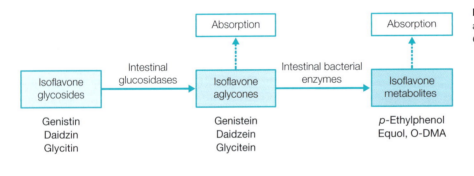

Figure 14.2. Summary of the absorption and metabolism of isoflavones. O-DMA, O-desmethylangolensin.

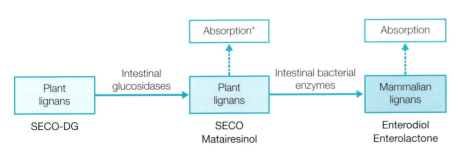

Figure 14.3. Summary of the absorption and metabolism of lignans. SECO, secoisolariciresinol; SECO-DG, secoisolariciresinol-diglucoside. *SECO and matairesinol have been detected in the urine, suggesting direct absorption.[12]

EFFECTS ON HUMAN HEALTH

There has been considerable scientific interest in the role of phyto-oestrogens in numerous aspects of human health. Of particular focus have been the prevalent Western diseases and/or conditions, including osteoporosis, breast cancer, prostate cancer, other types of cancer, cardiovascular disease and alleviation of menopausal symptoms. Research linking phyto-oestrogens to these conditions is continually growing, with common goals of determining the efficacy, safety and mechanisms involved.

OSTEOPOROSIS

Concerns regarding bone health and risk of osteoporosis is most relevant to post-menopausal women, since the decline in oestrogen production that occurs with menopause is thought to be a major contributing factor.[21] Although hormone replacement therapy (HRT) is able to ameliorate the loss of oestrogen at menopause and thereby address the concerns regarding osteoporosis,[22] there remains substantial interest in alternatives, particularly dietary alternatives, to HRT. It is in this regard that phyto-oestrogens have received considerable interest in relation to bone health.[23] Related to isoflavones in particular is research showing that ipriflavone, a synthetic isoflavone, effectively reduces bone loss in post-menopausal women,[24] although a larger, more recent study failed to find a significant effect of ipriflavone on bone mineral density (BMD) in post-menopausal women.[25]

Interest in the potential relation between phyto-oestrogens and osteoporosis risk was first generated from epidemiological observations of significantly lower numbers of hip fractures in Asian women (who consume relatively high amounts of soy), relative to Caucasian women (who consume relatively low amounts of soy).[26] The subsequent numerous observational studies that have related soy intake of pre- and post-menopausal women to BMD have generally reported significant positive associations,[27–29] with only some studies reporting no significant association.[30,31] Interestingly, some results appear dependent on ethnicity and menopausal status, with one study reporting significant positive associations observed between isoflavone intake and BMD within Japanese pre-menopausal women, but not within Japanese peri-menopausal or Chinese women,[32] and another study reporting a significant positive association between isoflavone intake and BMD within post-menopausal but not pre-menopausal women.[33]

Adding to the evidence from observational studies have been human intervention studies that have evaluated the effects of phyto-oestrogen consumption on BMD and/or biomarkers of bone metabolism. Some studies have found positive effects of soy and soy isoflavones on BMD of the lumbar spine[34 36] and bone mineral content of the hip,[37] while other research has not been able to demonstrate significant effects of isoflavone-rich soy protein on BMD of the lumbar spine or hip.[38] Studies evaluating biomarkers of bone metabolism have included endpoints that reflect both osteoblast and osteoclast activity, and as such are able to reflect effects prior to changes in BMD or incidence of fractures. These studies have been less consistent in their results, with some reporting beneficial effects with respect to bone health,[36,39–43] while others have reported no significant effects[44–47] or effects too small to be of clinical relevance.[48] One study that compared the effect of soy consumption directly to HRT in post-menopausal women found that while soy was not as effective as HRT in reducing bone turnover, it did stimulate osteoblastic activity.[49] Another related study concluded that the use of HRT influences the bone-sparing effect of soy, since they found that soy consumption was more effective at reducing bone resorption and urinary calcium excretion in post-menopausal women not on HRT relative to those on HRT.[50]

There are fewer data available concerning the relationship between lignans and bone health. Despite results of a recent epidemiological study showing a significant positive association between urinary enterolactone and BMD in Korean post-menopausal women,[51] intervention studies have reported that 3–12 months of flaxseed consumption resulted in no significant effects on BMD[52] or markers of bone turnover[53] and a non-significant increase in bone mineral content[54] in healthy post-menopausal American women.

BREAST CANCER

The epidemiological observation that Asian women have a significantly lower risk of breast cancer compared to Western women[55] has prompted the theory that high intake of isoflavone-rich soy by Asian women could contribute to this risk difference. Focused observational studies assessing cancer risk and diet have provided support for this theory through findings of significant inverse associations between breast cancer risk and soy isoflavones, both in relation to their consumption[56–59] and their urinary excretion.[60–62] Providing further support is the observation that Asian women who immigrate to the USA and adopt a Western diet lose their lower risk of breast cancer.[63]

Lignans have also received attention for their contribution toward reducing breast cancer risk through results of observational studies. Vegetarians, who have a low risk of breast cancer relative to omnivores, also have a significantly higher dietary intake and urinary excretion of lignans.[64] Furthermore, urinary enterodiol[65] and enterolactone[65,66] are significantly lower in post-menopausal breast cancer patients relative to controls. In addition, significant inverse correlations have been reported between breast cancer risk and dietary lignans,[67–69] serum enterolactone,[70,71] as well as urinary concentrations of enterolactone, enterodiol and total lignans.[62] Consistent with these data are studies showing that consumption of flax or purified lignans reduces risk of mammary cancer in rodents.[72]

Despite these supportive studies, the epidemiological studies relating breast cancer risk to intake and/or urinary excretion of phyto-oestrogens have not been consistent. There was no observed relationship between consumption of soy foods and breast cancer risk in a diet and cancer case–control study in Chinese women[73] or in a prospective study of Japanese women.[74] Similarly, breast cancer risk was not related to either isoflavone or lignan intake in a case–control study involving multi-ethnic American women[75] or a prospective study of Dutch women.[76] Finally, urinary genistein or enterolactone were not significantly associated with breast cancer risk in a prospective study of Dutch women,[77] and serum enterolactone was not related to breast cancer risk in either a case–control study conducted in Finland[78] or a larger prospective study conducted in New York.[79]

Substantial effort has been put toward uncovering potential mechanisms by which phyto-oestrogens may contribute toward a reduction in breast cancer risk. The relation of breast cancer to reproductive hormones,[80] the structural similarity of phyto-oestrogens to endogenous oestrogens (see Figure 14.1) and the ability of phyto-oestrogens to bind to the oestrogen receptor[81] have provided a rationale for evaluating the hormonal and anti-hormonal effects of phyto-oestrogens as one of these possibilities. Although results of human intervention studies evaluating effects of soy and soy isoflavone consumption on circulating reproductive hormone concentrations have been inconsistent,[82–84] effects on urinary hormones have revealed significant changes in oestrogen metabolites related to decreased breast cancer risk, including increases in the ratio of 2-hydroxyoestrone to 16α-hydroxyoestrone following soy[85,86] and flax[87,88] consumption. Other potential mechanisms by which phyto-oestrogens may protect against breast cancer risk are independent of the oestrogen receptor. In vitro studies have revealed that both isoflavones and lignans are able to inhibit enzymes involved in the synthesis of steroid hormones, including aromatase and 17β-hydroxysteroid dehydrogenase.[89,90] In addition, there is evidence that genistein is able to inhibit protein tyrosine kinases, DNA topoisomerases and angiogenesis, and exert antioxidant effects.[1]

Determining the mechanisms involved in the relation of phyto-oestrogens to breast cancer risk is complicated by numerous factors, one of which is age of exposure. Animal studies by Lamartiniere et al.[91] have demonstrated that the maximum protection against chemically induced breast cancer in adult rats is obtained from exposure to genistein pre-pubertally and again in adulthood. These results are consistent with two recent case–control studies reporting that exposure to isoflavone-rich soy foods in adolescence is associated with reduced breast cancer risk as an adult.[92,93]

> ### PRACTICE POINTS
>
> - Despite inconsistent data, many observational studies have shown an association between isoflavone-rich soy consumption and reduced breast cancer risk.
> - Early exposure to phyto-oestrogens may be necessary for breast cancer prevention.

> ### RESEARCH AGENDA
>
> - The impact of age of phyto-oestrogen exposure on the magnitude of potential breast cancer protection requires further exploration.

PROSTATE CANCER

Phyto-oestrogens have also been suggested to play a role in protection against prostate cancer, with most data focusing on soy isoflavones. Population studies report a worldwide discrepancy in clinical prostate cancer incidence, with rates lower in Asian men relative to Western men.[94] The high intake of phyto-oestrogens, particularly isoflavones, by Asian men is hypothesized to contribute toward their lower incidence of clinical prostate cancer.[95] A high intake of isoflavones by Asian men is evident by elevated concentrations of soy isoflavones detected in their blood,[96] urine[97] and prostatic fluid,[97] compared to their European and Western counterparts. Also providing evidence are results from an immigration study reporting an increased risk of developing prostate cancer when Asians are exposed to a Western diet.[98]

Epidemiological studies relating intake of isoflavone-rich soy and prostate cancer risk have been supportive, although not consistently. Two large prospective studies, one of Japanese-Hawaiian men[99] and one of California Seventh Day Adventist men,[100] reported that consumption of tofu[99] or soymilk[100] were associated with reductions in prostate cancer risk of 65% and 70% respectively, although the tofu relationship did not reach statistical significance ($P = 0.054$).[99] Also supportive are two US case–control studies, one of which found a significant inverse relationship between consumption of soy foods and prostate cancer risk,[101] and another which observed a trend toward an inverse association between daidzein intake and prostate cancer risk ($P = 0.07$).[102] Finally, Hebert et al.[103] reported a significant protective effect of soy consumption, four times as large as any other dietary factor, in a large ecological mortality study. In contrast, two case–control[104,105] and one prospective study,[106] all conducted in Asian countries, were unable to detect significant associations between soy consumption and prostate cancer risk. More recent epidemiological studies, however, have contributed more supportive evidence, with three case–control studies relating a reduction in prostate cancer risk with consumption of soy foods and isoflavones,[107] serum concentrations of genistein, daidzein and equol,[108] and the ability to produce equol.[109,110] There have been very few studies examining the association between lignans and prostate cancer, although a very recent large longitudinal case–control study reported no significant association between serum enterolactone and prostate cancer risk in Nordic men.[111]

Intervention studies designed to evaluate the role of phyto-oestrogens in modulating prostate cancer risk have primarily focused on serum prostate-specific antigen (PSA) as a primary outcome measure. No significant changes have been found in serum PSA of healthy men consuming isoflavone-rich soy protein,[112,113] and one study of elderly men with elevated PSA found no significant effects of isoflavone-rich soy protein on serum PSA or p105crB-2, another prostate cancer-related biomarker.[114] However, significant decreases in serum PSA have been observed in some, but not all, studies of men with prostate cancer consuming soy isoflavones or isoflavone-rich soy protein.[115–117] Also worth mention is a highly cited individual case study report that suggested phyto-oestrogens may cause prostate cancer tumour regression by documenting that 1 week of consumption of extracted phyto-oestrogens (160 mg/day), prior to prostatectomy, resulted in cancer cell death with no adverse side-effects.[118] Although there are less data regarding the role of lignans in prostate cancer, one intervention study did focus on lignan-rich flaxseed and assessed its effect on blood hormones, PSA and histopathic features before and after an average 34-day intervention in men who had been diagnosed with prostate cancer and were awaiting surgery.[119] When compared to historic controls, flaxseed consumption significantly reduced total testosterone and the free androgen index, significantly increased apoptotic cell death and tended to decrease tumour proliferation index ($P = 0.05$); however, there was no significant change in PSA. It should be noted that the intervention also included a low-fat diet, which cannot be separated from the effect of the flaxseed.[119]

Given that reproductive hormones are thought to play a role in prostate cancer[120] and that dietary genistein was recently shown to down-regulate androgen and oestrogen receptors in the rat prostate,[121] a potential mechanism by which soy isoflavones may reduce prostate cancer is through effects on blood reproductive hormones. Although epidemiological data indicate inverse associations between soy consumption and serum reproductive hormones in healthy men,[122] the few intervention studies completed have largely shown insignificant effects on serum hormones.[83] Evidence pertaining to other potential mechanisms for a role of soy isoflavones in prostate cancer protection include inhibition of 5α-reductase, the enzyme that converts testosterone to the more potent dihydrotestosterone,[123] inhibition of other enzymes involved in steroid hormone synthesis, including aromatase and 17β-hydroxysteroid dehydrogenase,[89,90] and induction of apoptosis in prostate cancer cells.[124]

PRACTICE POINTS

- Populations that consume large amounts of isoflavone-rich soy have low rates of clinical prostate cancer.

RESEARCH AGENDA

- There is a continued need for human intervention studies designed to evaluate the potential beneficial effects of isoflavone and lignan consumption on prostate cancer risk.

OTHER TYPES OF CANCER

There has also been research investigating the role of phyto-oestrogens in other cancers, such as gastric, colon, endometrial and others.[1] It is prudent to keep in mind that the majority of epidemiological studies relating phyto-oestrogens to these cancers were conducted prior to the hypothesis that phyto-oestrogens could protect against cancer.[125] As such, quantifying phyto-oestrogen intake was often not the focus, raising concern regarding the accuracy of the data.[125]

The relationship between consumption of soy foods and gastric cancer risk appears to depend on whether or not the soy food is fermented. A recent meta-analysis by Wu et al.[126] reported that soy consumption was significantly protective against stomach cancer, provided the analysis did not include studies with fermented soy foods, which actually resulted in a significantly increased risk of stomach cancer. The discrepant results could be due to the high salt content, N-nitroso compounds or other unidentified components of fermented foods;[126] however, the authors noted that the studies were not focused on the investigation of soy foods in particular and pointed out the existence of numerous other confounders, particularly intake of fruits and vegetables.[126]

Studies that have assessed the relationship between soy intake and risk of colon and rectal cancers have generally not been supportive of a protective effect.[125] For example, a large cross-cultural study involving 38 countries found no significant association between soy intake and colon cancer risk,[127] and another Japanese case–control study reported that miso significantly increased the risk of rectal cancer.[128] Studies that have reported a protective effect have often related the effect to low quantities of soy foods, thereby questioning the true effect.[125] A meta-analysis that summarized 19 epidemiological studies relating soy to colon cancer risk reported a general inverse association but noted that few of the associations were statistically significant.[129] Despite the unconvincing epidemiological data, this area warrants more investigation to provide clarity on the conflicting results regarding the relationship between soy foods and colorectal cancer.

Regarding other types of cancer, significant inverse associations have been observed between risk of endometrial cancer and consumption of soy products within Asians and non-Asians in a case–control study performed in Hawaii,[130] as well as consumption of soy protein and isoflavones within Chinese women in Shanghai.[131] In addition, a recent case–control study relating phyto-oestrogens to hepatocellular carcinoma found that cases had significantly lower intakes of genistein, but not daidzein, SECO or MAT.[132]

PRACTICE POINTS

- Consumption of soy isoflavones has the potential to decrease risk of several types of cancer; however, the limited studies preclude consistent conclusions.

- The role of isoflavones in gastric cancer appears to depend on whether the isoflavones are fermented in the soy food, although the high salt and other compounds of such foods may confound the relationship.

CARDIOVASCULAR DISEASE (CVD)

There have been several epidemiological observations supporting a protective role for phyto-oestrogens in modulating numerous markers of CVD risk. Consumption of soy products has been inversely associated with serum total cholesterol,[133] and consumption of both isoflavones and lignans has been significantly inversely associated with plasma triglycerides (TGs) and CVD risk metabolic score.[134] Other studies have observed significant inverse associations between dietary isoflavones and aortic stiffness,[135] dietary lignans and aortic pulse-wave velocity,[135] as well as serum enterolactone and risk of acute coronary events[136] and risk of CVD-related mortality.[137]

Intervention studies evaluating the effect of phyto-oestrogens on CVD risk have largely focused on blood lipid concentrations. A meta-analysis assessing the effects of isoflavone-rich soy protein on blood lipids reported overall reductions in total cholesterol by 9.3%, low-density lipoprotein (LDL) cholesterol by 12.9% and TGs by 10.5%, following an average soy protein intake of 47 grams/day.[138] This evidence contributed toward the approval of a health claim by the US Food and Drug Administration, allowing the food industry to promote soy protein for heart health on their products. Since then, a more recent meta-analysis also summarized a collection of studies that evaluated effects of isoflavone-rich soy protein on circulating lipids.[139] Consistent with the previously published meta-analysis,[138] the authors concluded that consumption of isoflavone-rich soy protein results in significant changes in serum lipids and that these effects are strongly related to gender, initial serum lipid concentrations and dietary pattern.[139]

Although these meta-analyses do not provide specific support for the isoflavone component of soy and the FDA health claim is for soy protein (not isoflavones), the hypothesis that isoflavones are the responsible component has been advanced.[138] This hypothesis is supported by results from clinical interventions designed to assess if isoflavones as part of the soy protein matrix are able to effectively decrease serum lipids.[140–143] Interestingly, clinical studies assessing effects of isoflavone extracted from the soybean matrix have found no significant effects on serum lipids,[144,145] suggesting that the efficacy of soy isoflavones depends on their presence in the soy protein matrix. Further complicating the relationship between isoflavones and soy protein is evidence from a monkey study showing that, although plasma lipids were lowered by isoflavone-rich soy protein but not by soy protein from which isoflavones were removed using alcohol, the lipid-lowering effects of soy protein were not restored when the alcohol-extracted isoflavones were added back to the soy protein matrix.[146] This observation raises the possibility that the alcohol extraction process may alter the quality of soy protein in a manner that compromises its lipid-lowering effects.[146]

Intervention studies assessing the effects of lignan-rich flaxseed on CVD risk have been fewer in number, but consistently report reductions in serum lipids. Jenkins et al.[147] found that serum concentrations of total and LDL cholesterol, as well as of apolipoproteins B and A-I, were significantly reduced following flaxseed consumption. Most recently, Lucas et al.[53] also observed a significant reduction in serum lipids, including total cholesterol and non-high-density lipoprotein (non-HDL) cholesterol, apolipoprotein B and apolipoprotein A-I, as a result of flaxseed consumption.

In addition to serum lipids, other potential beneficial effects have been studied that could provide a mechanism for the protection of phyto-oestrogen consumption against CVD.[148] Among these, antioxidant effects have received attention and are evident from intervention studies reporting an increase in LDL resistance to oxidation and a decrease in plasma F_2-isoprostanes following soy consumption,[149] as well as an observational study reporting a significant negative association between plasma F_2-isoprostanes and serum enterolactone.[150] Also receiving attention have been effects that phyto-oestrogens may exert on the vascular endothelium. Some studies have observed improved systemic arterial compliance in peri- and post-menopausal women consuming extracted isoflavones,[144,151] improved brachial arterial dilation in post-menopausal women consuming soy protein[152] and improved markers of endothelial function in post-menopausal women consuming genistein.[153] In contrast, a cross-sectional study was unable to detect significant associations between endothelial function and intakes of isoflavones or lignans,[154] and a recent 12-month intervention study found no significant effects of isoflavone-rich soy protein on endothelial function in post-menopausal women.[155]

PRACTICE POINTS

- Considerable evidence supports a role for soy protein in reducing blood lipids associated with CVD.
- Food products containing specific amounts of soy protein are authorized in the USA to include a health claim on the label promoting soy protein in the reduction of CVD risk.

RESEARCH AGENDA

- Further inquiry is necessary to understand why animal and human studies report that isoflavones extracted from the soybean do not exert the same beneficial effects as when isoflavones are part of the soy matrix.
- There is a need for further research to clarify the contribution of isoflavones to the lipid lowering effects of soy protein.
- Continued research is needed to understand potential cardio-protective mechanisms of action of phyto-oestrogens besides the reduction of circulating lipids.

MENOPAUSAL SYMPTOMS

The potential for phyto-oestrogens to alleviate symptoms associated with menopause, particularly hot flushes, is an area of active research and relates to the efficacy of isoflavone-rich soy or isoflavone supplements as a possible dietary alternative to HRT. It is well known that Asian women have considerably less menopausal symptoms than Western women and this difference has been hypothesized to possibly be due to their high phyto-oestrogen, particularly isoflavone, intake.[156] Soy intake has been significantly negatively correlated with number of hot flushes in cross-sectional[157] and prospective[158] studies of Japanese women.

Intervention studies in peri- and post-menopausal women have reported decreased hot flushes following consumption of soy; however, in many studies, these were not significantly greater than the decrease observed for the control group.[54,159–161] The apparently strong placebo effect is thought to be due to a true placebo effect and the normal decrease in vasomotor symptoms that naturally occurs over time.[162] Despite this, a few studies have found significant decreases in number[163] or severity[164,165] of hot flushes within the soy treatment group beyond placebo, although the clinical significance of some of the changes observed is debatable. Numerous intervention studies have also used isoflavone extracts and have revealed similarly inconsistent results, with some studies reporting significantly fewer hot flushes[39,166–168] and others reporting no significant effects secondary to an apparent placebo effect.[169–171] The effect of lignans on hot flushes has not been widely studied. Dalais et al.[54] included flaxseed as a treatment group in their intervention study evaluating the effects of phyto-oestrogens, and did find that it reduced the frequency of hot flushes; however, it was not significantly different from the soy or wheat groups. Flaxseed was also included as part of the intervention by Brzezinski et al.,[165] but the modest albeit statistically significant decrease in hot flushes observed could not be attributed directly to the flaxseed, as it was consumed in combination with soy products.

Overall, it appears there is some evidence to support a role for soy isoflavones in the management of menopausal hot flushes, but effects specifically due to soy isoflavones are modest in degree.

PRACTICE POINTS

- Numerous studies have shown that consumption of isoflavones, both as part of the soybean or extracted from the soybean, reduce menopausal symptoms, but this is largely due to a placebo effect.

SAFETY ISSUES

An important area regarding the safety of phyto-oestrogens relates to the widespread use of soy-based infant formula by infants who are intolerant to cow's milk-based formula.[172] Isoflavones from soy formula are well absorbed by infants and circulate at concentrations 13,000–22,000-fold higher than oestradiol,[173] generating considerable concern regarding their long-term health effects, particularly on endocrinological and reproductive outcomes. The most informative study addressing this issue is that of Strom et al.,[174] which involved a retrospective cohort design that examined the association between infant exposure to soy formula and numerous endocrinological and reproductive outcomes as adults aged 20–34 years. Results showed no statistically significant differences between exposed and non-exposed groups for more than 30 health outcomes, although women who had consumed soy formula reported slightly longer menstrual bleeding durations and greater discomfort with menstruation.[174] Although these data are encouraging, more research is clearly warranted and, as such, this topic remains an active area of investigation.[175]

An area of increasing interest relevant to the safety of isoflavones is their use in patients who have or have had breast cancer.[176] Much of this concern arises from studies of ovariectomized, athymic mice that have demonstrated the ability of genistein and soy protein to stimulate the grown of breast cancer cells in a dose-dependent manner,[177,178] as well as the ability of genistein to antagonize the inhibitory breast cancer growth effects of tamoxifen,[179] both at concentrations achievable by humans. Whether these effects would occur in humans is not clear, although there have been human studies reporting stimulatory[180] effects of isoflavone-rich soy protein on the breast tissue of healthy pre- and post-menopausal women and oestrogenic effects of isoflavone-rich soy protein on the breast tissue of the normal breast of pre-menopausal breast cancer patients.[181] It is noteworthy that these studies were of relatively short duration (2 weeks to 1 month) and one did not include a control group.[180]

A final issue worth discussing is the widespread availability of extracted isoflavones in dietary supplement form. The concerns include not only the ease at which high doses could be consumed using these supplements, but also the lack of data regarding their pharmacokinetics and efficacy.[182] Setchell et al.[182] demonstrated that isoflavone extracts are absorbed rapidly and efficiently and that the supplements vary considerably in their pharmacokinetics, dependent on factors such as the starting material, isoflavone profile and isoflavone concentration. Interestingly, deconjugation of the glucosidic linkages of isoflavones present in the soy matrix appears to be rate-limiting for their absorption,[183,184] resulting in a curvilinear relationship between intake of isoflavones in soy foods and their plasma concentrations and apparent bioavailability.[183] This suggests that absorption from isoflavones from food is saturable, possibly making it more difficult to obtain pharmacological blood levels that would raise health concerns.[183,184] Whether this occurs with isoflavone supplements is not as clear, although a recent study assessing the acute pharmacokinetics of one specific formulation of an isoflavone extract reported minimal toxicity of doses up to 16 mg/kg body weight/day in healthy men.[185] Genistein and daidzein were rapidly cleared from the plasma and excreted in the urine, although there were observed elevations of lipoprotein lipase and hypophosphataemia.[185] The long-term effects of consuming high doses of extracted isoflavones are not yet known. In addition to safety, the efficacy of extracted isoflavones is of concern. It appears that extracted isoflavones are able to alleviate menopausal symptoms to a modest degree in some studies;[39,166,167] however, unlike isoflavone-rich soy foods, they do not appear to be able to effectively reduce blood lipids.[144,145] The continual growth of knowledge concerning the safety and efficacy of extracted isoflavone supplements remains a research priority, particularly due to their widespread availability and growing use.[182]

PRACTICE POINTS

- Infants consuming soy-based formula have high circulating concentrations of isoflavones.
- A large epidemiological trial reported minimal long-term adult health effects of consuming infant formula, but more studies are needed.
- Soy isoflavones can stimulate the growth of breast cancer cells in ovariectomized athymic mice.
- The safety and efficacy of isoflavones extracted from the soybean are not as well understood as isoflavones present in the soy matrix.

RESEARCH AGENDA

- Continual evaluation of the safety of extracted isoflavones is necessary.
- There is a need for evaluation of the efficacy of extracted isoflavones relative to isoflavones present in the soy matrix, with respect to various aspects of human health.

SUMMARY

Phyto-oestrogens are important biologically active components present in our diet. Isoflavones (found in highest concentrations in soybeans) and lignans (found in highest concentrations in flaxseed) have received considerable scientific attention regarding their absorption, metabolism and human health effects. Overall, research has been more focused on isoflavones, although the available data on lignans clearly justifies the need for more. Osteoporosis is an active area of research in which soy isoflavones appear to exert some benefit, although not similar in magnitude to that of HRT. Evidence for a protective role of isoflavone-rich soy in protecting against breast cancer is not entirely consistent and is complicated by the apparent impact of age of phyto-oestrogen exposure. The limited studies regarding phyto-oestrogens and prostate cancer preclude consistent conclusions, yet highlight the need for human intervention studies involving both soy isoflavones and lignans. It is apparent that phyto-oestrogens can modulate risks of other cancers, some of which include gastric, colon, rectal and endometrial, underscoring the breadth of their role in human health. A large body of evidence supporting a role of soy protein in reducing CVD risk has led to approval of a health claim for foods in the USA. The role of isoflavones as part of the soybean requires more clarification and more studies are needed to explore the potential benefits of lignans in cardiovascular health. Relevant to a potential alternative to HRT are reports of reduced hot flushes following consumption of soy isoflavones, although a strong placebo effect is also apparent. Related to all areas of phyto-oestrogen research is the need for more knowledge of the safety and efficacy of isoflavones extracted from soybeans. Overall, the wide depth and breadth of research exploring a role for phyto-oestrogens in human health clearly warrants their major contribution to the relationship between diet and human health. Future research designed to explore the outstanding questions and issues will continue to clarify this exciting relationship.

REFERENCES

1. Adlercreutz H. Phyto-oestrogens and cancer. *Lancet Oncol* 2002; **3**(6): 364–373.

2. Reinli K & Block G. Phytoestrogen content of foods – a compendium of literature values. *Nutr Cancer* 1996; **26**(2): 123–148.

3. Wang HJ & Murphy PA. Isoflavone content in commercial soybean foods. *J Agric Food Chem* 1994; **42**(1): 1666–1673.

4. Wang HJ & Murphy PA. Isoflavone composition of American and Japanese soybeans in Iowa: effects of variety, crop year, and location. *J Agric Food Chem* 1994; **42**(1): 1674–1677.

5. Wakai K, Egami I, Kato K et al. Dietary intake and sources of isoflavones among Japanese. *Nutr Cancer* 1999; **33**(2): 139–145.

6. Chen Z, Zheng W, Custer LJ et al. Usual dietary consumption of soy foods and its correlation with the excretion rate of isoflavonoids in overnight urine samples among Chinese women in Shanghai. *Nutr Cancer* 1999; **33**(1): 82–87.

7. De Kleijn MJ, van der Schouw YT, Wilson PW et al. Intake of dietary phytoestrogens is low in postmenopausal women in the United States: the Framingham study. *J Nutr* 2001; **131**(6): 1826–1832.

8. Thompson LU, Robb P, Serraino M et al. Mammalian lignan production from various foods. *Nutr Cancer* 1991; **16**(1): 43–52.

9. Thompson LU, Rickard SE, Cheung F et al. Variability in anticancer lignan levels in flaxseed. *Nutr Cancer* 1997; **27**(1): 26–30.

10. Setchell KD. Phytoestrogens: the biochemistry, physiology, and implications for human health of soy isoflavones. *Am J Clin Nutr* 1998; **68**(6, Suppl.): 1333S–1346S.

11. Setchell KD & Cassidy A. Dietary isoflavones: biological effects and relevance to human health. *J Nutr* 1999; **129**(3): 758S–767S.

12. Setchell KDR & Adlercreutz H. Mammalian lignans and phyto-estrogens. Recent studies on their formation, metabolism and biological role in health and disease. In: *Role of the Gut Flora in Toxicity and Cancer*. Academic Press, 1988.

13. Adlercreutz H, Fotsis T, Lampe J et al. Quantitative determination of lignans and isoflavonoids in plasma of omnivorous and vegetarian women by isotope dilution gas chromatography–mass spectrometry. *Scand J Clin Lab Invest Suppl* 1993; **215**: 5–18.

14. Adlercreutz H, van der Wildt J, Kinzel J et al. Lignan and isoflavonoid conjugates in human urine. *J Steroid Biochem Molec Biol* 1995; **52**(1): 97–103.

15. Karr SC, Lampe JW, Hutchins AM et al. Urinary isoflavonoid excretion in humans is dose dependent at low to moderate levels of soy-protein consumption. *Am J Clin Nutr* 1997; **66**(1): 46–51.

16. Lampe JW, Martini MC, Kurzer MS et al. Urinary lignan and isoflavonoid excretion in premenopausal women consuming flaxseed powder. *Am J Clin Nutr* 1994; **60**(1): 122–128.

17. Nesbitt PD, Lam Y & Thompson LU. Human metabolism of mammalian lignan precursors in raw and processed flaxseed. *Am J Clin Nutr* 1999; **69**(3): 549–555.

18. Jacobs DR Jr, Pereira MA, Stumpf K et al. Whole grain food intake elevates serum enterolactone. *Br J Nutr* 2002; **88**(2): 111–116.

19. Mazur WM, Uehara M, Wahala K et al. Phyto-oestrogen content of berries, and plasma concentrations and urinary excretion of enterolactone after a single strawberry-meal in human subjects. *Br J Nutr* 2000; **83**(4): 381–387.

20. Horner NK, Kristal AR, Prunty J et al. Dietary determinants of plasma enterolactone. *Cancer Epidemiol Biomarkers Prev* 2002; **11**(1): 121–126.

21. Amonkar MM & Mody R. Developing profiles of postmenopausal women being prescribed estrogen therapy to prevent osteoporosis. *J Community Health* 2002; **27**(5): 335–350.

22. Gupta G & Aronow WS. Hormone replacement therapy. An analysis of efficacy based on evidence. *Geriatrics* 2002; **57**(8): 18–20, 23–24.

23. Messina M & Messina V. Soyfoods, soybean isoflavones, and bone health: a brief overview. *J Ren Nutr* 2000; **10**(2): 63–68.

24. Gennari C, Agnusdei D, Crepaldi G et al. Effect of ipriflavone – a synthetic derivative of natural isoflavones – on bone mass loss in the early years after menopause. *Menopause* 1998; **5**(1): 9–15.

25. Alexandersen P, Toussaint A, Christiansen C et al. Ipriflavone in the treatment of postmenopausal osteoporosis: a randomized controlled trial. *JAMA* 2001; **285**(11): 1482–1488.

26. Lauderdale DS, Jacobsen SJ, Furner SE et al. Hip fracture incidence among elderly Asian-American populations. *Am J Epidemiol* 1997; **146**(6): 502–509.

27. Tsuchida K, Mizushima S, Toba M et al. Dietary soybeans intake and bone mineral density among 995 middle-aged women in Yokohama. *J Epidemiol* 1999; **9**(1): 14–19.

28. Horiuchi T, Onouchi T, Takahashi M et al. Effect of soy protein on bone metabolism in postmenopausal Japanese women. *Osteoporosis Int* 2000; **11**(8): 721–724.

29. Kritz-Silverstein D & Goodman-Gruen DL. Usual dietary isoflavone intake, bone mineral density, and bone metabolism in postmenopausal women. *J Women's Health Gend Based Med* 2002; **11**(1): 69–78.

30. Kardinaal AF, Morton MS, Bruggemann-Rotgans IE et al. Phyto-oestrogen excretion and rate of bone loss in postmenopausal women. *Eur J Clin Nutr* 1998; **52**(11): 850–855.

31. Nagata C, Shimizu H, Takami R et al. Soy product intake and serum isoflavonoid and estradiol concentrations in relation to bone mineral density in postmenopausal Japanese women. *Osteoporosis Int* 2002; **13**(3): 200–204.

32. Greendale GA, FitzGerald G, Huang MH et al. Dietary soy isoflavones and bone mineral density: results from the study of women's health across the nation. *Am J Epidemiol* 2002; **155**(8): 746–754.

33. Mei J, Yeung SS & Kung AW. High dietary phytoestrogen intake is associated with higher bone mineral density in postmenopausal but not premenopausal women. *J Clin Endocrinol Metab* 2001; **86**(11): 5217–5221.

34. Potter SM, Baum JA, Teng H et al. Soy protein and isoflavones: their effects on blood lipids and bone density in postmenopausal women. *Am J Clin Nutr* 1998; **68**(6, Suppl.): 1375S–1379S.

35. Alekel DL, Germain AS, Peterson CT et al. Isoflavone-rich soy protein isolate attenuates bone loss in the lumbar spine of perimenopausal women. *Am J Clin Nutr* 2000; **72**(3): 844–852.

36. Harkness LS, Fiedler K, Sehgal AR et al. Decreased bone resorption with soy isoflavone supplementation in postmenopausal women. *J Women's Health (Larchmt)* 2004; **13**(9): 1000–1007.

37. Chen YM, Ho SC, Lam SS et al. Soy isoflavones have a favorable effect on bone loss in Chinese postmenopausal women with lower bone mass: a double-blind, randomized, controlled trial. *J Clin Endocrinol Metab* 2003; **88**(10): 4740–4747.

38. Kreijkamp-Kaspers S, Kok L, Grobbee DE et al. Effect of soy protein containing isoflavones on cognitive function, bone mineral density, and plasma lipids in postmenopausal women: a randomized controlled trial. *JAMA* 2004; **292**(1): 65–74.

39. Scambia G, Mango D, Signorile PG et al. Clinical effects of a standardized soy extract in postmenopausal women: a pilot study. *Menopause* 2000; **7**(2): 105–111.

40. Scheiber MD, Liu JH, Subbiah MT et al. Dietary inclusion of whole soy foods results in significant reductions in clinical risk factors for osteoporosis and cardiovascular disease in normal postmenopausal women. *Menopause* 2001; **8**(5): 384–392.

41. Uesugi S, Watanabe S, Ishiwata N et al. Effects of isoflavone supplements on bone metabolic markers and climacteric symptoms in Japanese women. *Biofactors* 2004; **22**(1–4): 221–228.

42. Crisafulli A, Altavilla D, Squadrito G et al. Effects of the phytoestrogen genistein on the circulating soluble receptor activator of nuclear factor kappaB ligand–osteoprotegerin system in early postmenopausal women. *J Clin Endocrinol Metab* 2004; **89**(1): 188–192.

43. Nikander E, Metsa-Heikkila M, Ylikorkala O et al. Effects of phytoestrogens on bone turnover in postmenopausal women with a history of breast cancer. *J Clin Endocrinol Metab* 2004; **89**(3): 1207–1212.

44. Murkies AL, Lombard C, Strauss BJ et al. Dietary flour supplementation decreases post-menopausal hot flushes: effect of soy and wheat. *Maturitas* 1995; **21**(3): 189–195.

45. Hsu CS, Shen WW, Hsueh YM et al. Soy isoflavone supplementation in post-menopausal women. Effects on plasma lipids, antioxidant enzyme activities and bone density. *J Reprod Med* 2001; **46**(3): 221–226.

46. Dalais FS, Ebeling PR, Kotsopoulos D et al. The effects of soy protein containing isoflavones on lipids and indices of bone resorption in post-menopausal women. *Clin Endocrinol (Oxford)* 2003; **58**(6): 704–709.

47. Roughead ZK, Hunt JR, Johnson LK et al. Controlled substitution of soy protein for meat protein: effects on calcium retention, bone, and cardiovascular health indices in postmenopausal women. *J Clin Endocrinol Metab* 2005; **90**(1): 181–189.

48. Wangen KE, Duncan AM, Merz-Demlow BE et al. Effects of soy isoflavones on markers of bone turnover in premenopausal and postmenopausal women. *J Clin Endocrinol Metab* 2000; **85**(9): 3043–3048.

49. Chiechi L, Secreto G, D'Amore M et al. Efficacy of a soy rich diet in preventing postmenopausal osteoporosis: the Menfis randomized trial. *Maturitas* 2002; **42**(4): 295–300.

50. Arjmandi BH, Khalil DA, Smith BJ et al. Soy protein has a greater effect on bone in postmenopausal women not on hormone replacement therapy, as evidenced by reducing bone resorption and urinary calcium excretion. *J Clin Endocrinol Metab* 2003; **88**(3): 1048–1054.

51. Kim MK, Chung BC, Yu VY et al. Relationships of urinary phyto-oestrogen excretion to BMD in postmenopausal women. *Clin Endocrinol (Oxford)* 2002; **56**(3): 321–328.

52. Dodin S, Lemay A, Jacques H et al. The effects of flaxseed dietary supplement on lipid profile, bone mineral density, and symptoms in menopausal women: a randomized, double-blind, wheat germ placebo-controlled clinical trial. *J Clin Endocrinol Metab* 2005; **90**(3): 1390–1397.

53. Lucas EA, Wild RD, Hammond LJ et al. Flaxseed improves lipid profile without altering biomarkers of bone metabolism in postmenopausal women. *J Clin Endocrinol Metab* 2002; **87**(4): 1527–1532.

54. Dalais FS, Rice GE, Wahlqvist ML et al. Effects of dietary phytoestrogens in postmenopausal women. *Climacteric* 1998; **1**(2): 124–129.

55. Parkin DM. Cancers of the breast, endometrium and ovary: geographic correlations. *Eur J Cancer Clin Oncol* 1989; **25**(12): 1917–1925.

56. Lee HP, Gourley L, Duffy SW et al. Dietary effects on breast-cancer risk in Singapore. *Lancet* 1991; **337**(8751): 1197–1200.

57. Hirose K, Tajima K, Hamajima N et al. A large-scale, hospital-based case-control study of risk factors of breast cancer according to menopausal status. *Jpn J Cancer Res* 1995; **86**(2): 146–154.

58. Dai Q, Shu XO, Jin F et al. Population-based case–control study of soyfood intake and breast cancer risk in Shanghai. *Br J Cancer* 2001; **85**(3): 372–378.

59. Wu AH, Ziegler RG, Horn-Ross PL et al. Tofu and risk of breast cancer in Asian-Americans. *Cancer Epidemiol Biomarkers Prev* 1996; **5**(11): 901–906.

60. Murkies A, Dalais FS, Briganti EM et al. Phytoestrogens and breast cancer in postmenopausal women: a case control study. *Menopause* 2000; **7**(5): 289–296.

61. Zheng W, Dai Q, Custer LJ et al. Urinary excretion of isoflavonoids and the risk of breast cancer. *Cancer Epidemiol Biomarkers Prev* 1999; **8**(1): 35–40.

62. Dai Q, Franke AA, Jin F et al. Urinary excretion of phytoestrogens and risk of breast cancer among Chinese women in Shanghai. *Cancer Epidemiol Biomarkers Prev* 2002; **11**(9): 815–821.

63. Ziegler RG, Hoover RN, Pike MC et al. Migration patterns and breast cancer risk in Asian-American women. *J Natl Cancer Inst* 1993; **85**(22): 1819–1827.

64. Adlercreutz H, Fotsis T, Bannwart C et al. Determination of urinary lignans and phytoestrogen metabolites, potential antiestrogens and anticarcinogens, in urine of women on various habitual diets. *J Steroid Biochem* 1986; **25**(5B): 791–797.

65. Adlercreutz H, Fotsis T, Heikkinen R et al. Excretion of the lignans enterolactone and enterodiol and of equol in omnivorous and vegetarian postmenopausal women and in women with breast cancer. *Lancet* 1982; **2**(8311): 1295–1299.

66. Ingram D, Sanders K, Kolybaba M et al. Case–control study of phyto-oestrogens and breast cancer. *Lancet* 1997; **350**(9083): 990–994.

67. McCann SE, Moysich KB, Freudenheim JL et al. The risk of breast cancer associated with dietary lignans differs by CYP17 genotype in women. *J Nutr* 2002; **132**(10): 3036–3041.

68. Linseisen J, Piller R, Hermann S et al. Dietary phytoestrogen intake and pre-menopausal breast cancer risk in a German case–control study. *Int J Cancer* 2004; **110**(2): 284–290.

69. McCann SE, Muti P, Vito D et al. Dietary lignan intakes and risk of pre- and postmenopausal breast cancer. *Int J Cancer* 2004; **111**(3): 440–443.

70. Pietinen P, Stumpf K, Mannisto S et al. Serum enterolactone and risk of breast cancer: a case–control study in eastern Finland. *Cancer Epidemiol Biomarkers Prev* 2001; **10**(4): 339–344.

71. Hulten K, Winkvist A, Lenner P et al. An incident case-referent study on plasma enterolactone and breast cancer risk. *Eur J Nutr* 2002; **41**(4): 168–176.

72. Thompson LU. Experimental studies on lignans and cancer. *Baillieres Clin Endocrinol Metab* 1998; **12**(4): 691–705.

73. Yuan JM, Wang QS, Ross RK et al. Diet and breast cancer in Shanghai and Tianjin, China. *Br J Cancer* 1995; **71**(6): 1353–1358.

74. Key TJ, Sharp GB, Appleby PN et al. Soya foods and breast cancer risk: a prospective study in Hiroshima and Nagasaki, Japan. *Br J Cancer* 1999; **81**(7): 1248–1256.

75. Horn-Ross PL, John EM, Lee M et al. Phytoestrogen consumption and breast cancer risk in a multiethnic population: the Bay Area Breast Cancer Study. *Am J Epidemiol* 2001; **154**(5): 434–441.

76. Keinan-Boker L, van Der Schouw YT, Grobbee DE et al. Dietary phytoestrogens and breast cancer risk. *Am J Clin Nutr* 2004; **79**(2): 282–288.

77. Den Tonkelaar I, Keinan-Boker L, Veer PV et al. Urinary phytoestrogens and postmenopausal breast cancer risk. *Cancer Epidemiol Biomarkers Prev* 2001; **10**(3): 223–228.

78. Kilkkinen A, Virtamo J, Vartiainen E et al. Serum enterolactone concentration is not associated with breast cancer risk in a nested case–control study. *Int J Cancer* 2004; **108**(2): 277–280.

79. Zeleniuch-Jacquotte A, Adlercreutz H, Shore RE et al. Circulating enterolactone and risk of breast cancer: a prospective study in New York. *Br J Cancer* 2004; **91**(1): 99–105.

80. Clemons M & Goss P. Estrogen and the risk of breast cancer. *N Engl J Med* 2001; **344**(4): 276–285.

81. Shutt DA & Cox RI. Steroid and phyto-oestrogen binding to sheep uterine receptors in vitro. *J Endocrinol* 1972; **52**(2): 299–310.

82. Kurzer MS. Hormonal effects of soy isoflavones: studies in premenopausal and postmenopausal women. *J Nutr* 2000; **130**(3): 660S–661S.

83. Kurzer MS. Hormonal effects of soy in premenopausal women and men. *J Nutr* 2002; **132**(3): 570S–573S.

84. Maskarinec G, Williams AE, Inouye JS et al. A randomized isoflavone intervention among premenopausal women. *Cancer Epidemiol Biomarkers Prev* 2002; **11**(2): 195–201.

85. Xu X, Duncan AM, Merz BE et al. Effects of soy isoflavones on estrogen and phytoestrogen metabolism in premenopausal women. *Cancer Epidemiol Biomarkers Prev* 1998; **7**(12): 1101–1108.

86. Xu X, Duncan AM, Wangen KE et al. Soy consumption alters endogenous estrogen metabolism in postmenopausal women. *Cancer Epidemiol Biomarkers Prev* 2000; **9**(8): 781–786.

87. Haggans CJ, Hutchins AM, Olson BA et al. Effect of flaxseed consumption on urinary estrogen metabolites in postmenopausal women. *Nutr Cancer* 1999; **33**(2): 188–195.

88. Haggans CJ, Travelli EJ, Thomas W et al. The effect of flaxseed and wheat bran consumption on urinary estrogen metabolites in premenopausal women. *Cancer Epidemiol Biomarkers Prev* 2000; **9**(7): 719–725.

89. Adlercreutz H, Bannwart C, Wahala K et al. Inhibition of human aromatase by mammalian lignans and isoflavonoid phytoestrogens. *J Steroid Biochem Molec Biol* 1993; **44**(2): 147–153.

90. Krazeisen A, Breitling R, Moller G et al. Phytoestrogens inhibit human 17beta-hydroxysteroid dehydrogenase type 5. *Molec Cell Endocrinol* 2001; **171**(1–2): 151–162.

91. Lamartiniere CA, Cotroneo MS, Fritz WA et al. Genistein chemoprevention: timing and mechanisms of action in murine mammary and prostate. *J Nutr* 2002; **132**(3): 552S–558S.

92. Shu XO, Jin F, Dai Q et al. Soyfood intake during adolescence and subsequent risk of breast cancer among Chinese women. *Cancer Epidemiol Biomarkers Prev* 2001; **10**(5): 483–488.

93. Wu AH, Wan P, Hankin J et al. Adolescent and adult soy intake and risk of breast cancer in Asian-Americans. *Carcinogenesis* 2002; **23**(9): 1491–1496.

94. Pienta KJ, Goodson JA & Esper PS. Epidemiology of prostate cancer: molecular and environmental clues. *Urology* 1996; **48**(5): 676–683.

95. Adlercreutz H. Phytoestrogens: epidemiology and a possible role in cancer protection. *Environ Health Perspect* 1995; **103**(Suppl. 7): 103–112.

96. Adlercreutz H, Markkanen H & Watanabe S. Plasma concentrations of phyto-oestrogens in Japanese men. *Lancet* 1993; **342**(8881): 1209–1210.

97. Morton MS, Chan PS, Cheng C et al. Lignans and isoflavonoids in plasma and prostatic fluid in men: samples from Portugal, Hong Kong, and the United Kingdom. *Prostate* 1997; **32**(2): 122–128.

98. Shimizu H, Ross RK, Bernstein L et al. Cancers of the prostate and breast among Japanese and white immigrants in Los Angeles County. *Br J Cancer* 1991; **63**(6): 963–966.

99. Severson RK, Nomura AM, Grove JS et al. A prospective study of demographics, diet, and prostate cancer among men of Japanese ancestry in Hawaii. *Cancer Res* 1989; **49**(7): 1857–1860.

100. Jacobsen BK, Knutsen SF & Fraser GE. Does high soy milk intake reduce prostate cancer incidence? The Adventist Health Study (United States). *Cancer Causes Control* 1998; **9**(6): 553–557.

101. Kolonel LN, Hankin JH, Whittemore AS et al. Vegetables, fruits, legumes and prostate cancer: a multiethnic case–control study. *Cancer Epidemiol Biomarkers Prev* 2000; **9**(8): 795–804.

102. Strom SS, Yamamura Y, Duphorne CM et al. Phytoestrogen intake and prostate cancer: a case–control study using a new database. *Nutr Cancer* 1999; **33**(1): 20–25.

103. Hebert JR, Hurley TG, Olendzki BC et al. Nutritional and socioeconomic factors in relation to prostate cancer mortality: a cross-national study. *J Natl Cancer Inst* 1998; **90**(21): 1637–1647.

104. Lee MM, Wang RT, Hsing AW et al. Case–control study of diet and prostate cancer in China. *Cancer Causes Control* 1998; **9**(6): 545–552.

105. Oishi K, Okada K, Yoshida O et al. A case–control study of prostatic cancer with reference to dietary habits. *Prostate* 1988; **12**(2): 179–190.

106. Hirayama T. Epidemiology of prostate cancer with special reference to the role of diet. *Natl Cancer Inst Monogr* 1979; **53**: 149–155.

107. Lee MM, Gomez SL, Chang JS et al. Soy and isoflavone consumption in relation to prostate cancer risk in China. *Cancer Epidemiol Biomarkers Prev* 2003; 12(7): 665–668.

108. Ozasa K, Nakao M, Watanabe Y et al. Serum phytoestrogens and prostate cancer risk in a nested case–control study among Japanese men. *Cancer Sci* 2004; **95**(1): 65–71.

109. Akaza H, Miyanaga N, Takashima N et al. Comparisons of percent equol producers between prostate cancer patients and controls: case-controlled studies of isoflavones in Japanese, Korean and American residents. *Jpn J Clin Oncol* 2004; **34**(2): 86–89.

110. Akaza H, Miyanaga N, Takashima N et al. Is daidzein non-metabolizer a high risk for prostate cancer? A case-controlled study of serum soybean isoflavone concentration. *Jpn J Clin Oncol* 2002; **32**(8): 296–300.

111. Stattin P, Adlercreutz H, Tenkanen L et al. Circulating enterolactone and prostate cancer risk: a Nordic nested case–control study. *Int J Cancer* 2002; **99**(1): 124–129.

112. Jenkins DJ, Kendall CW, D'Costa MA et al. Soy consumption and phytoestrogens: effect on serum prostate specific antigen when blood lipids and oxidized low-density lipoprotein are reduced in hyperlipidemic men. *J Urol* 2003; **169**(2): 507–511.

113. Adams KF, Chen C, Newton KM et al. Soy isoflavones do not modulate prostate-specific antigen concentrations in older men in a randomized controlled trial. *Cancer Epidemiol Biomarkers Prev* 2004; **13**(4): 644–648.

114. Urban D, Irwin W, Kirk M et al. The effect of isolated soy protein on plasma biomarkers in elderly men with elevated serum prostate specific antigen. *J Urol* 2001; **165**(1): 294–300.

115. Hussain M, Banerjee M, Sarkar FH et al. Soy isoflavones in the treatment of prostate cancer. *Nutr Cancer* 2003; **47**(2): 111–117.

116. DeVere White RW, Hackman RM, Soares SE et al. Effects of a genistein-rich extract on PSA levels in men with a history of prostate cancer. *Urology* 2004; **63**(2): 259–263.

117. Kumar NB, Cantor A, Allen K et al. The specific role of isoflavones in reducing prostate cancer risk. *Prostate* 2004; **59**(2): 141–147.

118. Stephens FO. Phytoestrogens and prostate cancer: possible preventive role. *Med J Aust* 1997; **167**(3): 138–140.

119. Demark-Wahnefried W, Price DT, Polascik TJ et al. Pilot study of dietary fat restriction and flaxseed supplementation in men with prostate cancer before surgery: exploring the effects on hormonal levels, prostate-specific antigen, and histopathologic features. *Urology* 2001; **58**(1): 47–52.

120. Lopez-Otin C & Diamandis EP. Breast and prostate cancer: an analysis of common epidemiological, genetic, and biochemical features. *Endocr Rev* 1998; **19**(4): 365–396.

121. Fritz WA, Wang J, Eltoum IE et al. Dietary genistein down-regulates androgen and estrogen receptor expression in the rat prostate. *Molec Cell Endocrinol* 2002; **186**(1): 89–99.

122. Nagata C, Inaba S, Kawakami N et al. Inverse association of soy product intake with serum androgen and estrogen concentrations in Japanese men. *Nutr Cancer* 2000; **36**(1): 14–18.

123. Evans BA, Griffiths K & Morton MS. Inhibition of 5 alpha-reductase in genital skin fibroblasts and prostate tissue by dietary lignans and isoflavonoids. *J Endocrinol* 1995; **147**(2): 295–302.

124. Onozawa M, Fukuda K, Ohtani M et al. Effects of soybean isoflavones on cell growth and apoptosis of the human prostatic cancer cell line LNCaP. *Jpn J Clin Oncol* 1998; **28**(6): 360–363.

125. Messina M & Bennink M. Soyfoods, isoflavones and risk of colonic cancer: a review of the in vitro and in vivo data. *Baillieres Clin Endocrinol Metab* 1998; **12**(4): 707–728.

126. Wu AH, Yang D & Pike MC. A meta-analysis of soyfoods and risk of stomach cancer: the problem of potential confounders. *Cancer Epidemiol Biomarkers Prev* 2000; **9**(10): 1051–1058.

127. McKeown-Eyssen GE & Bright-See E. Dietary factors in colon cancer: international relationships. *Nutr Cancer* 1984; **6**(3): 160–170.

128. Tajima K & Tominaga S. Dietary habits and gastro-intestinal cancers: a comparative case–control study of stomach and large intestinal cancers in Nagoya, Japan. *Jpn J Cancer Res* 1985; **76**(8): 705–716.

129. Spector D, Anthony M, Alexander D et al. Soy consumption and colorectal cancer. *Nutr Cancer* 2003; **47**(1): 1–12.

130. Goodman MT, Wilkens LR, Hankin JH et al. Association of soy and fiber consumption with the risk of endometrial cancer. *Am J Epidemiol* 1997; **146**(4): 294–306.

131. Xu WH, Zheng W, Xiang YB et al. Soya food intake and risk of endometrial cancer among Chinese women in Shanghai: population based case control study. *BMJ* 2004; **328**(7451): 1285.

132. Lei B, Roncaglia V, Vigano R et al. Phytoestrogens and liver disease. *Molec Cell Endocrinol* 2002; **193**(1–2): 81–84.

133. Nagata C, Takatsuka N, Kurisu Y et al. Decreased serum total cholesterol concentration is associated with high intake of soy products in Japanese men and women. *J Nutr* 1998; **128**(2): 209–213.

134. De Kleijn MJ, van der Schouw YT, Wilson PW et al. Dietary intake of phytoestrogens is associated with a favorable metabolic cardiovascular risk profile in postmenopausal U.S. women: the Framingham study. *J Nutr* 2002; **132**(2): 276–282.

135. Van der Schouw YT, Pijpe A, Lebrun CE et al. Higher usual dietary intake of phytoestrogens is associated with lower aortic stiffness in postmenopausal women. *Arterioscler Thromb Vasc Biol* 2002; **22**(8): 1316–1322.

136. Vanharanta M, Voutilainen S, Lakka TA et al. Risk of acute coronary events according to serum concentrations of enterolactone: a prospective population-based case–control study. *Lancet* 1999; **354**(9196): 2112–2115.

137. Vanharanta M, Voutilainen S, Rissanen TH et al. Risk of cardiovascular disease-related and all-cause death according to serum concentrations of enterolactone: Kuopio Ischaemic Heart Disease Risk Factor Study. *Arch Intern Med* 2003; **163**(9): 1099–1104.

138. Anderson JW, Johnstone BM & Cook-Newell ME. Meta-analysis of the effects of soy protein intake on serum lipids. *N Engl J Med* 1995; **333**(5): 276–282.

139. Zhan S & Ho SC. Meta-analysis of the effects of soy protein containing isoflavones on the lipid profile. *Am J Clin Nutr* 2005; **81**(2): 397–408.

140. Crouse JR III, Morgan T, Terry JG et al. A randomized trial comparing the effect of casein with that of soy protein containing varying amounts of isoflavones on plasma concentrations of lipids and lipoproteins. *Arch Intern Med* 1999; **159**(17): 2070–2076.

141. Merz-Demlow BE, Duncan AM, Wangen KE et al. Soy isoflavones improve plasma lipids in normocholesterolemic, premenopausal women. *Am J Clin Nutr* 2000; **71**(6): 1462–1469.

142. Wangen KE, Duncan AM, Xu X et al. Soy isoflavones improve plasma lipids in normocholesterolemic and mildly hypercholesterolemic postmenopausal women. *Am J Clin Nutr* 2001; **73**(2): 225–231.

143. Gardner CD, Newell KA, Cherin R et al. The effect of soy protein with or without isoflavones relative to milk protein on plasma lipids in hypercholesterolemic postmenopausal women. *Am J Clin Nutr* 2001; **73**(4): 728–735.

144. Nestel PJ, Pomeroy S, Kay S et al. Isoflavones from red clover improve systemic arterial compliance but not plasma lipids in menopausal women. *J Clin Endocrinol Metab* 1999; **84**(3): 895–898.

145. Dewell A, Hollenbeck CB & Bruce B. The effects of soy-derived phytoestrogens on serum lipids and lipoproteins in moderately hypercholesterolemic postmenopausal women. *J Clin Endocrinol Metab* 2002; **87**(1): 118–121.

146. Clarkson TB. Soy, soy phytoestrogens and cardiovascular disease. *J Nutr* 2002; **132**(3): 566S–569S.

147. Jenkins DJ, Kendall CW, Vidgen E et al. Health aspects of partially defatted flaxseed, including effects on serum lipids, oxidative measures, and ex vivo androgen and progestin activity: a controlled crossover trial. *Am J Clin Nutr* 1999; **69**(3): 395–402.

148. Anthony MS, Clarkson TB & Williams JK. Effects of soy isoflavones on atherosclerosis: potential mechanisms. *Am J Clin Nutr* 1998; **68**(6, Suppl.): 1390S–1393S.

149. Wiseman H, O'Reilly JD, Adlercreutz H et al. Isoflavone phytoestrogens consumed in soy decrease F(2)-isoprostane concentrations and increase resistance of low-density lipoprotein to oxidation in humans. *Am J Clin Nutr* 2000; **72**(2): 395–400.

150. Vanharanta M, Voutilainen S, Nurmi T et al. Association between low serum enterolactone and increased plasma F2-isoprostanes, a measure of lipid peroxidation. *Atherosclerosis* 2002; **160**(2): 465–469.

151. Nestel PJ, Yamashita T, Sasahara T et al. Soy isoflavones improve systemic arterial compliance but not plasma lipids in menopausal and perimenopausal women. *Arterioscler Thromb Vasc Biol* 1997; **17**(12): 3392–3398.

152. Steinberg FM, Guthrie NL, Villablanca AC et al. Soy protein with isoflavones has favorable effects on endothelial function that are independent of lipid and antioxidant effects in healthy postmenopausal women. *Am J Clin Nutr* 2003; **78**(1): 123–130.

153. Squadrito F, Altavilla D, Crisafulli A et al. Effect of genistein on endothelial function in postmenopausal women: a randomized, double-blind, controlled study. *Am J Med* 2003; **114**(6): 470–476.

154. Kreijkamp-Kaspers S, Kok L, Bots ML et al. Dietary phytoestrogens and vascular function in postmenopausal women: a cross-sectional study. *J Hypertens* 2004; **22**(7): 1381–1388.

155. Kreijkamp-Kaspers S, Kok L, Bots ML et al. Randomized controlled trial of the effects of soy protein containing isoflavones on vascular function in postmenopausal women. *Am J Clin Nutr* 2005; **81**(1): 189–195.

156. Adlercreutz H, Hamalainen E, Gorbach S et al. Dietary phyto-oestrogens and the menopause in Japan. *Lancet* 1992; **339**(8803): 1233.

157. Nagata C, Shimizu H, Takami R et al. Hot flushes and other menopausal symptoms in relation to soy product intake in Japanese women. *Climacteric* 1999; **2**(1): 6–12.

158. Nagata C, Takatsuka N, Kawakami N et al. Soy product intake and hot flashes in Japanese women: results from a community-based prospective study. *Am J Epidemiol* 2001; **153**(8): 790–793.

159. Murkies AL, Wilcox G & Davis SR. Clinical review 92: Phytoestrogens. *J Clin Endocrinol Metab* 1998; **83**(2): 297–303.

160. Knight DC, Howes JB, Eden JA et al. Effects on menopausal symptoms and acceptability of isoflavone-containing soy powder dietary supplementation. *Climacteric* 2001; **4**(1): 13–18.

161. Van Patten CL, Olivotto IA, Chambers GK et al. Effect of soy phytoestrogens on hot flashes in postmenopausal women with breast cancer: a randomized, controlled clinical trial. *J Clin Oncol* 2002; **20**(6): 1449–1455.

162. Davis SR. Phytoestrogen therapy for menopausal symptoms? *BMJ* 2001; **323**(7309): 354–355.

163. Albertazzi P, Pansini F, Bonaccorsi G et al. The effect of dietary soy supplementation on hot flushes. *Obstet Gynecol* 1998; **91**(1): 6–11.

164. Washburn S, Burke GL, Morgan T et al. Effect of soy protein supplementation on serum lipoproteins, blood pressure, and menopausal symptoms in perimenopausal women. *Menopause* 1999; **6**(1): 7–13.

165. Brzezinski A, Adlercreutz H, Shaoul R et al. Short-term effects of phytoestrogen-rich diet on postmenopausal women. *J North Am Menopause Soc* 1997; **4**(2): 89–94.

166. Faure ED, Chantre P & Mares P. Effects of a standardized soy extract on hot flushes: a multicenter, double-blind, randomized, placebo-controlled study. *Menopause* 2002; **9**(5): 329–334.

167. Han KK, Soares JM Jr, Haidar MA et al. Benefits of soy isoflavone therapeutic regimen on menopausal symptoms. *Obstet Gynecol* 2002; **99**(3): 389–394.

168. Crisafulli A, Marini H, Bitto A et al. Effects of genistein on hot flushes in early postmenopausal women: a randomized, double-blind EPT- and placebo-controlled study. *Menopause* 2004; **11**(4): 400–404.

169. Baber RJ, Templeman C, Morton T et al. Randomized placebo-controlled trial of an isoflavone supplement and menopausal symptoms in women. *Climacteric* 1999; **2**(2): 85–92.

170. Knight DC, Howes JB & Eden JA. The effect of Promensil, an isoflavone extract, on menopausal symptoms. *Climacteric* 1999; **2**(2): 79–84.

171. Quella SK, Loprinzi CL, Barton DL et al. Evaluation of soy phytoestrogens for the treatment of hot flashes in breast cancer survivors: a North Central Cancer Treatment Group Trial. *J Clin Oncol* 2000; **18**(5): 1068–1074.

172. Mendez MA, Anthony MS & Arab L. Soy-based formulae and infant growth and development: a review. *J Nutr* 2002; **132**(8): 2127–2130.

173. Setchell KD, Zimmer-Nechemias L, Cai J et al. Isoflavone content of infant formulas and the metabolic fate of these phytoestrogens in early life. *Am J Clin Nutr* 1998; **68**(6, Suppl): 1453S–1461S.

174. Strom BL, Schinnar R, Ziegler EE et al. Exposure to soy-based formula in infancy and endocrinological and reproductive outcomes in young adulthood. *JAMA* 2001; **286**(7): 807–814.

175. Badger TM, Ronis MJ, Hakkak R et al. The health consequences of early soy consumption. *J Nutr* 2002; **132**(3): 559S–565S.

176. Messina MJ & Loprinzi CL. Soy for breast cancer survivors: a critical review of the literature. *J Nutr* 2001; **131**(11, Suppl.): 3095S–3108S.

177. Allred CD, Allred KF, Ju YH et al. Soy diets containing varying amounts of genistein stimulate growth of estrogen-dependent (MCF-7) tumors in a dose-dependent manner. *Cancer Res* 2001; **61**(13): 5045–5050.

178. Ju YH, Allred CD, Allred KF et al. Physiological concentrations of dietary genistein dose-dependently stimulate growth of estrogen-dependent human breast cancer (MCF-7) tumors implanted in athymic nude mice. *J Nutr* 2001; **131**(11): 2957–2962.

179. Ju YH, Doerge DR, Allred KF et al. Dietary genistein negates the inhibitory effect of tamoxifen on growth of estrogen-dependent human breast cancer (MCF-7) cells implanted in athymic mice. *Cancer Res* 2002; **62**(9): 2474–2477.

180. Petrakis NL, Barnes S, King EB et al. Stimulatory influence of soy protein isolate on breast secretion in pre- and postmenopausal women. *Cancer Epidemiol Biomarkers Prev* 1996; **5**(10): 785–794.

181. Hargreaves DF, Potten CS, Harding C et al. Two-week dietary soy supplementation has an estrogenic effect on normal premenopausal breast. *J Clin Endocrinol Metab* 1999; **84**(11): 4017–4024.

182. Setchell KD, Brown NM, Desai P et al. Bioavailability of pure isoflavones in healthy humans and analysis of commercial soy isoflavone supplements. *J Nutr* 2001; **131**(4, Suppl.): 1362S–1375S.

183. Setchell KD. Absorption and metabolism of soy isoflavones – from food to dietary supplements and adults to infants. *J Nutr* 2000; **130**(3): 654S–655S.

184. Setchell KD, Brown NM, Zimmer-Nechemias L et al. Evidence for lack of absorption of soy isoflavone glycosides in humans, supporting the crucial role of intestinal metabolism for bioavailability. *Am J Clin Nutr* 2002; **76**(2): 447–453.

185. Busby MG, Jeffcoat AR, Bloedon LT et al. Clinical characteristics and pharmacokinetics of purified soy isoflavones: single-dose administration to healthy men. *Am J Clin Nutr* 2002; **75**(1): 126–136.

Chapter 15

Oestrogen and selective oestrogen receptor modulators (SERMs): current roles in the prevention and treatment of osteoporosis

David W. Purdie

Human female fertility, declining from age >30, reaches a relatively abrupt halt at around the age of 45–50 years, when the impact of senescence on most other systems is yet small. In the animal kingdom only chimpanzees and macaques experience an event similar to the human menopause, although data are few and the pathophysiology is far less clear-cut. In humans, the evolution of programmed ovarian failure and the consequent menopause must have conferred an evolutionary survival advantage, perhaps in releasing grandmothers to assist daughters in the rearing of offspring through the decade-long human childhood.[1] However, with female life expectancy now at a mean of 82 years in the UK, the menopause at its modal age of 51 years is now a midlife event and is followed by some 30 years of obligatory oestrogen deficiency. Trabecular bone loss, already under way in both sexes during the fifth decade, is accelerated by oestradiol withdrawal for around a decade, after which loss rates decline, but continue through the remainder of life. Life expectancy is not matched by health expectancy. The rapid secular increase in the aged population and in the age-specific incidence of fragility fractures mandates that the early detection of osteoporosis and the prevention of fractures is now a major public health issue.

Since the post-menopause is by definition a state of oestrogen deprivation, oestrogen replacement therapy would therefore seem to be the most obvious solution. However, problems with adherence due to adverse effects and regulatory caution in the wake of safety concerns from randomized trial data have inhibited its use. For the prevention of osteoporosis, treatment has to be continued long term and adherence to hormone replacement theory (HRT) regimens is less than ideal, with only some 20% of women prescribed HRT still taking it after 6 months. Women reject the return of monthly bleeding in particular and fear an increased risk of breast cancer. Hence the urgent search for agents that can only target the oestrogen receptor in specified tissues where an oestrogenic effect is desirable and which will hence function more specifically. Ideally, these drugs should confer all the benefits of HRT on bone without adverse effects on the breast and uterus. The pharmaceutical sector is working to provide such drugs and a new class of drug – the selective oestrogen receptor modulators (SERMs) – has arisen.

In the following, an outline is given of how successful the quest has been for a more patient-acceptable form of therapy in post-menopausal osteoporosis.

THE BONE REMODELLING UNIT AND OESTROGEN

Bone remodelling occurs throughout life at discrete microscopic sites within the skeleton and proceeds in an orderly fashion, with initial bone resorption being followed by bone formation, a phenomenon referred to as coupling. This maintenance programme is necessary for both metabolic and mechanical skeletal functions.

Although this sequence occurs in both cortical and cancellous bone,[2] in the post-menopause, the bone remodelling unit (BRU) frequency is highest in the 20% of the skeleton which is cancellous or trabecular bone, i.e. the part of the skeleton in proximity to red marrow. These are the sites that consequently are more responsive to metabolic perturbation or pharmacological intervention. By contrast, the area of the skeleton in which marrow is principally fat is primarily designed to maintain biomechanical competence, although obviously the whole skeleton carries out this purpose. Vertebrae, the femoral neck and the distal arm bones are sites that are particularly rich in trabecular bone, and consequently are the preferential sites for osteoporosis and potential fractures.

The cyclic process of bone resorption followed by synthesis of bone matrix and its subsequent mineralization takes up to 6 months. If the processes of bone resorption and bone formation are not matched there is a remodelling imbalance, and such an imbalance is magnified when the rate of initiation of new cycles of bone remodelling increases. This occurs in post-menopausal women in whom, at any time, some bone will have been resorbed and not yet replaced. This is referred to as the remodelling space. Menopausal oestrogen decline reduces bone mass through at least two mechanisms. On the one hand, it increases the rate at which remodelling sites are activated, while on the other it decouples the remodelling cycle in such a way that the amount of new bone synthesized by osteoblasts falls below the amount previously removed by the osteoclast team. Whether this results from excessive osteoclast action or inefficient osteoblast activity remains unclear, although the general opinion is that the excessive osteoclast activity is responsible. The net result, however, is a moderate reduction of bone mass that can be arrested by reintroducing oestrogen. If, however, the process is allowed to continue, it may result in progressive thinning and then disconnection – through perforation – of trabeculae. This loss of template upon which new bone can no longer be built will result in a permanent deficit of mass and structure.[3] Oestrogen replacement therapy prevents postmenopausal bone loss. Its principal action is to reduce bone resorption by decreasing the rate of initiation of new remodelling cycles and recoupling, i.e. rebalancing, bone resorption and formation. This results in fewer remodelling sites and a decrease in the remodelling space. The 5–10% increase in bone mineral density observed in the first few years of treatment is due to the filling-in of the remodelling space produced by oestrogen. This process usually takes 2 or 3 years, after which bone density changes very little. Oestrogens play a further role in the bone remodelling process by indirectly affecting calcium homeostasis through promotion of intestinal calcium absorption and by stimulating renal production of 1,25-dihydroxyvitamin D – the hormonally active form of the vitamin that promotes the conservation of calcium.

OESTROGEN RECEPTORS; EXPRESSION AND FUNCTION IN BONE

Oestrogen is important for the development, maturation and maintenance of the skeleton, and has significant effects on bone in both males and females. Oestrogen appears to have effects on both osteoblasts and osteoclasts. 17β-Oestradiol (E2) has been reported to both stimulate and inhibit osteoblast proliferation, probably depending on cell density.[4] There are several ways in which oestrogen can exert its effects. One of the most important is probably through the oestrogen receptors. The oestrogen receptors belong to the steroid receptor superfamily, which comprises the glucocorticoid, vitamin D, thyroid hormone, androgen and retinoid receptors, and whose modular construction with its highly conserved DNA-binding domains bespeaks a common evolutionary origin for these complex proteins.

Originally, oestrogens were believed to act via a single nuclear receptor, now denoted oestrogen receptor-α (ERα). Recently, a second receptor (ERβ) has been cloned.[5] The two ERs have an almost identical DNA-binding domain (Figure 15.1), and studies in vitro have demonstrated that the two receptors have similar affinities for oestrogen compounds, similar tissue distributions but different levels of expression. They also have different affinities for oestrogen and the oestrogen antagonist.[6] Although both ER types have been identified in bone cells in culture, in particular on the osteoblast, there is no definite evidence that these cells represent the target cells for oestrogen in vivo. Most of the data currently available seem to support the evidence that ERα is the main ER in bone and in organs associated with calcium homeostasis. This is confirmed in oestrogen receptor-α knockout (ERKO) human and mice models, where ERβ alone cannot prevent failure of growth plate closure and osteoporosis.[7] Other potential target cells of oestrogens are stromal cells and cells of the haemopoietic immune system in bone mrrow. These, together with bone cells, may be implicated in the production of substances defined as second messengers that may also influence bone formation and resorption. These include interleukins (IL-1, IL-6, IL-11), prostaglandins, tumour

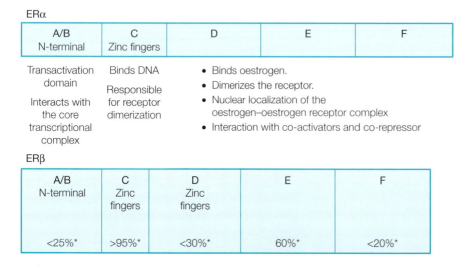

Figure 15.1. Schematic representation of the α and β oestrogen receptors, each with six domains (A–F). *Percentage of amino acid identities shared with ERα.

necrosis factor (TNF-α), transforming growth factors (TGF-β) and the insulin growth factor (IGF) system.[8] Recent evidence suggests that a central mechanism is that oestrogen deficiency promotes TNF-α release from T-cells, which then stimulates osteoclast maturation and longevity.

HRT IN OSTEOPOROSIS PREVENTION

Different oestrogens appear to exert similar effects on bone turnover and the bone protective doses that are commonly recommended are listed in Table 15.1.

In North America unopposed oestrogen alone is still sometimes used, but the general view is that the addition of at least 12 days of a progestational agent is mandatory to ensure adequate endometrial protection. These sequential HRT formulations often produce regular withdrawal bleeding. Continuous combined HRT consists of an oestrogen and progestogen formulation given on a daily basis and aims to produce amenorrhoea through endometrial atrophy. These HRT regimens maintain bone density adequately and there is some evidence that they may do so to a greater extent than sequential regimens.[9] Continuous combined preparations are becoming increasingly popular with patients. They suit women wishing to avoid regular withdrawal bleeding and, in low doses, are particularly useful in women who are many years beyond menopause.

The dose and type of oestrogen preparation need to be titrated against the patients' response. Women who experience a premature menopause (<45 years) either spontaneously or as a result of either surgical or medical interventions often need a higher dose of oestrogen both for bone conservation and for climacteric symptom control. By contrast, women who are many years past their last menstrual period may experience fewer side-effects – in particular mastalgia or bleeding – if they are started on a lower dose of oestrogen replacement. These doses can be increased if necessary, but there is increasing evidence that, even at these low doses, oestrogen may conserve bone, particularly in older women.[10]

At least seven studies have shown a bone-sparing effect of low-dose oestrogen. Recker et al.[11] used a daily dose of 0.3 mg of conjugated equine oestrogen (CEE) plus 2.5 mg of medroxyprogesterone acetate (MPA) in elderly women, and showed a significant increase both in hip (+1.6%) and spine (+5%) bone mineral density (BMD) when HRT was associated with a dose of vitamin D that kept serum vitamin D levels above 75 nmol/L. The percentage increase in BMD was similar to that obtained with a similar HRT containing twice the amount of oestrogen (CEE, 0.625 mg). Genant et al.[12] reported that spine BMD increased by 1.76% in response to continuous unopposed 0.3 mg/day esterified oestrogen. Ettinger et al.[13] found that 0.3 mg of CEE per day with a calcium supplement of 1000 mg/day prevented spinal bone loss even in the immediate post-menopausal period. Continuous combined CEE (0.3 mg/day) and MPA (2.5 mg/day) has been reported to maintain both forearm[14] and spine BMD.[15] Gallagher et al.[16] found that cyclical administration of a daily dose of 0.3 mg of CEE plus 10 mg/day of MPA coupled with high-dose calcium carbonate prevented bone loss in the spine.

The dose of oestrogen used, however, appears to be critical for the BMD increment observed with HRT. Studd et al.[17] described a significant correlation between serum oestradiol and percentage increase in bone density. Wahab et al.[18] described a considerable average increase in bone mass of 45.5% at the spine and 39.9% in the hip in women treated long term with high-dose oestradiol implants versus matched untreated controls. From these data it is plausible to extrapolate that high doses of oestrogens may exert a stimulatory action on osteoblastic function that in turn will translate into a substantial increase in BMD, while conventional doses will only suppress bone resorption. High-dose oestrogen therapy is not recommended on safety grounds.

Tibolone

Tibolone is a steroid molecule that is inert itself, but which, on absorption, is converted to metabolites that have oestrogenic, progestogenic and androgenic properties, and appears to be as efficacious as other forms of HRT on climacteric symptoms. It does not cause withdrawal bleeding when used in women with at least 1 year of amenorrhoea and it causes less breast tenderness compared to other forms of HRT. Furthermore, the androgenic

Table 15.1. Regimens of oestrogen that will arrest bone loss.

Agent	Route	Daily dose	Low dose
Oestradiol	Oral	2 mg	1 mg + norethisterone (0.5 mg)
Conjugated equine oestrogen	Oral	0.625 mg	0.3 mg + calcium
Oestradiol	Transdermal patch either weekly or twice weekly patches	50 μg release/day	25 μg
Oestradiol	Transdermal gel	1 g	
Oestradiol	Subcutaneous	50 mg every 6 months	
Tibolone	Oral	2.5 mg	

action of tibolone may also improve depression and libido.[19] Tibolone has been shown to compare favourably with other forms of HRT in both bone effects and tolerability.[20] It is now described by its manufacturers as a STEAR – a selective targeted oestrogen activity regulator.

SELECTIVE OESTROGEN RECEPTOR MODULATORS (SERMS)

The adverse effect of oestrogen on breast and endometrium have prompted studies on the design of drugs that would retain desirable oestrogenic effects while selectively blocking the unwanted effects of oestrogen. In other words, selective oestrogen receptor modulation was the objective and agents fulfilling the role are termed SERMs (Figure 15.2).

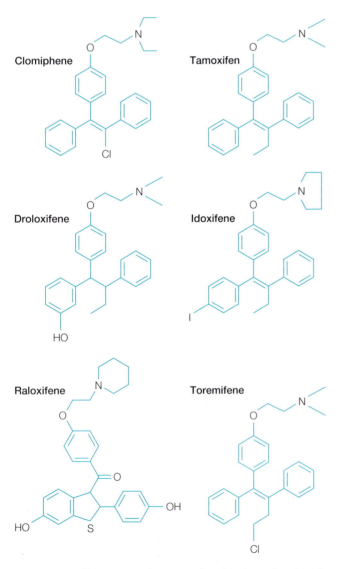

Figure 15.2. Different types of SERMs either already used in clinical practice or still in development.

First generation SERMs: clomiphene and tamoxifen

Compounds known as the first generation SERMs were originally classed as anti-oestrogens until it was found that their actions were more complex and contained an admixture of agonist and antagonist activities. Clomiphene citrate, a triphenylethylene, was synthesized in 1956 and was found by Greenblatt et al.[21] in 1961 to be capable of inducing ovulation in infertile women, a clinical role which it still performs. The central action of clomiphene is to block the negative feedback of oestrogen and induce, through positive feedback, a follicle-stimulating hormone (FSH) surge from the gonadotrophs of the anterior pituitary. In 1984 it was observed that clomiphene attenuated bone loss in the oophorectomized (OVX) rat.[22] This was most interesting since, intuitively, an anti-oestrogen would have been expected to promote rather than retard bone loss in this animal model. However, clomiphene is not a purely chemical entity but a combination of two geometric isomers. The *trans* isomer, enclomiphene, is a partial oestrogen whereas the *cis* isomer, zuclomiphene, is a pure oestrogen. The molecular species responsible for clomiphene's remarkable effect on rat bone could thus not be immediately ascertained.

Subsequently, another triphenylethylene, tamoxifen, was similarly shown to prevent bone loss in the OVX rat and it subsequently became clear that this agent, now in general use as adjunctive therapy in breast cancer, was also operating as an oestrogen agonist in the skeleton and in the cardiovascular system.[23,24] Clomiphene and tamoxifen were thus exposed as selective oestrogens and it was immediately apparent that such compounds could be of great potential benefit in supplying oestrogenic action in such tissues as bone while antagonizing oestrogenic action in the breast and uterus. In post-menopausal women, tamoxifen has been shown to have a bone-sparing action.[25] Increases in BMD are modest, however, and are in the region of 1–2% at both hip and spine. Nevertheless, a significant decrease in fracture incidence has been observed both at the hip and wrist in treated women.[26] In pre-menopausal women, tamoxifen has no bone-sparing effect, and bone loss is observed with long-term treatment.

Tamoxifen has been conclusively shown to decrease the risk of recurrent and contralateral breast cancer, and death from disease. Tamoxifen does not cause an excess of endometrial cancer in pre-menopausal women but is associated with a three- to four-fold increased risk of endometrial cancer in post-menopausal women,[27] an effect that is irrespective of dose and duration of use. A bothersome vaginal discharge may also occur in post-menopausal women, in whom tamoxifen has an oestrogen-like action on the vaginal epithelium with an increase in secretion and in the maturation index.

Second generation SERM: raloxifene

Raloxifene, originally called keoxifene, was first synthesized as one of an array of benzothiophenes being developed for potential use in the treatment of breast cancer.[28] The crystallization of the ligand-binding domain of the two ERs, when the receptor has bound either oestradiol or raloxifene, has provided an

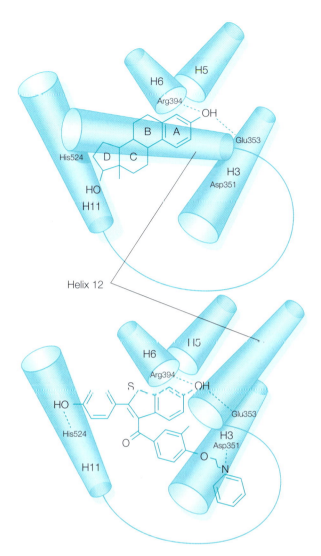

Figure 15.3. Oestradiol (A) and raloxifene (B) in the ligand-binding domain. Effect on the positioning of helix 12. Modified from Jordan and Morrow.[30]

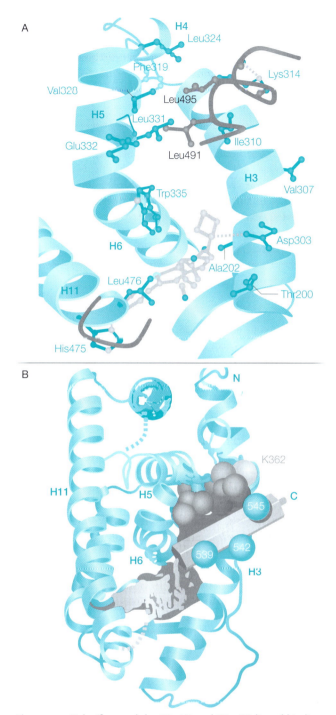

Figure 15.4. Raloxifene and the ERβ (A) and ERα (B) ligand-binding domain complex. (A) Reproduced with permission from: Pike ACW et al. *EMBO J* 1999; **18**: 74608–74618.[32] (B) Reproduced with permission from: Brzozowski et al. *Nature* 1997; **389**: 753–758.[29]

important insight into the conformational changes that occur in the receptor when an oestrogen or an anti-oestrogen enters the hydrophobic binding pocket. In the normal course of events, when oestrogen binds to ERα, it causes helix 12 to rotate, thereby sealing the ligand inside the pocket of the ligand-binding domain. By contrast, the binding of raloxifene prevents helix 12 from sealing the pocket and gene transcription cannot proceed because the essential co-activators cannot bind. This splinting effect of raloxifene on the ER thus prevents the rotation of helix 12 and disables the AF-2 domain of ERα, ultimately preventing the activation of RNA polymerase II (Figure 15.3).[29,30]

The amino acid residue (aspartate) at position 351 in the ERα helix 3 structure, as well as the alkylaminoethoxy side-chain of the raloxifene molecule, are of key importance for the anti-oestrogenic effect. Levenson and Jordan[31] showed that a natural mutation of aspartate 351 to tyrosine 351 reversed the antagonism to oestrogen agonism of raloxifene in human breast cancer cells. The amino acid 351 mechanism appears to be specific to the anti-oestrogenic effect of raloxifene and does not apply to other anti-oestrogens such as ICI (Imperial Chemical Industries) 182,780.

A similar mechanism of action to that described for ERα also seems to apply to ERβ. The bulky side-chain of raloxifene also protrudes from the cavity of the ligand-binding domain and physically prevents the alignment of helix 12 over the bound ligand,[32] resulting in the differential modulation of certain responsive genes in target tissues (Figure 15.4).

Nevertheless, this two-dimensional model that describes oestrogenic and anti-oestrogenic action is too simple to encompass all of the complexities of target-site-specific action of the anti-oestrogens or SERMs. Furthermore, the crystallization data do not include conformational information about the other sectors, the A, B, C, or F domains (Figure 15.1), of the ER, which control the interaction with transcription factors and binding to DNA. The finding that an anti-oestrogen ER complex could become increasingly oestrogenic in different cell contexts has raised the possibility that the contribution of a variety of co-activators and co-repressors modulate the effect of raloxifene and other SERMs in different tissues such as bone or breast.

Partial agonist activity of SERMs through ERα is thought to be dependent on the AF-1 transactivation domain. However the AF-1 domain of ERβ is devoid of this function and SERMs act as pure antagonists via this receptor.[33]

Furthermore, it is possible that the anti-oestrogen ER complex might bind to alternative DNA promoter region sites in order to initiate transcription. A different response element for raloxifene has in fact been identified.[34] Finally, a novel protein–protein interaction between ERβ and the AP-1 (Fos and Jun) signalling pathway has been identified. This is capable of activating a reported gene in the presence of an anti-oestrogen such as raloxifene but not oestradiol.[35]

Effects of raloxifene on bone

Using the ^{45}Ca isotope, Heaney and Draper[36] found that raloxifene at a dose of 60 mg/day significantly reduced urinary calcium excretion without significant change in calcium absorption from the gut. These data indicated a significant fall in calcium of bony origin being presented to the kidneys. In other words, bone resorption had been restrained. No change in bone formation by raloxifene was found. Support for the notion that raloxifene reduced bone resorption came from the work of Draper et al.,[37] who reported an 8-week study of healthy post-menopausal women. They found that raloxifene induced a significant reduction in the bone-specific markers alkaline phosphatase and osteocalcin (which reflect bone formation), and a reduction in urinary hydroxyproline and pyridinoline cross-links, which reflect bone resorption. This suggestion of a raloxifene-induced reduction in turnover was supported by Delmas et al.[38] in a larger, randomized, placebo-controlled study of 601 post-menopausal non-osteoporotic women. Raloxifene, at a dose of 60 mg/day, induced a significant fall in alkaline phosphatase, osteocalcin and urinary Type I collagen C-telopeptide, the latter reflecting bone resorption, over a 24-month period. The translation of reduced turnover into maintenance of BMD was also examined in this study and it was shown that raloxifene-treated patients exhibited, at 24 months, a percentage BMD gain of 2.4 (±0.4) at the spine and of 2.4 (±0.4) at the hip. Although these gains in BMD were not as impressive as those obtained with either oestrogen or bisphosphonates (approximately 5%), they were associated with a reduction in spinal fracture by 40%.[38] Ettinger et al.[39] reported on 3 years' experience with raloxifene

in the Multiple Outcomes of Raloxifene Evaluation (MORE) study, which enrolled 7705 osteoporotic women, randomized to receive placebo, raloxifene (60 mg) or raloxifene (120 mg/day). All participants received calcium/vitamin D supplements. Bone density measurement was by dual-energy X-ray absorptiometry (DEXA) at 12-month intervals, and vertebral deformation and fracture were assessed blindly on a semi-quantitative scale. Overall, the relative risk (RR) of a first vertebral fracture in a raloxifene-treated patient receiving 60 mg/day was 0.70 (95% confidence interval (CI): 0.50–0.80). Protection was present whether or not patients had a pre-existing vertebral fracture. When such a fracture was present the risk of a subsequent fracture was 0.70 (95% CI: 0.60–9.90), and when it was not present the risk fell to 0.50 (95% CI: 0.40–0.80). The 60 mg/day raloxifene regime increased BMD at the femoral neck by 2.1%, which was significant compared to controls ($P < 0.001$), but neither at this nor at any other non-spine site was any difference in fracture incidence found (RR: 0.9; 95% CI: 0.8–1.1). The vertebral fracture protection data are encouraging, but it remains to be seen if the all-important long-term effect of femoral neck fracture prevention will be achieved. The maintenance of bone quality during interventions is of high importance and hence the observations of Susan Ott and colleagues on bone histomorphometry were of interest.[40] The purpose of this study was to examine the effects of raloxifene on bone tissue by studying bone biopsy specimens before and after 2 years of raloxifene or placebo therapy in the MORE trial. None of the biopsy specimens showed evidence of toxic effects on bone or bone cells or met criteria for osteomalacia. The results from this study suggest that raloxifene has actions on bone tissue that are similar to those observed with oestrogen. Interestingly, the depressive effects on bone remodelling were less marked than those seen with alendronate.

Since the long-term economic implications of treatment with raloxifene are unknown, Kanis et al.[41] recently reported the use of a previously developed computer simulation model to estimate the cost-effectiveness of treatment benefits. The model was populated with epidemiological data and cost data relevant for a UK female population, with clinical outcome data from the MORE study. The analysis showed that raloxifene is cost-effective in the treatment of post-menopausal women at an increased risk of vertebral fractures.

SERMs: further development

A number of preparations have been tested in the hope of finding the best combination of oestrogenic and anti-oestrogenic action. One triphenylethylenetamoxifen derivative, droloxifene, is in phase III trials for osteoporosis prevention and treatment. Two other agents, levomeloxifene and idoxifene, have been withdrawn from clinical trials because of adverse events, principally endometrial stimulation and, in the case of idoxifene, an excess of cases of uterovaginal prolapse. Toremifene, a chlorinated derivative of tamoxifen having a similar action on uterine and breast tissue, has been approved for the treatment of breast cancer as an alternative to tamoxifen.

WHEN TO START TREATMENT?

HRT

Although it is generally accepted that HRT should be started in the early post-menopausal period in order to prevent osteoporosis,[42–44] there are now several studies that have shown that HRT is able to halt or possibly reverse bone loss even when started long after the menopause in elderly women. Even when started at age 60 or 70, HRT has been shown to produce an increase in BMD of 5–12%, particularly during the first year of treatment. Ettinger and Grady[45] argued that starting HRT later in life would provide as much protection against osteoporotic fractures as starting at menopause, while reducing the potential risks associated with very long oestrogen therapy such as breast cancer. They concluded that women who begin therapy at menopause and stop at age 65 have only a small (8%) increase in bone density at age 75–85, when the risk of hip fracture is highest. Women who begin treatment at menopause and continue for the remainder of their life were predicted to have the highest mean bone density at age 75–85, and greater fracture prevention. But women who began HRT at age 65 showed an increase in bone density and a decrease in fracture incidence that was almost as great. Two further studies support this data. Quigley et al.[46] found that HRT determined a similar rate of reduced bone loss irrespective of age in 397 post-menopausal women aged 51–80. Schneider et al.[47] found no significant difference in BMD values between women who had started HRT immediately after the menopause (mean duration of 20 years) and those who started treatment at age 65 (mean duration 9 years).

Further data on late-starting HRT derives from a prospective study[48] that has suggested that bone loss after menopause may not be as great as previously thought from cross-sectional studies, but it may accelerate with ageing. Starting treatment at age 65 may be relevant, since at that age densitometry can more precisely estimate the subsequent risk of hip fracture and treatment may be targeted more effectively. However, in the light of randomized trial results from the Women's Health Initiative (WHI) study and elsewhere, it is likely that oestrogen therapy for bone protection will be largely confined to symptomatic women in their sixth decade.

SERMs

While HRT is the drug of choice in symptomatic peri- and post-menopausal women, since it also reduces or abolishes vasomotor and psychological effects of oestrogen withdrawal, SERMs preferably need to be started later in life, when climacteric symptoms have subsided and when complete lack of withdrawal bleeding with treatment is particularly desirable. Raloxifene has no stimulatory effects on the breast and thus it does not cause breast enlargement, mastalgia or increased radiographic density. It would therefore be the drug of choice in those elderly women with vertebral osteoporosis intolerant of bisphosphonates.

Adverse effects of treatment

Raloxifene is generally well tolerated. In the MORE study,[49] fewer than one in 10 of the participants withdrew due to an adverse event, although it should be noted that in the study of Delmas et al.[38] the drop-out rate was 25%, the reasons for which were not specified by the authors. Experience in the MORE study was that side-effects were usually mild and transient, the most common being vasomotor symptoms, hot flushes and sweats, calf cramps, and peripheral oedema. More significant was the incidence of venous thrombo-embolic phenomena. In the MORE study there were 18 deep vein thromboses and 10 pulmonary embolisms among the group receiving 60 mg raloxifene, the numbers among the placebo group being five and three respectively. Overall, the relative risk of deep vein thrombosis (DTE) in the raloxifene group compared to the placebo group was 3.1 (95% CI: 1.5–6.2), an increase that is comparable to that consistently found with conventional HRT. Given that raloxifene reduces plasma fibrinogen and does not appear to inhibit fibrinolysis, no explanation for these data is presently available and is urgently required. A study of adverse effects of raloxifene when in General Practice use in England, reported in 2005 by Layton et al.,[50] confirmed that the drug was safe overall, the most common adverse effect – and reason for discontinuation – being vasomotor flushing.

WHAT ARE THE RISKS AND BENEFITS OF LONG-TERM TREATMENT?

The HERS trial[51] focused on the use of equine oestrogens plus MPA as secondary prevention for cardiovascular disease and its result challenged the previous findings of benefit found in observational studies, which are now ascribed to the 'well patient' effect. New cardiovascular events increased during the first year of use and no overall benefit was observed over the whole 5 years of study. Thus, the balance of risks and benefits for hormone use in healthy post-menopausal women remained uncertain. The Women's Health Initiative (WHI) study reported on 16,608 post-menopausal women aged 50–79 years with an intact uterus at baseline, recruited by 40 centres in 1993–1998.[52] Participants received conjugated equine oestrogen (CEE; 0.625 mg/day), plus medroxyprogesterone acetate (MPA; 2.5 mg/day) ($n = 8506$) or placebo ($n = 8102$). The primary outcome was coronary heart disease (CHD; non-fatal myocardial infarction and CHD death), with invasive breast cancer as the primary adverse outcome. After a mean of 5.2 years of follow-up, the study was halted when the 95% CI for breast cancer in the HRT group, preset by the DSMB, trespassed to the lower limit, which was 1.00. The hazard ratios (HRs) (nominal 95% CIs) were: CHD, 1.29 (1.02–1.63); breast cancer, 1.26 (1.00–1.59); stroke, 1.41 (1.07–1.85). Interestingly, the fracture data showed protection, although the population studied had not been selected on the basis of low BMD or prior fractures. The HRs (95% CI) were 0.66 (0.45–0.98) for hip fracture and 0.76 (0.69–0.85) for combined fractures. Overall mortality was unchanged at an HR of 0.98 (95% CI: 0.82–1.18). Absolute excess risks per 10,000 person-years attributable to oestrogen plus progestin were seven more CHD events, eight more strokes, eight more Peps and eight more invasive breast cancers, while absolute risk reductions per 10,000 person-years were six fewer colorectal cancers and five fewer hip fractures. The authors concluded that CEE plus MPA should not be utilized for cardiovascular system (CVS) protection in the population studied. This was a US population of average age 64, i.e. significantly older than the population generally in receipt of HRT in the UK. Subsequently, the WHI writing group reported that the use of CEE alone, i.e. without a progestogen, over an average of 6.8 years, increased the risk of stroke but decreased the risk of hip fracture, and did not affect CHD incidence in post-menopausal women with prior hysterectomy. There was a reduction in breast cancer risk which, though it failed to reach statistical significance, clearly requires further investigation. The burden of incident disease events was equivalent in the CEE and placebo groups, indicating no overall benefit. Further long-term primary prevention studies are needed to clarify this issue. Though it has no effect on established Alzheimer's disease, there is observational evidence of a reduced incidence of Alzheimer's disease in treated women even after adjustment for the Apo E4 genotype and years of education.[53]

Raloxifene appears to improve risk factors for cardiovascular disease such as the lipid profile, although to a lesser extent compared to oestrogen. In the study of Delmas et al.,[38] the 60 mg raloxifene/day regimen, given to some 152 women over 2 years, produced a similar picture with a significant reduction in low-density-lipoprotein cholesterol (LDL-C) and no change in high-density-lipoprotein cholesterol (HDL-C) and triglycerides. Further long-term data are, however, needed since no human studies have yet had sufficient power to detect changes in clinical cardiovascular end-points. No statement can yet be made as to whether the lipid change observed with raloxifene will translate into a clinically useful effect. In the MORE study, all causes of mortality did not differ between the raloxifene-treated and control groups.[49] Raloxifene does not appear to have any adverse effects on the endometrium, and data on its effect on the central nervous system are scarce.

In many studies one of the prime disincentives to the acceptance of, or long-term continuation of, conventional HRT is the perceived risk of breast cancer, the most common malignancy in UK females.

HRT and breast cancer risk

The largest observational study addressing this issue was the Million Women Study (MWS), which reported in 2003.[54] It investigated the effects of specific types of HRT on incident and fatal breast cancer. Some 1,084,110 UK women aged 50–64 years, recruited between 1996 and 2001, provided information about their HRT exposure and were followed up for breast cancer incidence and death. Half the women had used HRT. There were 9364 incident invasive breast cancers and 637 breast cancer deaths after an average of 2.6 and 4.1 years of follow-up respectively. Current users of HRT were more likely than those who had never undergone this therapy to develop breast cancer (adjusted RR: 1.66; 95% CI: 1.58–1.75; $P < 0.0001$) and die from it (adjusted RR: 1.22; 95% CI: 1.00–1.48; $P = 0.05$). Past users of HRT were, however, not at an increased risk. Incidence was significantly increased not only for those using oestrogen only

(adjusted RR: 1.30; 95% CI: 1.21–1.40; $P < 0.0001$), but also for oestrogen–progestogen (adjusted RR: 2.00; 95% CI: 1.88–2.12; $P < 0.0001$) and tibolone (adjusted RR: 1.45; 95% CI: 1.25–1.68; $P < 0.0001$). The increased risk applied to all forms of oestrogen therapy, to all routes of delivery, and was exposure related. Ten-year exposure was calculated to result in five (95% CI: 3–7) additional breast cancers per 1000 users of oestrogen-only preparations and 19 (95% CI: 15–23) additional cancers per 1000 users of oestrogen–progestogen combinations.

Prior to the appearance of the WHI and Million Women Study data, the largest meta-analysis of HRT studies had shown a continuing increase in incidence of breast cancer among women taking HRT.[55] The use of HRT for 5 years appeared to be associated with an estimated cumulative excess of two cancers/1000 users over a 20-year period, while use for 10 years would lead to six excess cases for every 1000 users. Mortality from the disease, however, was not increased, but was in fact found to be at least 10% lower among oestrogen users compared with non-users. It should be noted, however, that all the data available so far on this issue are derived from either cohort or case–control studies. Prospective data from randomized placebo-controlled studies are still lacking and this might have led to possible biases introduced by differences in breast cancer risk factors in those women that chose to take oestrogen compared with non-users.

Effects of raloxifene on the breast

Cummings et al.[49] reported that among the 5129 women in the MORE trial[39] randomized to receive raloxifene, 13 developed invasive breast cancer over the first 3 years of the trial. Among the 2576 placebo-treated controls, 27 cases of invasive breast cancer developed. The overall RR of breast cancer in raloxifene-treated women was 0.24 (95% CI: 0.13–0.44).

Four-year data from the MORE trial relating raloxifene use to breast cancer incidence were reported in 2001 by Cauley et al.[56] A total of 61 invasive breast cancers were reported and were confirmed by the adjudication board. Among raloxifene-treated women there was a 72% risk reduction (RR: 0.28; 95% CI: 0.17–0.46) in invasive breast cancer. Some 93 osteoporotic women would need to be treated with raloxifene for 4 years to prevent one case of invasive breast cancer. Raloxifene reduced the risk of oestrogen receptor-positive invasive breast cancer by 84% (RR: 0.16; 95% CI: 0.09–0.30). These data have now been augmented by the report of Martino et al.,[57] who conducted the Continuing Outcomes Relevant to Evista (CORE) trial. Its central purpose was to examine the effect of 4 additional years of raloxifene therapy on the incidence of invasive breast cancer in women in MORE who agreed to continue in CORE. During the CORE trial, the 4-year incidences of invasive breast cancer and oestrogen receptor (ER)-positive invasive breast cancer were reduced by 59% (HR: 0.41; 95% CI: 0.24–0.71) and 66% (HR: 0.34; 95% CI: 0.18–0.66) respectively, in the raloxifene group compared with the placebo group. There was no difference between the two groups in incidence of ER-negative invasive breast cancer. Over the total of 8 years of the two sequential trials, the incidences of invasive breast cancer and ER-positive invasive breast cancer in the raloxifene group were reduced by 66% (HR: 0.34; 95% CI: 0.22–0.50) and 76% (HR: 0.24; 95% CI: 0.15–0.40) respectively.

As with tamoxifen, the anti-tumour effect appears to be concentrated against the more common ER-positive cancers, with ER-negative cancers showing no change. Since mammograms of raloxifene-treated patients do not show the increase in radio-opacity found with conventional HRT regimes, it is unlikely that any observational or test bias is operating. It should be understood that breast cancer prevention was a secondary, and not a primary, end-point of MORE and the study population, being osteoporotic, were at no excess risk for the disease. However, the incidence of invasive breast cancer in the control group was no different than that expected for this population and it would appear, prima facie, that a useful effect is present. Given that breast tumours are present for months or even years before coming to clinical notice, it is likely that the raloxifene effect is one of suppression rather than primary prevention. Hence, it will be necessary to follow-up, with adequate statistical power, a significant number of patients exiting the study to ensure that no rebound phenomenon occurs.

Raloxifene has already been found not to cause breast enlargement, tenderness[38] and relative mammographic opacity, which occur with HRT treatment. Its ability to reduce the incidence of invasive breast cancer in a group of women at high risk is now being explored in the Study of Tamoxifen And Raloxifene (STAR), which is now recruiting in North America.

WHO SHOULD USE HRT OR SERMS?

It is some 6 years now since the first of the second generation SERMs was licensed for use in the European Union. Raloxifene, however, appears to be well tolerated and the general absence of breast and uterine adverse events is a significant advantage. Patients do not, however, achieve a reduction in menopausal symptoms, and where these are a clinical problem, conventional HRT must retain the central role. Similarly, there are as yet no data on the ability of raloxifene to control the vaginal dryness and associated dyspareunia that can be so distressing to post-menopausal women, and here again systemic or local oestrogen therapy is indicated. Future studies with SERMs will need to address the issues of cardiovascular protection, cognitive function and neuronal degeneration.

The patient in whom the use of an SERM is indicated is a post-menopausal woman at risk of osteoporosis-related vertebral fracture. These agents will be of particular value in patients who have experienced adverse events during HRT therapy or who are unable to accept bleeding or the small but quantifiable increased risk for breast cancer. For the present, in a patient at risk for osteoporosis, and especially afflicted by menopausal symptoms, a general schedule for oestrogen use after menopause might involve the use of conventional HRT initially, followed by an actuarial assessment of future fracture risk using validated clinical risk factors and BMD measurement by DEXA of the hip and spine. In patients showing a significant risk of fracture – the risk roughly doubles for each standard deviation fall in BMD – the options would be to switch to an SERM or to use a bisphosphonate. Densitometric follow-up will be required and all women at risk should make any necessary lifestyle adjustments to take a diet that is rich in calcium/vitamin D and an activity pattern producing adequate weight-bearing exercise.

The SERMs are a major step forward in therapeutics. They are the fruit of our new understanding of the complexity of oestrogen receptor structure and function, a complexity which has been correctly seen not as an obstacle but as an opportunity. These purpose-designed agents will, with increasing sophistication, maintain oestrogenic action wherever in physiology the hormone and its receptor have been adopted as a signal transduction system, while dispensing with those reproductive actions that become redundant with menopause and whose reactivation is, at best, an encumbrance and, at worst, a clinical hazard.

HOW LONG SHOULD TREATMENT CONTINUE AND IS THE BENEFIT LOST?

How long the benefit of HRT or raloxifene is retained following cessation of medication remains unknown. It has been calculated that 5- to 10-year HRT treatment continuation has a transient effect, since discontinuation produces an accelerated reduction of bone mass. Six or more years after stopping treatment the risk of hip fracture becomes close to what it was before starting HRT, independent of the duration of use. Targeting intervention at the age of 70, were a safe and acceptable regimen to be available, may thus prevent more hip fractures than intervention at the time of the menopause. However, while most authors support the view that current oestrogen use seems to be critical, at least for reducing the incidence of hip fracture, other authors maintain that HRT protects against hip fracture even after treatment has been stopped, suggesting a permanent persistent effect of oestrogen on bone.

WHAT IS THE COST-EFFECTIVENESS?

A review by Torgerson and Iglesias[58] identified 15 economic evaluations of HRT. Short-term HRT treatment is all that is normally used for the treatment of climacteric symptoms. This is clearly cost-effective, so much so that women were prepared to pay more for the relief of menopausal symptoms than the actual cost of HRT itself. Current published evaluations suggest that treatment beyond 1–2 years is cost-effective on the assumption of cardiovascular disease, as well as osteoporosis, prevention. However, since the majority of these evaluations were published some of the key epidemiological assumptions, such as cardiovascular disease prevention, on which they were based have been undermined.

It had been assumed that 5–10 years of HRT use after the menopause would delay the peak incidence of hip fracture by a corresponding number of years. But 5–10 years of HRT use soon after the menopause does not confer sufficient fracture protection 30 years later. To be effective, lifelong HRT use is required. This would have a number of cost and health implications. The

Table 15.2. Comparison of HRT and raloxifene.

	Vertebral fractures	Non-vertebral fractures	Annual costs (£)	Side-effects
HRT	↓ 60%	↓ 30–50%	23–168	↑ Breast cancer, breast pain, unwanted bleeding
SERMs – raloxifene	↓ 50%		238	↑ Menopausal symptoms, ? ↓ risk of breast cancer

Source: modified from Torgerson and Iglesias.[58]

increased risk of breast cancer might not outweigh the benefits for fracture risk, particularly since the long-term effect on cardiovascular disease is adverse. The long-term effect of raloxifene on organs such as the cardiovascular system and the breast has still to be evaluated. Clearly the cost of treatment is a very important variable; Table 15.2 shows a comparison between the two treatment classes. Unfortunately, there are no directly comparable trials that would enable us to judge which is the more effective treatment, let alone which is most cost-effective. These data need further evaluation.

SUMMARY

Oestrogen therapy begun at the time of menopause and continued for the remainder of life would be, if safe, the optimal treatment for post-menopausal women at risk of osteoporosis. However, the relegation by the Committee on Safety of Medicines of oestrogen to a subsidiary role has ruled out such an approach – at least until an acceptable regimen is found.

Also, many women are reluctant to embark on long-term HRT, mainly due to the fear of breast cancer. Raloxifene may be a viable alternative for these women provided that they do not suffer from oestrogen deficiency symptoms. Oestrogen protection wanes with discontinuation and current use seems to be critical for fracture prevention, particularly that of the hip. Low-dose continuous-combined oestrogen preparations, or tibolone, may be of value in older women, since they will reduce the incidence of mastalgia and withdrawal bleeding, thus improving treatment acceptability. Raloxifene could thus be an alternative in those women at risk of vertebral fracture, as well as in younger women who particularly fear the risk of breast cancer with HRT. How long bone protection will last after stopping raloxifene treatment is unknown. Similarly, further studies are under way to assess whether raloxifene can be used in women who are at increased risk of breast cancer or heart disease.

The trail leading to the ideal HRT will be long and difficult. The advent of licensed SERMs is, however, a major second step along the road.

PRACTICE POINTS

- No HRT unless clinically indicated – and then only with low dose and short exposure times.
- Advise patients of the HRT–breast cancer connection using absolute not relative risks.
- Switch patients from cyclic to no-fixed-bleed regimes at around age 55 unless contraindicated.
- Consider SERM therapy where the spine is affected or at risk and when the patient is fearful of breast cancer.
- No long-term gain without long-term treatment.
- Remember, patients are more than a skeleton with a heart and brain.

RESEARCH AGENDA

- Are oestrogens, or tibolone, safe in patients with a prior history of breast cancer?
- How do we advise parents/teachers on maximizing bone gain in childhood?
- How do we ensure that all non-pregnant amenorrhoeic women are checked for oestrogen deficiency?
- Does HRT exposure cause an excess of CHD in women in their fifties?
- Are the SERMs cardioprotective clinically?
- How do we build in symptom control to the osteoprotective action of SERMs?

REFERENCES

1. Hayrick L. The future of ageing. *Nature* 2000; **408**: 267–269.
2. Parfit AM, Mundy GR, Roodman GD et al. A new model for the regulation of bone resorption, with particular reference to the effects of bisphosphonates. *J Bone Miner Res* 1996; **11**: 150–159.
3. Parfitt AM. Morphologic basis of bone mineral measurement: transient and steady state effects of treatment in osteoporosis. *Miner Electrolyte Metab* 1980; **4**: 273–287.
4. Bland R. Steroid hormone receptor expression and action in bone. *Clin Sci* 2000; **98**: 217–240.
5. Kuipper GG, Enmark E, Peto-Huikko M et al. Cloning of a novel receptor expressed in rat prostate and ovary. *Proc Natl Acad Sci USA* 1996; **93**: 5925–5930.
6. Kuiper GGJM, Carlsson B, Grandien K et al. Comparison of the ligand binding specificity and transcript tissue distribution of estrogen receptors α and β. *Endocrinology* 1997; **132**: 195–199.
7. Smith EP, Boyd J, Frank GR et al. Estrogen resistance caused by a mutation in the estrogen-receptor gene in man. *N Engl J Med* 1994; **331**: 1056–1061.
8. Pacifici R. Postmenopausal osteoporosis: how the hormonal changes of menopause cause bone loss. In: Marcus R, Feldman D & Kelsey J, eds. *Osteoporosis*. San Diego: Academic Press, 1996; 315–329.
9. Nielsen SP, Brenholdt O, Hermansen F et al. Magnitude and pattern of skeletal response to continuous and cyclical sequential oestrogen/progestin treatment. *Br J Obstet Gynaecol* 1994; **101**: 319–324.
10. Ettinger B, Genant HK, Steiger P et al. Low-dosage micronized 17β-estradiol prevents bone loss on postmenopausal women. *Am J Obstet Gynecol* 1992; **166**: 479–488.
11. Recker RR, Davies MK, Dowd RM et al. The effects of low-dose continuous estrogen and progesterone therapy with calcium and vitamin D on bone in elderly women: a randomized controlled trial. *Ann Intern Med* 1999; **130**: 897–904.
12. Genant HK, Lucas J, Weiss S et al. Low-dose esterified estrogen therapy: effects on bone, plasma estradiol concentrations, endometrium, and lipid levels. Estratab/Osteoporosis Study Group. *Arch Intern Med* 1997; **157**: 2609–2615.
13. Ettinger B, Genant HK & Cann CE. Postmenopausal bone loss is prevented by treatment with low dosage estrogen with calcium. *Ann Intern Med* 1987; **106**: 40–45.
14. MacLennan AH, MacLennan A, Wenzel S et al. Continuous low dose oestrogen and progestogen hormone replacement therapy: a randomised trial. *Med J Aust* 1993; **159**: 102–106.
15. Webber CE, Blake JM, Chambers LF et al. Effects of 2 years of hormone replacement upon bone mass, serum lipids and lipoproteins. *Maturitas* 1994; **19**: 13–23.
16. Gallagher JC. Kable WT & Goldgar D. Effect of progestin therapy on cortical and trabecular bone; comparison with estrogen. *Am J Med* 1991; **90**: 171–178.
17. Studd J, Savvas M, Watson N et al. The relationship between plasma estradiol and the increase in bone density in postmenopausal women after treatment with subcutaneous implants. *Am J Obstet Gynecol* 1990; **163**: 1474–1479.
18. Wahab M, Ballard P, Purdie DP et al. The effect of long term oestrodiol implantation on bone mineral density in postmenopausal women who have undergone hysterectomy and bilateral oophorectomy. *Br J Obstet Gynaecol* 1997; **104**: 728–731.
19. Albertazzi P, Di Micco R & Zanardi E. Tibolone: a review. *Maturitas* 1998; **30**: 295–305.
20. Beardsworth SA, Kearney CE & Purdie DW. Prevention of postmenopausal bone loss at lumbar spine and upper femur with tibolone: a two-year randomised controlled trial. *Br J Obstet Gynaecol* 1999; **106**: 678–683.
21. Greenblatt RB, Barfield WE, Jungck EC et al. Induction of ovulation with MRI-41. *JAMA* 1961; **178**: 101–106.
22. Beall PT, Misra KL, Young RL et al. Clomiphene protects against osteoporosis in the mature ovariectomized rat. *Calcif Tissue Int* 1985; **36**: 123–135.
23. Jordan VC, Phelps E & Lindgren JU. Effects of anti-estrogens on bone in castrated and intact female rats. *Breast Cancer Res Treat* 1987; **10**: 31–35.
24. Love RR, Barden HS, Mazess RB et al. Effect of tamoxifen on lumbar spine bone mineral density in postmenopausal women after 5 years. *Arch Intern Med* 1994; **154**: 2585–2588.
25. Cosman F & Linsday R. Selective estrogen receptor modulators: clinical spectrum. *Endocr Rev* 1999; **20**: 418–434.
26. Fisher B, Whickerham DL, Costantino JP et al. Tamoxifen for the prevention of breast cancer: report of the National Surgical Adjuvant Breast and Bowel Project P-1 study. *J Natl Cancer Inst* 1998; **90**: 1372–1388.
27. Ismail SM. Effect of tamoxifen on the uterus. *Lancet* 1994; **344**: 622–623.
28. Draper MW, Flowers DE, Neild JA et al. Antiestrogenic properties of raloxifene. *Pharmacology* 1995; **50**: 209–217.
29. Brzozowski AM, Pike ACW, Dauter Z et al. Molecular basis of agonism and antagonism in the oestrogen receptor. *Nature* 1997; **389**: 753–758.
30. Jordan C & Morrow M. Tamoxifen, raloxifen, and the prevention of breast cancer. *Endocr Rev* 1999; **20**: 253–278.
31. Levenson AS & Jordan VC. The key to the antiestrogenic mechanism of raloxifene is amino acid 351 (aspartate) in the estrogen receptor. *Cancer Res* 1998; **58**: 1872–1875.
32. Pike ACW, Brzozowski AM, Hubbard RE et al. Structure of the ligand-binding domain of oestrogen receptor beta in the presence of a partial agonist and full antagonist. *EMBO J* 1999; **18**: 74608–74618.
33. Barkhem T, Carlsson B, Nilsson Y et al. Differential response of estrogen receptor α and estrogen receptor β to partial estrogen agonist/antagonist. *Molec Pharmacol* 1998; **54**: 105–112.
34. Yang NN, Venugopalan M, Hardikar S et al. Identification of an oestrogen response element activated by metabolite of 17β-estradiol and raloxifen. *Science* 1996; **273**: 1222–1225.
35. Paech K, Webb P, Kuiper GG et al. Differential ligand activation of estrogen receptor ERα and ERβ at Ap-1 sites. *Science* 1997; **277**: 1508–1510.
36. Heaney RP & Draper MW. Raloxifene and estrogen: comparative bone-remodeling kinetics. *J Clin Endocrinol Metab* 1997; **82**: 3425–3429.
37. Draper MW, Flowers DE, Huster WJ et al. A controlled trial of raloxifene (LY139481) HCl: impact on bone turnover and serum lipid profile in healthy postmenopausal women. *J Bone Miner Res* 1996; **11**: 835–842.
38. Delmas PD, Bjarnason NH, Mitlak BH et al. Effects of raloxifene on bone mineral density, serum cholesterol concentrations and uterine endometrium in postmenopausal women. *N Engl J Med* 1997; **337**: 1641–1647.
39. Ettinger B, Black DM, Mitlak BH et al. Reduction of vertebral fracture risk in postmenopausal women with osteoporosis treated with raloxifene. *JAMA* 1999; **282**: 637–645.
40. Ott S, Oleksik A, Lu Y et al. Bone histomorphometric and biochemical marker results of a 2-year placebo-controlled trial of raloxifene in postmenopausal women. *J Bone Miner Res* 2002; **17**: 341–348.
41. Kanis J, Borgstrom F & Johnell O. Cost effectiveness of raloxifene in the UK. *Osteoporosis Int* 2005; **16**: 15–25.
42. Cauley JA, Seeley DG, Ensrud K et al. Estrogen replacement therapy and fractures in older women: study of Osteoporotic Fracture Research Group. *Ann Intern Med* 1995; **122**: 9–16.
43. Weiss N, Ure C, Ballard J et al. Decreased risk of fracture of hip and lower forearm with postmenopausal use of estrogen. *N Engl J Med* 1980; **303**: 1195–1198.
44. Naessen T, Person Y, Adami H et al. Hormone replacement therapy and the risk for the first hip fracture. *Ann Intern Med* 1990; **113**: 95–103.
45. Ettinger B & Grady D. Maximising the benefit of estrogen therapy for prevention of osteoporosis. *Menopause* 1994; **1**: 19–24.
46. Quigley MET, Martin PL, Burnier AM et al. Estrogen therapy arrests bone loss in elderly women. *Am J Obstet Gynecol* 1987; **156**: 1516–1523.
47. Schneider D, Barret-Connor E & Morton D. Timing of postmenopausal estrogen for optimal bone mineral density: the Rancho Bernardo Study. *JAMA* 1997; **277**: 543–547.
48. Jones G, Nguyen T, Sanbrook P et al. Progressive loss of bone in the femoral neck in elderly people: longitudinal findings from Dubbo osteoporosis epidemiology study. *BMJ* 1994; **309**: 691–695.
49. Cummings SR, Eckert S, Krueger KA et al. The effect of raloxifene on risk of breast cancer in postmenopausal women. Results from the MORE randomized trial. *JAMA* 1999; **281**: 2189–2197.
50. Layton D, Wilton LV & Shakir SA. Safety profile of raloxifene as used in general practice in England: results of a prescription-event monitoring study. *Osteoporosis Int* 2005; **16**(5): 490–500.
51. Hulley SB, Grady D, Bush T et al. Randomized trial of oestrogen plus progestin for secondary prevention of coronary heart disease in postmenopausal women. Heart and Estrogen/Progestin Replacement Study (HERS) Research Group. *JAMA* 1998; **280**: 605–613.

52. Rossouw J, Anderson G, Prentice R et al. Risks and benefits of estrogen plus progestin in healthy postmenopausal women: principal results from the Women's Health Initiative randomized controlled trial. *JAMA* 2002; **288**: 321–333.

53. Tang MX, Jacobs D, Stern Y et al. Effect of oestrogen during menopause on risk and age at onset of Alzheimer's Disease. *Lancet* 1996; **348**: 429–432.

54. Beral V & Million Women Study Collaborators. Breast cancer and hormone-replacement therapy in the Million Women Study. *Lancet* 2003; **362**: 419–427.

55. Collaborative Group on Hormonal Factors in Breast Cancer. Breast cancer and hormonal replacement tharapy: collaborative reanalysis of data from 51 epidemiological studies of 52,705 women with breast cancer and 108,411 without breast cancer. *Lancet* 1997; **350**: 1047–1059.

56. Cauley J, Norton L & Lippman M. Continued breast cancer risk reduction in postmenopausal women treated with raloxifene: 4-year results from the MORE (Multiple Outcomes of Raloxifene Evaluation) trial. *Breast Cancer Res Treat* 2001; **65**: 125–134.

57. Martino S, Cauley J & Barrett-Connor E. Continuing outcomes relevant to Evista: breast cancer incidence in postmenopausal osteoporotic women in a randomized trial of raloxifene. *J Natl Cancer Inst* 2004; **96**: 1751–1761.

58. Torgerson DJ & Iglesias CP. The economics and management of osteoporosis in post-menopausal women. *J Br Menopause Soc* 1999; 67–71.

Chapter 16

Role of bisphosphonates and calcitonin in the prevention and treatment of osteoporosis

Tricia K. W. Woo and Jonathan D. Adachi

INTRODUCTION

Osteoporosis is a major health concern, affecting a growing number of individuals worldwide. The disorder is characterized by low bone mass and bone fragility, resulting in an increased risk of fracture. Vertebral fractures are synonymous with the diagnosis of osteoporosis since its characterization as a metabolic bone disease. Bone mass is commonly quantified using dual-energy X-ray absorptiometry, typically of the spine and hip. Normal bone density is within 1 standard deviation (SD) of the mean of young adults. If the bone density is between 1 and 2.5 SDs below the normal reference range then it is osteopoenic, and if it is less than 2.5 SDs it is osteoporosis. Based on these criteria, it has been estimated that about 30% of post-menopausal women have osteoporosis.

The prevention of fractures is the primary goal of osteoporosis treatment. Several anti-resorptive agents have been successfully used for the treatment of post-menopausal osteoporosis with recent trials of calcitonin and the bisphosphonates.

BISPHOSPHONATES

The bisphosphonates are a class of drugs that have revolutionized the therapy of bone diseases. Several bisphosphonates are available for a wide variety of clinical applications, including the treatment of Paget's disease, hypercalcaemia of malignancy, bone metastases and osteoporosis.

In the 1960s, Fleisch showed that inorganic pyrophosphate, a naturally occurring polyphosphate, was present in serum and urine and could prevent calcification by binding to newly forming crystals of hydroxyapatite. The bisphosphonates are the stable analogues of naturally occurring pyrophosphate.[1,2] The anti-resorptive effects of bisphosphonates are due to inhibition of bone resorption by osteoclasts, rather than by purely physicochemical mechanisms. Bisphosphonates inhibit osteoclast-mediated bone resorption in a variety of ways, and they interfere with osteoclast recruitment, differentiation and action.[2] Bisphosphonates can be classified into at least two groups based on different modes of action. Those that most closely resemble pyrophosphate, such as clodronate and etidronate, are incorporated into cytotoxic ATP analogues. The more potent nitrogen-containing bisphosphonates such as alendronate and risedronate interfere with protein prenylation through their effects on the mevalonate pathway, and therefore may affect the intracellular trafficking of key regulatory proteins. There is clear evidence that the dominant mechanism of action of some bisphosphonates involves the inhibition of the mevalonate pathway, rather than other mechanisms such as inhibition of protein phosphatases. The grouping of bisphosphonates into two classes may help to explain some of their pharmacological differences.

Bisphosphonates are accepted as the most potent clinical inhibitors of bone resorption and are a mainstay of the treatment of osteoporosis. Currently, the most widely available forms of bisphosphonates include ICT-etidronate, alendronate and risedronate. Oral absorption of bisphosphonates is poor (1–5% absorption), even when taken on an empty stomach. The plasma half-life is 1 h, with 80% clearance by the kidneys. The most common side-effect of bisphosphonate treatment is gastrointestinal upset. Caution should be exercised in patients with underlying renal insufficiency. Bisphosphonates also reduce serum calcium concentration, which can cause symptomatic hypocalcaemia in patients with vitamin D deficiency.[1]

Etidronate

Etidronate is a first generation bisphosphonate that was shown to benefit patients with osteoporosis. It is available in oral and intravenous forms and is generally well tolerated, with few reports of gastrointestinal upset. If administered continuously for prolonged periods, etidronate has been shown to cause impaired mineralization of bone. Due to this narrow therapeutic index, etidronate is given in an intermittent cyclic fashion. Typically, a dose of 400 mg/day for 2 weeks every 3 months is recommended.

Several studies have examined the anti-fracture efficacy of cyclical etidronate in post-menopausal women with prevalent vertebral fractures.[3,4] Storm et al.[3] conducted a study in 66 women with post-menopausal osteoporosis using ICT-etidronate. The patients were randomly assigned to receive oral etidronate (400 mg/day) or placebo for 2 weeks, followed by a 13-week period with no drugs. This sequence was repeated 10 times, for a total of 150 weeks. Supplementation with calcium and vitamin D was given to both groups. Vertebral bone mineral content increased significantly ($P < 0.01$) after 150 weeks of ICT-etidronate (5.3%; 95% confidence interval (CI): 2.0–8.6%) but decreased with placebo (–2.7%; 95% CI: –7.3% to –1.9%). The rates of fracture were significantly different from week 60 to week 150 between the etidronate and placebo groups (6 versus 54 fractures/100 patient-years; $P = 0.023$). They concluded that ICT-etidronate therapy significantly increased vertebral bone mineral content and decreased the rate of new vertebral fractures.

Watts et al.[4] also determined the effects of ICT-etidronate on post-menopausal osteoporosis by studying 429 women who had one to four vertebral compression fractures plus radiographic evidence of osteopoenia. The patients were randomly assigned to one of four groups; with ICT-etidronate (400 mg) or 2/2 with placebo daily on days 4–17, and supplemental calcium (500 mg) daily on days 18–91. After 2 years, patients receiving ICT-etidronate had significantly increased their mean (±SE) spinal bone density (4.2 ± 0.8% and 5.2 ± 0.7% respectively; $P < 0.017$). The rate of new vertebral fractures was reduced by half in the etidronate-treated patients compared with the patients on placebo (29.5 versus 62.9 fractures/1000 patient-years; $P = 0.043$). The effect of treatment was most striking in the subgroup of patients with lowest spinal bone mineral density at baseline, in whom fracture rates were reduced by two-thirds (42.3 versus 132.7 fractures/1000 patient-years; $P = 0.004$). They concluded that ICT-etidronate for 2 years significantly increases spinal bone mass and reduces the incidence of new vertebral fractures in women with post-menopausal osteoporosis.

Despite methodological problems in fracture assessment and limited statistical power, the combined results indicated that this form of treatment was effective in preventing new vertebral fractures in post-menopausal women with low bone mass and multiple prevalent vertebral fractures. There was no randomized controlled trial (RCT) evidence of the effect of ICT-etidronate on hip fracture risk, but a post-marketing survey suggested that its use was associated with decreased risk of non-vertebral fracture, including those of the hip.[5]

The Food and Drug Administration in the USA allows etidronate to be used in Paget's disease and hypercalcaemia due to malignancy. It has not been approved for use in osteoporosis in the USA, but has been approved in 22 other countries.[1]

Cyclic etidronate has also been used in combination with oestrogen in women. In a randomized study, Wimalawansa[6] gave post-menopausal women with no osteoporosis either oestrogen or etidronate alone, or in combination therapy or placebo. At the end of 4 years, patients who received the combination therapy had a 10.9% increase in bone mineral density (BMD) in the vertebra ($P = 0.001$) and a 7.25% increase ($P = 0.001$) in the femur, while placebo patients had an 8.58% decrease in the vertebrae and a 7.83% decrease in the femur. Patients on oestrogen alone showed 6.78% ($P = 0.001$) and 4.01% ($P = 0.01$) increases in the spine and hip, while those on etidronate only had 6.79% ($P = 0.001$) and 1.20% increases respectively ($P = 0.001$).

There is evidence that cyclical etidronate therapy maintains bone mass in the prevention and treatment of corticosteroid-treated patients.[7] One study examined 117 patients starting on corticosteroid therapy who were randomized to placebo or ICT-etidronate. Bone mass was maintained in the ICT-etidronate group. In the placebo group 15 fractures occurred in five subjects, while only five fractures occurred in four subjects in the ICT-etidronate group.[8] In another RCT of ICT-etidronate, 141 subjects were enrolled and significant differences were demonstrated in favour of ICT-etidronate treatment in the spine and trochanter. There were 22 fractures in 10 patients (15.4%) in the placebo group, and five patients in the ICT-etidronate group sustained multiple vertebral fractures. The relative risk of fractures in the ICT-etidronate compared to the placebo group was 0.57 (95% CI: 0.21–1.57). This is a 43% reduction of patients with new vertebral fractures. Fracture analysis in post-menopausal women showed that ICT-etidronate was associated with an 85% reduction in the proportion of patients with vertebral fractures (3.2% versus 21.9%; $P = 0.05$). There was only a trend in reduction in vertebral fractures in the whole study population and it was not statistically significant ($P = 0.19$).

Alendronate

Alendronate is a second generation bisphosphonate with a nitrogen-containing side-chain. It inhibits a rate-limiting step in the mevalonic acid pathway that is essential for proper osteoclast function. The drug has approximately 10-fold increase in anti-resorptive properties compared to etidronate and has a large therapeutic window.[1] It is available in both oral and intravenous forms. There are gastrointestinal complaints with alendronate and the intravenous form has been associated with transient flu-like symptoms. Alendronate is given continuously at a dose of 5 mg/day for the prevention of osteoporosis and 10 mg daily for treatment of established osteoporosis. Weekly dosing with alendronate (70 mg) has been shown to have comparable effects on BMD as daily dose regimen, but with fewer gastrointestinal side-effects.[9]

Alendronate is the most extensively studied pharmacological agent against osteoporosis.[9–12] In an initial 3-year study, when given in different doses to osteoporotic women (20% with prevalent vertebral deformities), alendronate significantly reduced the incidence of new vertebral deformities.[10] Its efficacy has since been re-examined in two large populations of post-menopausal women, one with and one without pre-existing vertebral fractures.[11,12] In both trials, supplemental calcium and vitamin D were given to all participants. In The Fracture Intervention Trial (FIT), 2027 women with a mean age of 71 years and with at least one vertebral fracture were treated with 5 mg daily for 2 years and 10 mg/day for the third year or with placebo for 3 years. Treatment with alendronate reduced the incidence of clinical spine, hip and wrist fractures by about 50%. Active treatment over 3 years also decreased the incidence of new radiographic vertebral fractures from 15% to 8% in the alendronate-treated group. Alendronate also reduced the risk of multiple vertebral fractures and the incidence of new hip fractures. This study was the first RCT to show hip fracture benefits in calcium- and vitamin D-replete osteoporotic women. The extension study of the Fracture Intervention Trial (FIT) showed that these benefits are maintained for up to 10 years.[13]

The anti-fracture efficacy of alendronate has also been examined in 4432 post-menopausal women with no prior vertebral fractures.[14] Women with a low hip BMD were treated with placebo or with 5 mg alendronate/day for 2 years and then 10 mg/day for the remainder of the 4-year trial. As in the other studies,[10,14] alendronate increased BMD at all measured sites. Treatment with alendronate significantly reduced radiographic vertebral fractures by 44% (risk ratio: 0.56; 95% CI = 0.39–0.80). The reduction in all clinical fractures was not statistically significant (risk ratio: 0.86; 95% CI: 0.73–1.01). A pre-planned subset analysis of the clinical fracture data, however, revealed that treatment significantly reduced fracture rates among women with initial T-scores below −2.5 (risk ratio: 0.64; 95% CI: 0.50–0.82) but not among women with T-scores of −2.5 and above (risk ratio: 1.08; 95% CI: 0.87–1.35). The Fosamax International Trial (FOSIT) study recently demonstrated a reduction in non-vertebral fracture incidence in post-menopausal women, with a T-score <−2.0 confirming that alendronate decreases clinical fracture rates in post-menopausal women with osteoporosis.[14] Alendronate prevents bone loss in normal post-menopausal women and its anti-fracture efficacy has not been demonstrated.

Long-term treatment with alendronate also suggested ongoing skeletal benefits to women with osteoporosis.[15] In a 7-year clinical trial, 235 post-menopausal women were treated with alendronate (10 mg/day) or placebo, and their BMD showed an increase in all skeletal sites and this remained stable for 7 years. In addition, there was a concomitant decrease in biochemical markers of bone turnover. Similar 10-year results are seen in the extension study of Bone et al.[16]

Lindsay et al.[17] compared the combined effects of alendronate and oestrogen in post-menopausal women. In this randomized trial, 428 post-menopausal women who had been receiving oestrogen replacement therapy for at least 1 year were randomized to either alendronate (10 mg/day) or placebo. After 12 months of treatment the patients on alendronate plus oestrogen produced significantly greater increases in BMD in the lumber spine (3.6% versus 1.0%; P < 0.001) and hip trochanter (2.7% versus 0.5%; P < 0.001). The results of this trial were supported by Bone et al.[18] It consisted of 425 post-menopausal women who were randomized to 2 years of placebo, alendronate

(10 mg daily), conjugated oestrogen or both treatments. The lumbar spine BMD in the placebo group had a 0.6% mean loss. The alendronate group showed a 6.0% gain (P < 0.001), conjugated oestrogen a 6.0% gain (P < 0.001) and the combined group an 8.3% gain (P < 0.001 versus placebo and oestrogen; P = 0.022 versus alendronate). These results suggest that the combination is more effective than either treatment alone.

Alendronate has also been studied for the treatment of osteoporosis in men.[19] Orwoll et al. randomized 241 men with osteoporosis to alendronate (10 mg/day) or placebo for 2 years. All patients received calcium and vitamin D supplements. One-third of the patients had baseline low serum free testosterone; the rest had levels within the normal range. The BMD of patients with alendronate had mean increases of 7.1 ± 0.3% (P < 0.001) at the lumbar spine and 2.5 ± 0.4% (P < 0.001) at the femoral neck. These increases were greater than those in the placebo group (P < 0.001). In addition, the incidence of vertebral fractures was lower in the alendronate group (0.8% versus 7.1%; P = 0.02). The conclusion was that alendronate not only significantly increased bone mineral density, but also helped to prevent vertebral fractures.

Alendronate may also reduce the risk of fractures in glucocorticoid-treated post-menopausal women. In an RCT of 477 corticosteroid-treated patients, alendronate demonstrated clinically relevant, statistically significant benefits at the spine, trochanter and femoral neck in doses of 5 and 10 mg/day.[20] All patients received between 800 and 1000 mg of calcium and between 250 and 500 IU of vitamin D per day. Over 48 weeks the mean increase in spine BMD was between 2% and 3% in the alendronate-treated groups (P < 0.001) and the decrease was 0.4% in the placebo-treated groups (P < 0.01). Significant differences in favour of alendronate therapy were also seen with trochanter and total body measurements. Alendronate was beneficial to all groups. It was effective in those who had recently commenced on corticosteroids as well as in those who had been on long-term therapy. Interestingly, in those post-menopausal women who were on HRT, there was an added benefit with alendronate therapy. There were proportionally fewer new vertebral fractures in the alendronate groups than in the placebo groups.

Alendronate is beneficial in the prevention of vertebral, hip and non-vertebral fractures in post-menopausal women and vertebral fractures in men. The increase in bone mass is sustained for as long as 10 years of therapy. It may be used in patients currently on oestrogen and in that population of patients it has an additive effect on increasing BMD. The drug is also effective in the prevention and treatment of corticosteroid-induced osteoporosis.

Risedronate

Risedronate is a third generation bisphosphonate with a pyridinyl side-chain. In vitro studies have suggested that risedronate is 1000 times more potent than etidronate as an anti-resorptive agent. It is well tolerated, as there are no serious adverse reactions; however, there are occasional reports of headache and diarrhoea in some patients.[21] Risedronate has been approved in several countries for the treatment of osteoporosis and Paget's disease of the bone.

Many randomized controlled trials have been conducted to evaluate the efficacy of risedronate for treating postmenopausal osteoporosis. The first study was conducted in North America,[22] while a second was performed in Europe and Australia (Multi-National).[23] The primary purpose of these trials was to determine the efficacy of risedronate in the prevention of vertebral fractures. A total of 2458 post-menopausal women with at least two vertebral fractures (or one vertebral fracture and a lumbar spine BMD T-score of –2.0 or lower) participated in the North American study, whereas the Multi-National trial involved 1226 post-menopausal women who had at least two osteoporotic vertebral fractures. Patients were randomly assigned to placebo or treatment with risedronate (2.5 or 5 mg/day). The 2.5 mg/day group was discontinued before the completion of the study because the new data from the 5 mg/day dose showed better results and a similar safety profile. All patients received 1000 mg/day of calcium and vitamin D supplement if baseline levels of the vitamin were low. Quantitative (15% loss in vertebral height) and semi-quantitative assessments were used to identify both prevalent and incident vertebral fractures. Regarding the number of patients who did not complete the full 3 years of follow-up, the rates were no higher than anticipated and there were no differences in dropouts between the treatment groups. Indeed, many of the non-completers were captured as they had reached the study end-point of fracture. Following 3 years of treatment, results indicated that risedronate (5 mg/day) reduced the incidence of vertebral fractures by 41% ($P = 0.003$) and 49% ($P < 0.001$), and non-vertebral fractures by 39% ($P = 0.02$) and 33% (NS; $P = 0.06$) in the North American and Multi-National studies respectively. Compared with placebo, treatment with risedronate (5 mg/day) reduced the incidence of vertebral fractures by 65% and 61% in the North American and Multi-National studies. There were no significant differences in adverse events between the groups.

These studies are also notable for what they tell us about osteoporotic vertebral fractures. The placebo group in the Multi-National study had more advanced osteoporosis at baseline (greater number of prevalent vertebral fractures and lower lumbar spine BMD) than in the North American study. This corresponded to a higher incidence of new vertebral fractures (13% and 29% over 1 and 3 years) in the Multi-National study compared with the North American study (6.4% and 16% over 1 and 3 years). This finding emphasizes that vertebral fracture risk increases in relation to the number of existing vertebral fractures. In conclusion, the clinical trials demonstrated that oral risedronate therapy, given over 3 years, is well tolerated and reduces the incidence of both vertebral and non-vertebral fractures in women with established post-menopausal osteoporosis. Furthermore, these studies are the first to show a rapid and clinically important reduction in the incidence of vertebral fractures following 1 year of therapy.

Researchers have also examined the role of risedronate therapy in corticosteroid-induced osteoporosis.[24,25] In a prevention study, 224 men and women who were beginning long-term corticosteroid treatment received either risedronate or placebo for 12 months.[24] The primary outcome was the percentage of change in lumbar spine BMD. Incidence of vertebral fractures was a secondary outcome. The results demonstrated no significant change in BMD decrease in patients receiving risedronate (–2.8 ± 0.5%; $P < 0.05$) compared to a decrease in the placebo group (–2.8 ± 0.5%; $P < 0.05$). There was a concomitant decrease in the incidence of vertebral fractures in the 5 mg risedronate group compared to placebo (5.7% compared to 17.3%; $P = 0.072$). The trial concluded that risedronate prevented bone loss in patients who had begun long-term corticosteroid therapy.

There were 290 patients with corticosteroid-induced osteoporosis in the Reid et al. study.[25] The mean lumbar spine difference between the 5 mg group and the placebo group was 2.68%. Risedronate (5 mg/day) for 12 months caused a statistically significant increase in lumbar spine BMD (2.90%). Mean differences between the two groups were between 1% and 2%, although the difference was only statistically significant at the femoral neck. Statistically significant increases from baseline were also seen in the BMD of the femoral neck (1.76%) and trochanter (2.43%) after 12 months of treatment with risedronate. Analysis of pooled data for the risedronate (5 mg) group from both studies showed a 70% reduction ($P = 0.016$) in the incidence of vertebral fractures compared to controls.[24]

In a recently published head-to-head trial,[26] 1053 post-menopausal women with osteoporosis were randomly assigned to receive once-weekly risedronate (35 mg) or alendronate (70 mg) for 12 months. Both groups had similar rates of adverse events. The alendronate group showed significantly greater increases in bone density at all sites after 12 months (treatment differences of 1.0%, 0.7% and 1.2% for total hip, femoral neck and lumbar spine respectively; $P < 0.001$). Significant reductions ($P < 0.001$) in all biochemical markers occurred with alendronate compared with risedronate by 3 months. Risk of fracture was not evaluated in this study.

Combination therapy of risedronate and conjugated oestrogens has also been examined in a 12-month prospective study of 524 post-menopausal women.[27] Patients were randomized to conjugated oestrogen alone or in combination with residronate. Femoral neck BMD increased significantly in the combination therapy group (2.7% versus 1.8%), whereas there was no difference in lumbar spine BMD (4.6% and 5.2%).

Ibandronate

Ibandronate is a highly potent nitrogen-containing bisphosphonate that has the potential to be administered intermittently with extended between-dose intervals. It was postulated that a longer therapy-free interval would improve long-term adherence to therapy. Chesnut et al.[28] studied its efficacy and safety in a randomized controlled trial of 2946 post-menopausal women with osteoporosis. Study participants were randomized to ibandronate either daily or intermittently with a dose-free interval of

>2 months or placebo for 3 years. Ibandronate was well tolerated, with side-effects no different than placebo. After 3 years, the rate of new vertebral fractures was lower with ibandronate (4.7%, 4.9% and 9.6% for daily ibandronate, intermittent ibandronate and placebo respectively). There was no difference in the rate of non-vertebral fractures.

BMD increased by 6.5%, 5.7% and 1.3% in the daily ibandronate, intermittent ibandronate and placebo groups respectively. Daily ibandronate has also been studied in early post-menopausal women without osteoporosis. McClung et al.[29] randomized 653 women to either 1 mg ibandronate, 2.5 mg ibandronate or placebo. All patients received calcium supplementation. After 2 years, 2.5 mg ibandronate produced statistically significant BMD gains at the spine and hip (3.8% and 1.8% respectively) compared to placebo. Monthly oral ibandronate is also being evaluated and to date has been shown to be well tolerated.[30] The daily ibandronate but not the intermittent regimen has been approved for use by the United States Food and Drug Administration.

Zoledronate

Zoledronate also appears to be effective for the treatment of post-menopausal osteoporosis. In a study[31] of five regimens of intravenous zoledronate infused over 5 minutes, lumbar spine bone density increased similarly in all five groups (4.3–5.1%). Thus, a single yearly infusion of this drug may be an effective for post-menopausal osteoporosis. Zoledronate is currently approved for treatment of malignancy-associated hypercalcaemia, multiple myeloma and for those with documented bone metastases from solid tumours. Recently, a trial by Reid et al.[32] demonstrated that a single infusion of zoledronic acid produced a more complete and sustained therapeutic response compared to daily resideronate for Paget's disease.

There have been reports of osteonecrosis of the jaw in those treated with IV bisphosphonates.[33] These were in patients who had confounding reasons for developing osteonecrosis of the jaw, including underlying malignancy, chemotherapy and corticosteroids. Those who seemed to be at highest risk were those who had periodonatal disease and recent tooth extraction. The vast majority were those who had malignancy. Therapy in these individuals is much greater, with zoledronate being given in doses of 4 mg IV monthly. In contrast, osteonecrosis of the jaw has not been reported in clinical trials of osteoporosis where the dose given is 5 mg IV once a year. Clinicians should be aware of this potential problem and should avoid its use in those with poor dental hygiene.

CALCITONIN

Calcitonin is a polypeptide produced by C-cells in the thyroid, with receptors in the osteoclasts, kidney, gastrointestinal tract and brain. It causes osteoclasts to become immobile and stop bone-resorbing activity. The hormone inhibits the rate of increase of bone turnover and is induced by parathyroid hormone. It is also known to act on the central nervous system, causing an analgesic effect. Post-menopausal women tend to have lower plasma calcitonin levels compared to age-matched men or pre-menopausal women.[34]

Calcitonin is available as a nasal spray, subcutaneous or intramuscular injections. Side-effects are generally dose related and consist of anorexia, nausea or facial flushing. These side-effects are more frequently associated with parenteral administration of the medication and are seldom seen with the nasal spray. A true allergic reaction, namely urticaria or anaphylaxis, is rare.[34] A long-term consequence of calcitonin usage is the development of antibodies and the potential for host resistance. The extent to which these antibodies may interfere with calcitonin action remains unresolved; however, long-term fracture efficacy data suggest that they are likely to be inconsequential.

Efficacy in treatment and prevention of osteoporosis

The efficacy of calcitonin and etidronate in the treatment of post-menopausal osteoporosis was examined in a meta-analysis study.[35] Eighteen clinical trials of calcitonin and six with etidronate were included in the meta-analysis. The studies indicated that pooled change in vertebral BMD was 1.97 (95% CI: 1.77–2.17) with calcitonin and 3.20 (95% CI: 2.92–3.48) with etidronate. The aggregated numbers of vertebral fractures that were prevented by the treatment were 59.2/1000 patient-years (95% CI: 55.1–63.3) for calcitonin and 28.3 (95% CI: −0.27–0.91) for etidronate. The authors could not establish superiority of either of the two drugs for the treatment of post-menopausal osteoporosis. They found that the clinical trials did not have data on hip fractures, the most important consequence of osteoporosis.

Chesnut et al.[36] conducted a 5-year, randomized trial to determine whether salmon calcitonin nasal spray reduced the risk of new vertebral fractures in post-menopausal women with osteoporosis. A total of 1255 post-menopausal women with established osteoporosis were assigned to receive salmon calcitonin nasal spray in doses of 100, 200 or 400 IU or placebo daily. All participants received elemental calcium and vitamin D supplements. The primary efficacy end-point was the risk of new vertebral fractures.

A total of 783 women completed 3 years of treatment and 511 completed 5 years. The 200 IU dose of salmon calcitonin nasal spray significantly reduced the risk of new vertebral fractures by 33% compared with placebo (relative risk (RR): 0.67; 95% CI: 0.47–0.97; $P = 0.03$). In the 817 women with one to five prevalent vertebral fractures on enrolment, the risk was reduced by 36% (RR: 0.64; 95% CI: 0.43–0.96; $P = 0.03$). The reductions in vertebral fractures in the 100 IU (RR: 0.85; 95% CI: 0.60–1.21) and 400 IU (RR: 0.84; 95% CI: 0.59–1.18) groups were not significantly different from the placebo group. Lumbar spine and BMD increased significantly from baseline (1–1.5%; $P < 0.01$) in all active treatment groups. The conclusion was that salmon calcitonin nasal spray at a dose of 200 IU daily significantly reduces the risk of new vertebral fractures in post-menopausal women with osteoporosis.

Unfortunately, the results of the Prevent Recurrence Of Osteoporotic Fractures (PROOF) study are open to some scepticism. Perhaps the greatest criticisms are on the large number of drop-outs, the lack of change in BMD and the lack of demonstrated treatment efficacy with doses other than 200 IU.

Cranney et al.[37] also conducted a meta-analysis on the efficacy of calcitonin in corticosteroid-induced osteoporosis. Nine trials were reviewed. The weighted mean difference in lumbar bone density was 2.8% (95% CI: 1.4–4.3%) and at 1 year it was 3.2% (95% CI: 0.3–6.1%). After 24 months of treatment, the lumbar spine density was not statistically significant compared to placebo. The RR was 0.71 (95% CI: 0.26–1.189) for vertebral fractures and 0.52 (95% CI: 0.14–1.96) for non-vertebral fractures, and neither was statistically significant. The conclusions were that calcitonin preserved bone mass in the first year of corticosteroid therapy at the lumbar spine but not at the femoral neck.

A recent open-label study[38] on idiopathic osteoporosis in men did suggest some benefit for intranasal calcitonin. A total of 71 men were randomized to 200 IU calcitonin nasal spray or a control group receiving calcium and vitamin D. After 18 months the treatment group showed an increased BMD at the lumbar spine (+3.5 ± 4.3% versus +0.83 ± 6.4%; $P = 0.04$) and the femoral neck (+1.4 ± 8.8% versus +1.4 ± 10.9%; $P = 0.98$). Treatment was well tolerated. Larger studies would be needed to confirm these results, as well as examine the effect of calcitonin on the incidence of fractures.

Calcitonin and bone pain

Several studies have demonstrated a short-term benefit in pain control in patients with sustained fracture. In one study, 56 women with osteoporosis who had an atraumatic fracture were assigned to either a placebo group or to 100 IU/day subcutaneous calcitonin for 2 weeks.[39] By the second day, there was a significant difference in the mean pain scores and analgesic use. Patients who received calcitonin not only had reduced pain, but also were able to sit, stand and gradually start to walk earlier than the control group. The mechanism of pain control is not known, but it has been hypothesized that calcitonin stimulated endorphin release.

Monitoring therapy and medication compliance

Monitoring anti-resorptive therapy is an important component of patient care. A recent paper[40] suggested that while BMD measurements are not correlated with fracture risk reduction, they could be useful at 2-year intervals to detect significant variations in post-menopausal osteoporosis. Biochemical markers for bone turnover such as osteocalcin, bone-specific alkaline phosphatase, C-telopeptide and N-telopeptide may be used 3 months after initiating therapy provided that intra-individual variability has been accounted for.

A study by McCombs et al.[41] examined compliance with drug therapies in the treatment of osteoporosis. Data from a health insurer were used to identify 58,109 osteoporosis patients who initiated drug therapy (hormone replacement therapy, bisphosphonate or raloxifene). One-year compliance rates were below 25% for all osteoporosis therapies, with a mean unadjusted duration of continuous therapy of 245 days for bisphosphonates (etidronate, alendronate and residronate). Compliance with therapy was associated with reduced risk of hip and vertebral fracture, as well as reduced use of hospital care.

SUMMARY

Fractures from osteoporosis are increasing in our ageing population. The addition of therapies such as the bisphosphonates alendronate and risedronate offer safer effective therapy for the prevention of fractures. Alendronate, risedronate and ibandronate should be considered drugs of choice for the treatment of osteoporosis, with etidronate and calcitonin being good alternatives.

PRACTICE POINTS

- The newer nitrogen-containing bisphosphonates – alendronate, ibandronate and risedronate – should be considered as first-line therapy for post-menopausal women with osteoporosis who are at high risk for fractures. There is good evidence that the drugs can prevent both vertebral and non-vertebral fractures, including hip fractures. Weekly dosing may lead to better patient adherence to therapy.

- The addition of alendronate to oestrogen therapy or to those on raloxifene may offer further benefits in increasing bone density. Whether this translates to fracture rate reduction has yet to be determined.

- The bisphosphonates are the only therapies that have proven fracture efficacy in post-menopausal women on corticosteroids.

- Calcitonin is an effective therapy for acute vertebral fracture pain.

- Calcitonin is not currently a first-line therapy for osteoporosis.

- Calcitonin may be used in conjunction with a bisphosphonate, oestrogen or raloxifene in women with severe osteoporosis or those with poor initial response to therapy.

RESEARCH AGENDA

- Demonstrate fracture prevention in men and pre-menopausal women with corticosteroid-induced osteoporosis.

- Determine the long-term safety of the bisphosphonates.

- Determine if the risk of osteonecrosis of the jaw occurs with oral bisphosphonates.

- Determine the long-term anti-fracture potential of calcitonin.

- Examine the role of calcitonin in men and pre-menopausal women.

- Issues surrounding possible calcitonin resistance in long-term osteoporosis treatment need to be examined.

REFERENCES

1. Fleish H. Bisphosphonates: mechanisms of action. *Endocr Rev* 1998; **19**: 80–100.

2. Russell RGG, Croucher PI & Rogers MJ. Bisphosphonates: pharmacology, mechanisms of action and clinical uses. *Osteoporosis Int* 1999; **10**(Suppl. 2): S66–S80.

3. Storm T, Thamsborg G, Steiniche T et al. Effect of intermittent cyclical etidronate therapy on bone mass and fracture rate in women with post-menopausal osteoprosis. *N Engl J Med* 1990; **322**: 1265–1271.

4. Watts NB, Harris ST, Genant HK et al. Intermittent cyclical etidronate treatment of postmenopausal osteoporosis. *N Engl J Med* 1990; **323**: 73–79.

5. Van Staa TP, Abenhaim L & Cooper C. Use of cyclical etidronate and prevention of non-vertebral fractures. *Br J Rheumatol* 1998; **37**: 87–94.

6. Wimalawansa SJ. Combined therapy with estrogen and etidronate has an additive effect on bone marrow density in the hip and vertebral bone: four year randomized study. *Am J Med* 1995; **99**: 36–42.

7. Adachi JD, Olszynski W, Hanley DA et al. Management of corticosteroid-induced osteoporosis. *Semin Arth Rheum* 2000; **29**: 228–251.

8. Adachi JD, Bensen WG, Brown J et al. Intermittent cyclical etidronate therapy in the prevention of corticosteroid-induced osteoporosis. *N Engl J Med* 1997; **337**: 382–387.

9. Schnitzer T, Bone HG, Crepaldi G et al. Therapeutic equivalence of alendronate 70 mg once-weekly and alendronate 10 mg daily in the treatment of osteoporosis. *Aging* 2000; **12**: 1–12.

10. Liberman UA, Weiss SR, Broll J et al. Effect of oral alendronate on bone mineral density and the incidence of fractures in postmenopausal osteoporosis. *N Engl J Med* 1995; **333**: 1437–1443.

11. Black DM, Cummings SR, Karpf DB et al. Randomized trial of effect of alendronate on risk of fracture in women with existing vertebral fractures. *Lancet* 1997; **348**: 1535–1541.

12. Cummings SR, Balck DM, Thompson DE et al. Effect of alendronate on risk of fracture in women with low bone density but without vertebral fractures: results from the Fracture Intervention Trial. *JAMA* 1998; **280**: 2077–2082.

13. Ensrud, KE, Barrett-Connor EL, Schwartz A et al. Randomized trial of effect of alendronate continuation versus discontinuation in women with low BMD: results from the Fracture Intervention Trial long-term extension. *J Bone Miner Res* 2004; **19**: 1259–1269.

14. Pols HA, Felsenberg D, Hanley DA et al. Multinational, placebo-controlled randomized trial of the effect of alendronate on bone density and fracture risk in postmenopausal women with low bone mass: results of the FOSIT study. *Osteoporosis Int* 1999; **9**: 461–468.

15. Tonino RP, Meunier PJ, Emkey R et al. Skeletal benefits of alendronate: 7 year treatment of postmenopausal osteoporotic women. *J Clin Endocrinol Metab* 2000; **85**: 3109–3115.

16. Bone HG, Hosking D, Devogelaer JP et al. Ten years' experience with alendronate for osteoporosis in postmenopausal women. *N Engl J Med* 2004; **350**: 1189–1199.

17. Lindsay R, Cosman F, Lobo RA et al. Addition of alendronate to ongoing hormone replacement therapy in the treatment of osteoporosis: a randomized controlled clinical trial. *J Clin Endocrinol Metab* 2000; **85**: 3109–3115.

18. Bone HG, Greenspan SL, McKeever C et al. Alendronate and estrogen effects in postmenopausal women with low bone density. *J Clin Endocrinol Metab* 1999; **84**: 3076–3081.

19. Orwoll E, Ettinger M, Weiss S et al. Alendronate for the treatment of osteoporosis in men. *N Engl J Med* 2000; **343**: 604–610.

20. Saag KG, Emkey R, Schnitzer TJ et al. Alendronate for the prevention and treatment of glucocorticoid-induced osteoporosis. *N Engl J Med* 1998; **339**: 292–299.

21. Licata AA. Risedronate, a novel pyridinyl bisphosphonate for the treatment of osteoporosis and Paget's disease of bone. *Expert Opin Invest Drugs* 1999; **8**: 1093–1102.

22. Harris ST, Watts N, Genant HK et al. Effects of risedronate treatment on vertebral and nonvertebral fractures in women with postmenopausal osteoporosis. *JAMA* 1999; **282**: 1344–1352.

23. Reginster JY, Minne W, Sorensen OH et al. Randomized trial of the effects of risedronate on vertebral fractures in women with established postmenopausal osteoporosis. *Osteoporosis Int* 2000; **11**: 83–91.

24. Cohen S, Levy RM, Keller M et al. Risedronate therapy prevents corticosteroid-induced bone loss: a twelve-month, multicentre, randomized double-blind, placebo-controlled, parallel-group study. *Arthritis Rheum* 1999; **42**: 2309–2318.

25. Reid D, Hughes RA, Laan RFJM et al. Efficacy and safety of daily risedronate in the treatment of corticosteroid-induced osteoporosis in men and women: a randomized trial. *J Bone Miner Res* 2000; **15**: 1006–1013.

26. Rosen CJ, Hochberg MC, Bonnick SL et al. Treatment with once-weekly alendronate 70 mg compared with once-weekly risedronate 35 mg in women with postmenopausal osteoporosis: a randomized double-blind study. *J Bone Miner Res* 2005; **20**: 141–151.

27. Harris ST, Eriksen EF, Davidson M et al. Effect of combined risedronate and hormone replacement therapies on bone mineral density in postmenopausal women. *J Clin Endocrinol Metab* 2001; **86**: 1890–1897.

28. Chestnut CH, Skag A, Christiansen C et al. Effects of oral ibandronate administered daily or intermittently on fracture risk in postmenopausal osteoporosis. *J Bone Miner Res* 2004; **19**: 1241–1248.

29. McClung MR, Wasnich RD, Recker R et al. Oral daily ibandronate prevents bone loss in early postmenopausal women without osteoporosis. *J Bone Miner Res* 2004; **19**: 11–17.

30. Reginster JY, Wilson KM, Dumont E et al. Monthly oral ibandronate is well tolerated and efficacious in postmenopausal women: results from the monthly oral pilot study. *J Clin Endocrinol Metab* 2005; **90**: 5018–5024.

31. Reid IR, Brown JP, Burckhardt P et al. Intravenous zoledronic acid in postmenopausal women with low bone mineral density. *N Engl J Med* 2002; **346**: 653–661.

32.   Reid, IR, Miller P, Lyles K et al. Comparison of a single infusion of zoledronic acid with risedronate for Paget's disease. *N Engl J Med* 2005; **353**: 898–908.

33.   Ruggiero SL, Mehrotra B, Rosenberg TJ et al. Osteonecrosis of the jaws associated with the use of bisphosphonates: a review of 63 cases. *J Oral Maxillofac Surg* 2004; **62**: 527–534.

34.   Simonski K & Josse RG. Calcitonin in the treatment of osteoporosis. *CMAJ* 1996; **155**: 962–965.

35.   Cardona JM & Pastor E. Calcitonin versus etidronate for the treatment of postmenopausal osteoporosis: a meta-analysis of published clinical trials. *Osteoporosis Int* 1997; **7**: 165–174.

36.   Chesnut CH III, Silverman S, Andriano K et al. A randomized trial of nasal spray salmon calcitonin in postmenopausal women with established osteoporosis: the prevention recurrence of osteoporotic fractures study. *Am J Med* 2000; **109**: 267–276.

37.   Cranney A, Welch V, Adachi JD et al. Calcitonin for the treatment and prevention of corticosteroid-induced osteoporosis. *Cochrane Database Syst Rev* 2000; CD001983.

38.   Toth E, Csupor E, Meszaros S et al. The effect of intranasal salmon calcitonin therapy on bone mineral density in idiopathic male osteoporosis without vertebral fractures – an open label study. *Bone* 2005; **36**: 47–51.

39.   Lyritis GP, Tsakalakos N, Magiasis B et al. Analgesic effect of salmon calcitonin in osteoporotic vertebral fractures: a double-blind placebo-controlled clinical study. *Calcif Tissue Int* 1991; **49**: 369–372.

40.   Roux C, Garnero P, Thomas T et al. Recommendations for monitoring antiresorptive therapies in postmenopausal osteoporosis. *Joint Bone Spine* 2005; **72**: 26–31.

41.   McCombs JS, Thiebaud P, McLaughlin-Miley C et al. Compliance with drug therapies for the treatment and prevention of osteoporosis. *Maturitas* 2004; **48**: 271–287.

Chapter 17

Anabolic bone-binding agents: parathyroid hormone analogues and strontium ranelate

Christine Manette and Jean-Yves Reginster

INTRODUCTION

Osteoporosis is characterized by a decrease in bone mass and a deterioration in skeletal microarchitecture, leading to an increased fragility and susceptibility to fractures. In treating established osteoporosis, the objective is to prevent further skeletal deterioration, improve bone mass and/or bone microarchitecture to provide a documented reduction of the risk of vertebral and/or peripheral fractures. Caregivers often face complicated situations with women consulting for the first time at later stages of the disease, namely after the diagnosis of the osteoporosis has already been made on the basis of random radiographs, densitometry measurement or, even worse, a fracture. Unfortunately, none of the anti-resorptive medications has unequivocally demonstrated the ability to prevent fully the occurrence of new vertebral or peripheral osteoporotic fractures once the disease is established. Although promising results have been reported with inhibitors of bone resorption,[1–5] patients treated with these drugs usually achieve modest increases in bone mass that translate into a partial reduction of incident fractures when compared with the rate observed in subjects receiving a placebo or treated with calcium alone. Therefore, there is an urgent need for the development of medications that stimulate osteoblast activity to such an extent that bone strength can be restored to values observed in normal subjects.

PEPTIDES FROM THE PARATHYROID HORMONE FAMILY

Although secondary hyperparathyroidism resulting from decreased calcium absorption and subsequent increases in bone resorption is considered a major determinant of hip fractures in the elderly,[6] more recent evidence suggests that parathyroid hormone (PTH) may also have an anabolic action on the skeleton.[7,8] Early animal studies showed that the anabolic effects of PTH on bone are more likely to occur after intermittent exposures to high blood concentrations than after sustained exposure to moderately increased blood levels, such as occurs in human hyperparathyroidism.[9]

In vitro studies in rats and human cells have greatly improved our understanding of the mechanisms underlying the anabolic effects of PTH on bone. Local production of insulin-like growth factor-1 (IGF-1) and subsequent synthesis of collagen occur in intermittent treatment but are inhibited during continuous administration.[10,11] Other actions include modulation of paracrine mediators (transforming growth factor-beta), enzymes (ornithine decarboxylase), and substances (prostaglandins) involved in cell replication and the stimulation of bone formation.[11] PTH might have the potential to increase osteoblast number by concomitantly increasing their replication rate and decreasing their programmed removal from bone by apoptosis.[11] In ovariectomized[12,13] or aged rats,[14] treatment with PTH increases the bone mass and bone strength of the vertebral bodies and the femoral neck in a highly significant manner. This effect is more pronounced than that seen with oestrogens or bisphosphonates.[12,13]

In early human studies, PTH fragment administration has increased trabecular bone mass, whereas cortical bone mass has remained unchanged or even decreased.[15] Studies claiming a benefit of the 1–34 PTH fragment (hPTH 1–34) were conducted with dosages in the range of 400–800 U/day. PTH stimulus had to be given for a period in excess of 2 weeks to result in increased bone mass.[16,17] The best regimen of administration seems to be uninterrupted daily injections.[11] In young women with oestrogen deficiency caused by treatment with gonadotropin-releasing hormone analogues, hPTH 1–34 prevented bone loss in the lumbar spine.[18] Beneficial effects on bone density observed during PTH treatment were shown to persist subsequent to stopping PTH therapy in patients receiving anti-resorptive substances such as oestrogens and bisphosphonates.[19,20]

In order to assess the effects of the 1–34 amino-terminal fragment of PTH on fractures, 1637 post-menopausal women with prior vertebral fractures were randomly assigned to receive 20 or 40 µg of PTH (1–34) or placebo, self-administered subcutaneously daily. Vertebral radiographs were obtained at baseline and at the end of the study (median duration of observation: 21 months) and serial measurements of bone mass were performed by dual-energy X-ray absorptiometry.

New vertebral fractures occurred in 14% of the women in the placebo group and in 5% and 4% respectively of the women in the 20- and 40-µg dose groups; the relative risks (RRs) of fracture as compared with the placebo group were 0.35 and 0.31 (95% CI: 0.22–0.55 and 0.19–0.50) respectively. New non-vertebral fragility fractures occurred in 6% of the women in the placebo group and 3% of those in each PTH-treated group (RR: 0.47 and 0.46; 95% CI: 0.25–0.88 and 0.25–0.86). As compared with placebo, the 20- and 40-µg doses of PTH increased bone mineral density by 9% and 13% in the lumbar spine and by 3% and 6% in the femoral neck; the 40-µg dose decreased bone mineral density at the shaft of the radius by 2%. Both doses increased total body bone mineral by 2–4% more points than did placebo. Parathyroid hormone had only minor side-effects (occasional nausea and headache).[21]

The anti-fracture efficacy of PTH on spinal fracture was not modulated by the age of the subjects (<65 years, 65–75 years or >75 years), prevalent spinal bone mineral density (BMD) values (T-score <–2.5 or >–2.5) or number of prevalent fractures (one, two or more fractures).[22]

At the end of this trial, patients were followed for an additional 18-month period, without PTH, during which there were allowed to use any anti-osteoporotic medication considered appropriate by their caregiver. While the proportion of patients having received an inhibitor of bone resorption was slightly higher in patients previously in the placebo group than in the patients having received 20 µg/day PTH, the reduction of vertebral fractures observed in this particular group during the initial trial was confirmed during this 18-month period of follow-up (RR: 0.59; 95% CI: 0.42–0.85).[23]

The relationship between previous fractures and risk of new fractures was evaluated in 931 post-menopausal women with prevalent vertebral fractures randomized to daily placebo or teriparatide (20 µg) in the Fracture Prevention trial. The number and severity of prevalent vertebral fractures independently predicted the risk for new vertebral fractures, and the number of previous non-vertebral fractures predicted the risk for new non-vertebral fractures in placebo patients. However, in teriparatide-treated patients, the increased fracture risk associated with previous number and severity of fracture was not observed.[24]

In direct comparison with alendronate, during 14 months, in osteoporotic women, a high dose (40 µg/day) of PTH induces a statistically more pronounced increase in lumbar BMD (12.2% versus 5.6%). This effect was also observed at the level of the femoral or total body BMD but, at the level of the distal radius, containing mainly cortical bone, BMD reached lower values on PTH than on alendronate. In this relatively small study, the incidence of non-vertebral fractures was lower in the PTH group (4.1%) compared to the alendronate group (13.4%).[25]

An important issue is whether the use of an anti-resorptive agent and an anabolic drug such as PTH together would provide a therapeutic advantage by combining different mechanisms for the reduction of risk of fracture. While several trials reported the addition of PTH to ongoing oestrogens/hormone replacement therapy (HRT),[26–29] fewer data are available for the use of anti-resorptive agents together with PTH from the start of therapy in previously untreated patients.

After 14 months' open, uncontrolled administration of 1–38 PTH (720–750 U/day) and intermittent nasal salmon calcitonin, eight patients (six males and two females), selected on the basis of bone mass (quantitative computed tomography) 'near the empirical fracture threshold' presented a 12–89% increase in spinal trabecular bone mass without significant changes at the forearm.[30] In a much more rigorous trial, patients receiving 28-day courses of 1–34 PTH (800 U/day), every 3 months, were randomized to be given calcitonin (75 U/day salmon calcitonin) or placebo for 42 days at the end of each PTH cycle. After 2 years of treatment, lumbar spine BMD was not significantly different between the two treatment groups, but those patients receiving calcitonin injections gained bone mass at a consistently slower rate. The authors concluded that there was no evidence that anti-resorptive therapy with calcitonin was of any benefit over that conferred by cyclical PTH alone.[31] Histomorphometry performed on iliac crest biopsies of patients with vertebral osteoporotic fractures receiving co-therapy of HRT and 1–34 PTH revealed substantial increases in cancellous bone volume, mainly through an increase in the width of packets of new cancellous bone, with consequent increases in the width of trabecular plates, compared to pre-treatment values.[32,33]

The Parathyroid Hormone and Alendronate Study (PATH) addressed this question by following up, for 12 months, 238 post-menopausal women (who were not using bisphosphonates), with low BMD at the hip or spine. They were randomly assigned to daily treatment with PTH (1–84, 100 µg/day), alendrolate (10 mg/day), or both. The areal BMD at the spine (dual X-ray absorption) increased in all the treatment groups, and there was no significant difference in the increase between the PTH and the PTH–alendronate group. The volumetric density quantitative computed tomography of the trabecular bone at the spine increased substantially in all groups, but the increase in the PTH-alone group was about twice that found in either of the other groups. Bone formation of amino-terminal propeptide of Type I collagen increased markedly in the PTH group but not in the combination therapy group. Bone resorption of serum C-telopeptide of type I collagen decreased in the combination therapy group and the alendronate group. The authors concluded that there was no evidence of synergy between PTH and alendronate. They considered that the changes in the volumetric density of trabecular bone, the cortical volume at the hip (significantly increased in the PTH group but not in the other treatment groups) and the levels of bone markers suggested that the concurrent use of alendronate may reduce the anabolic effects of PTH.[34] These results were in close agreement with those observed in men treated with alendronate (10 mg/day for 30 months), PTH (1–34, 40 µg/day begun at month 6) or both. BMD of the lumbar spine and femoral neck (dual X ray absorption) increased significantly more in men treated with PTH alone than in those in the other groups. At 12 months, changes in bone-specific alkaline phosphatase were significantly greater in the PTH group than in the alendronate or PTH–alendronate groups. The authors concluded that alendronate impairs the ability of PTH to increase BMD at the lumbar spine and the femoral neck in men, through an attenuation of PTH-induced stimulation of bone formation by alendronate.[35] These results suggest that if therapy with PTH is contemplated, it should be used alone and not with alendronate.[36] Whether this can be extrapolated to other bisphosphonates or other anti-resorptive agents remains unclear and will only be concluded after the appropriate study (ideally including fracture end-points) has been performed. The proposed explanation for the attenuation of the effects of PTH by alendronate is that the inhibition of overall bone turnover by alendronate impairs the anabolic activity of PTH. PTH appears to act primarily on mature osteoblasts to enhance their functions, their lifespan or both. PTH may also promote the differentiation of cells in the osteoblastic lineage, but it does not appear to expand the overall pool of uncommitted or pre-osteoblastic cells. Thus, if bone turnover and, subsequently, bone formation is reduced (after alendronate therapy), PTH may be less effective, since there are fewer osteoblasts for it to work on.[36]

STRONTIUM RANELATE

In 1910, the first elaborate investigation of the effects of stable strontium on bone suggested that it greatly stimulates the formation of osteoid tissues and tends to repress the resorptive process in bone. A comprehensive review of strontium was published in 1964. Strontium can substitute for calcium in many physiological processes. It is a trace element in the body, but administered strontium is almost exclusively deposited in bone. Long-term studies show that after incorporation in bone, strontium and calcium behave almost identically. Calcium deposition in bone was shown in 1952 to be enhanced when strontium is administered, a finding that first hinted at the potential of strontium in the treatment of osteoporosis.[37] Strontium ranelate is composed of an organic moiety, ranelic acid, and two atoms of stable, non-radioactive strontium. The effects of strontium ranelate on bone cell replication and bone formation were examined in vitro.[38] Strontium ranelate (1 mM) increased DNA synthesis in cell populations enriched with fibroblast and pre-osteoblastic cells, suggesting increased cell replication; this effect was less pronounced in cell populations enriched with mature osteoblasts. Conversely, at this dose strontium ranelate increased collagen and non-collagenic protein synthesis by 34% in mature osteoblast-enriched cells, indicting increased bone formation rates. The effects of strontium ranelate on bone formation (evaluated in calvariae cultures by autoradiography and

histomorphometry) were confirmed. In rats exposed to strontium ranelate (1 mM) for 24–96 h, pre-osteoblastic cell replication was enhanced. This effect was specific to pre-osteoblastic cells, as there was no change in the numbers of osteoblasts or periosteal cells. These effects appeared to be specific to strontium ranelate, as neither calcium ranelate nor sodium ranelate at the same concentration were able to induce similar effects.[38] Stimulation by strontium ranelate of the replication of osteoprogenitor cells and collagen as well as non-collagen protein synthesis in osteoblasts provides substantial evidence to categorize strontium ranelate as a bone-forming agent. In in vitro studies, strontium ranelate does not affect matrix mineralization.[39] Strontium ranelate markedly inhibited ^{45}Ca release from mouse pre-labelled bone, both in control cultures and in cultures treated with vitamin D_3. The inhibitory effects of strontium ranelate were close to those of salmon calcitonin in this model.[40] In addition, the electron microscopic features of osteoclasts were examined in foetal long bones treated with vitamin D_3 or strontium ranelate. Vitamin D_3-treated osteoclasts exhibited well-developed ruffled borders and clear zones, while strontium ranelate-treated osteoclasts had only clear zones facing the bone surface, and failed to form ruffled borders. That the structure of clear zones was not significantly affected by treating cells with the drug suggests that the attachment of osteoclasts to bone is not affected by strontium ranelate. The presence of ruffled borders indicates the active resorption phase of the osteoclasts, so these findings suggest that strontium ranelate has a direct inhibitory effect on the bone-resorbing activity of the pre-existing osteoclasts. This hypothesis is supported by another finding of this study that strontium ranelate inhibited the pit-forming activity of mature osteoclasts placed on dentine slices.[40]

In an isolated rat osteoclast assay, pre-incubation of bone slices with strontium ranelate (0.1–1 mM) induced a dose-dependent inhibition of the bone-resorbing activity of untreated rat osteoclasts (32–66% respectively).[41] Neither calcium nor sodium ranelate had significant effect in this assay. At the highest dose tested, the effect was similar to that following addition of salmon calcitonin (0.6 nM) to the culture medium. The effect of strontium ranelate on osteoclast differentiation was indirectly assessed on 1,25-dihydroxyvitamin D_3-induced expression of the osteoclast markers carbonic anhydrase-II (CA-II) and the vitronectin receptor (VNR) in chicken bone marrow culture.[41] After 6 days of treatment, strontium ranelate (0.1 1mM) dose-dependently inhibited the 1,25-dihydroxyvitamin D_3-induced increase in the expression of osteoclast differentiation markers. Expression of both CA-II and the α_v subunit of VNR were reduced by 40–45% at a concentration of 1 mM. These results show that strontium ranelate significantly inhibits bone resorption by direct and/or matrix-mediated inhibition of osteoclast activity and differentiation, which is compatible with the profile of anti-resorptive drugs.[41]

Thus, in vitro results indicate that strontium ranelate has a profile characterized by the stimulation of bone formation and the inhibition of bone resorption, suggesting that, for the first time, a chemical entity used in the treatment of osteoporosis could be targeted to the uncoupling of the bone remodelling process. It is also of note that strontium ranelate has demonstrated a beneficial effect on cartilage matrix formation in vitro,[42] suggesting a potential additional role for the drug in osteoarthritis. In vivo studies also support the concept that strontium ranelate increases bone formation and reduces bone loss.

Bone mass, dimensions and mechanical properties were assessed in the femur and fourth lumbar vertebra (L4) of female rats treated with strontium ranelate (225, 450 or 900 mg/kg/day, p.o.) for 2 years. Histomorphometric analysis of trabecular and cortical bone was carried out on the tibia. At the highest dose (900 mg/kg/day), strontium ranelate significantly increased the volume of the vertebral body by 6.4% and the diameter of the midshaft femur by 4.3% compared with controls. Bone mass of both the lumbar vertebra and the femur increased dose dependently, as did bone strontium concentration. The compression test was used to determine the mechanical properties of bone following 2 years of drug treatment. At the highest dose, there were significant increases in maximal load and total energy without affecting bone stiffness for both vertebral and femoral bone.[43] Histomorphometric analysis of the tibio-fibular junction and the proximal tibia metaphysis showed dose-dependent increases in trabecular bone volume due to increased trabecular number and thickness. There was no variation in osteoid thickness or volume, suggesting that the drug does not affect mineralization. With respect to cortical bone, total bone area, cortical bone area and periosteal perimeter were significantly increased at the highest dose tested in female rats, while cortical bone porosity was not affected.

Strontium ranelate has been investigated in a large phase III programme, which was initiated in 1996.[44] The goal of the 3-year phase III programme was to test whether strontium ranelate (2000 mg/day) reduces the risk of fracture in women with post-menopausal osteoporosis. The programme consisted of three international studies. The Spinal Osteoporosis Therapeutic Intervention (SOTI) study was aimed at assessing the effect of strontium ranelate on the risk of vertebral fractures, and the Treatment Of Peripheral Osteoporosis (TROPOS) trial aimed to evaluate the effect of strontium ranelate on peripheral (non-spinal) fractures. Both were randomized, double-blind and placebo-controlled, multicentre trials. All patients included in these two studies had previously participated in a run-in study, the Fracture International Run-in Strontium Ranelate Trials (FIRST), aimed at normalizing the calcium and vitamin D status of all patients prior to trial entry into either SOTI or TROPOS, according to the inclusion criteria of each study. Patients received a calcium/vitamin D supplement throughout the studies, which was individually adapted according to their deficiencies (0, 500 or 1000 mg of calcium, and 400 or 800 IU of vitamin D_3).[44] Patients entering FIRST had to be ambulatory with osteoporosis, with high risk of fracture. Of more than 9000 post-menopausal women with osteoporosis who took part in FIRST,[44] 1649 patients, with a mean age of 70 years, were included in SOTI[45] and 5091

patients, with a mean age of 77, were included in TROPOS.[46] In these two studies, the main statistical analysis was performed in the intent-to-treat population (ITT; patients who took at least one sachet of study treatment and with baseline and post-baseline evaluation of the main criteria). The primary end-point of SOTI and TROPOS was reduction in incidence over time of patients experiencing a new vertebral or non-vertebral fracture respectively.[44-46]

The results of the SOTI study showed that treatment with strontium ranelate for 3 years was associated with a 41% reduction in relative risk of experiencing a new vertebral fracture (semi-quantitative assessment) compared with placebo. In the treatment group, 139 patients experienced a new vertebral fracture compared with 222 in the placebo group (RR: 0.59; 95% CI: 0.48–0.73; $P < 0.001$) in the ITT population. The relative risk of experiencing a new vertebral fracture was also significantly reduced (by 49%) in the strontium ranelate group compared with the placebo group at the end of the first year of treatment (RR: 0.51; 95% CI: 0.36–0.74; $P < 0.001$). The proportion of patients with more than one new vertebral fracture over the 3-year period was 6.4% in the strontium ranelate group and 9.8% in the placebo group. Bone-specific alkaline phosphatase increased in the strontium ranelate group, while serum Type I collagen C-telopeptide cross-links decreased. Lumbar BMD increased from baseline in the treated group by 12.7% at the lumbar spine, 7.2% at the femoral neck and 8.6% at the total hip. BMD adjusted for strontium content increased by 6.8% from baseline at the lumbar spine after 3 years compared with a decrease of 1.3% in the placebo group. Strontium ranelate was well tolerated without any specific adverse events.[45]

TROPOS, a randomized, double-blind, placebo-controlled clinical trial, was designed to assess the effectiveness of strontium ranelate in preventing non-vertebral fractures in post-menopausal women with osteoporosis and also to assess its tolerability. Ambulatory post-menopausal women were eligible for the study if they had femoral neck BMD corresponding to a T-score <−2.5 and were ≥74 years, or aged between 70 and 74 years but with one additional fracture risk factor. All enrolled women received daily supplements of up to 1000 mg of elemental calcium adapted to their needs according to their dietary intake and vitamin D according to their serum 25-hydroxyvitamin D levels.

In the 5091 patients initially recruited, strontium ranelate was associated with a 16% relative risk (RR) reduction in all non-vertebral fractures over a 3-year follow-up period (RR: 0.84; 95% CI: 0.702–0.995; $P = 0.04$). Strontium ranelate treatment was associated with a 19% reduction in risk of major non-vertebral osteoporotic fractures (RR: 0.81; 95% CI: 0.66–0.98; $P = 0.031$). In the high-risk fracture subgroup (women ≥74 years and with femoral neck BMD T-score ≤−3), treatment was associated with a 36% reduction in risk of hip fracture (RR: 0.64; 95% CI: 0.412–0.997; $P = 0.046$). Yearly vertebral X-rays were performed in 3640 patients; a reduction in the RR of new vertebral fracture of 39% over 3 years was observed in the strontium ranelate group (RR: 0.61; 95% CI: 0.51–0.73; $P < 0.001$), the value being 45% (RR: 0.55; 95% CI: 0.39–0.77; $P < 0.001$) over the first year of treatment. In these 3640 patients, 66.4% had no prevalent vertebral fracture at inclusion. The risk of experiencing a first vertebral fracture in these patients was reduced by 45% (RR: 0.55; 95% CI: 0.42–0.72; $P < 0.001$). In the subgroup of patients with at least one prevalent fracture ($n = 1224$), the risk of experiencing a first vertebral fracture was reduced by 32% (RR: 0.68; 95% CI: 0.53–0.85; $P < 0.001$).

Femoral neck BMD and total hip BMD significantly increased from 6 months onwards in the strontium ranelate group. At 3 years, the BMD in the strontium ranelate group had increased from baseline by 5.7% at the femoral neck and 7.1% at the total hip ($P < 0.001$ for both comparisons with baseline values) corresponding to differences between the placebo and treatment groups at 3 years of 8.2% (95% CI: 7.7–8.7; $P < 0.001$) and 9.8% (95% CI: 9.3–10.4; $P < 0.001$) respectively.

Treatment was well tolerated: the incidence of adverse events (AEs) was well balanced between the two groups (87.9% in the strontium ranelate group and 88.9% in the placebo group), as were the serious AEs (24.7% in the strontium ranelate group and 24.4% in the placebo group) and withdrawals due to AEs (24.2% in the strontium ranelate group and 21.6% in the placebo group). Upper gastrointestinal symptoms were comparable between the two groups (incidence of gastritis: 2.3% in the strontium ranelate group and 2.7 % in the placebo group).[46]

CONCLUSION

During the last 5 years, a new paradigm has emerged in the treatment of osteoporosis. While the anti-catabolic agents were the option of choice for more than three decades, it is now clear that agents aiming at building new bone are able to concomitantly improve bone density and bone quality, ultimately resulting in a significant improvement of bone strengths. Teriparatide has unequivocally demonstrated its ability to reduce vertebral and non-vertebral fractures in women with low bone mineral density and prevalent vertebral fractures. This compound is characterized by an outstanding effect on the occurrence of new severe vertebral fractures, resulting in a decrease in back pain in osteoporotic subjects. Whereas its concomitant use with an inhibitor of bone resorption has not been shown to improve the properties of teriparatide alone, there is a strong rationale to consider the prescription of an anti-catabolic drug once teripartide is withdrawn. Strontium ranelate is one of the most exciting concepts observed in the field of osteoporosis during the last 20 years. This substance has a unique mode of action, concomitantly inhibiting bone resorption and stimulating bone formation. From pre-clinical results, it is clear that strontium ranelate is able to increase bone mass and bone strength. In human subjects, recent publications have confirmed that this effect results in a reduction of vertebral, non-vertebral and hip fractures. Anti-fracture efficacy has been documented in women with osteopoenia, osteoporosis

and severe osteoporosis, as well as in very elderly subjects. Both teriparatide and strontium ranelate have an excellent profile of tolerance, generating a very positive risk/benefit ratio, making them a first-line option for the management of osteoporosis, in the populations where they have shown anti-fracture efficacy.

REFERENCES

1. Black DM, Cummings SR, Karpf DB et al. Randomised trial of effect of alendronate on risk of fracture in women with existing vertebral fractures. *Lancet* 1996; **348**: 1535–1541.

2. Reginster JY, Minne HW, Sorensen OH et al. Randomized trial of the effects of risedronate on vertebral fractures in women with established postmenopausal osteoporosis. *Osteoporosis Int* 2000; **11**: 83–91.

3. Liberman U, Weiss SR, Broll J et al. Effect of oral alendronate on bone mineral density and the incidence in fractures in postmenopausal osteoporosis. *N Engl J Med* 1995; **333**: 1437–1443.

4. Overgaard K, Hansen MA, Jensen SB et al. Effect of salcatonin given intranasally on bone mass and fracture rates in established osteoporosis: a dose–response study. *BMJ* 1992; **305**: 556–561.

5. Delmas PD, Ensrud KE, Adachi JD et al. Efficacy of raloxifene on vertebral fracture risk reduction in postmenopausal women with osteoporosis: four-year results from a randomized clinical trial. *J Clin Endocrinol Metab* 2002; **87**: 3609–3617.

6. Riggs BL & Melton LJ. Involutional osteoporosis. *N Engl J Med* 1986; **314**: 1676–1684.

7. Dempster DW, Cosman F, Parisien M et al. Anabolic actions of parathyroid hormone on bone. *Endocr Rev* 1993; **14**: 690–709.

8. Pugsley LI & Selye H. The histological changes in the bone responsible for the action of parathyroid hormone on the calcium metabolism of the rat. *J Physiol* 1993; **79**: 113–117.

9. Podbesek R, Edouard C, Meunier PJ et al. Effects of two treatment regimens with synthetic human parathyroid hormone fragment on bone formation and the tissue balance of trabecular bone in greyhounds. *Endocrinology* 1983; **112**: 1000–1005.

10. Canalis E, McCarthy TL & Centrella M. Differential effects of continuous and transient treatment with parathyroid hormone related peptide (PTHrP) on bone collagen synthesis. *Endocrinology* 1990; **126**: 1806–1812.

11. Reeve J. PTH: a future role in the management of osteoporosis? *J Bone Miner Res* 1996; **11**: 440–445.

12. Mosekilde L, Sogaard CH, McOsker JE et al. PTH has a more pronounced effect on vertebral bone mass and biomechanical competence than antiresorptive agents (estrogen and bisphosphonate) assessed in sexually mature, ovariectomized rats. *Bone* 1994; **15**: 401–408.

13. Sogaard CH, Wronski TJ, McOsker JE et al. The positive effect of parathyroid hormone on femoral neck bone strength in ovariectomized rats is more pronounced than that of estrogen or bisphosphonates. *Endocrinology* 1994; **134**: 650–657.

14. Ejersted C, Andreassen TT, Nilsson MHL et al. Human parathyroid hormone (1–34) increases bone formation and strength of cortical bone in aged rats. *Eur J Endocrinol* 1994; **130**: 201–207.

15. Eriksen EF, Melsen F & Mosekilde L. *Drug Therapy: Formation-stimulating Regimens. Osteoporosis: Etiology, Diagnosis and Management.* Philadelphia: Lippincott-Raven, 1995; 403–434.

16. Reeve J, Arlot ME, Price TR et al. Periodic courses of human 1–34 parathyroid peptide alternating with calcitriol paradoxically reduce bone remodeling in spinal osteoporosis. *Eur J Clin Invest* 1987; **17**: 421–428.

17. Slovik DM, Neer RM & Potts JT. Short-term effects of synthetic human parathyroid hormone (1–34) administration on bone mineral metabolism in osteoporotic patients. *J Clin Invest* 1981; **68**: 1261–1271.

18. Finkelstein JS, Klibanski A, Schaefer EH et al. Parathyroid hormone for the prevention of bone loss induced by estrogen deficiency. *N Engl J Med* 1994; **331**: 1618–1623.

19. Hodsman A, Fraher L & Adachi J. A clinical trial of cyclical clodronate as maintenance therapy following withdrawal of parathyroid hormone in the treatment of postmenopausal osteoporosis. *J Bone Miner Res* 1995; **10**: S200.

20. Lindsay R, Cosman F, Shen V et al. Bone mass increments induced by PTH treatment can be maintained by estrogen. *J Bone Miner Res* 1995; **10**: S200.

21. Neer RM, Arnaud CD, Zanchetta JR et al. Effect of parathyroid hormone (1–34) on fractures and bone mineral density in postmenopausal women with osteoporosis. *N Engl J Med* 2001; **344**: 1434–1441.

22. Marcus R, Wang O, Satterwhite J et al. The skeletal response to teriparatide is largely independent of age, initial bone mineral density, and prevalent vertebral fractures in postmenopausal women with osteoporosis. *J Bone Miner Res* 2003; **18**: 18–23.

23. Lindsay R, Scheels WH, Neer R et al. Sustained vertebral fracture risk reduction after withdrawal of teriparatide (recombinant human parathyroid hormone (1–34)) in postmenopausal women with osteoporosis. *Arch Intern Med* 2004; **164**: 2024–2030.

24. Gallagher JC, Genant HK, Crans GG et al. Teriparatide reduces the fracture risk associated with increasing number and severity of osteoporotic fractures. *J Clin Endocrinol Metab* 2005; **90**: 1583–1587.

25. Body JJ, Gaich GA, Scheele WH et al. A randomized double-blind trial to compare the efficacy of teriparatide (recombinant human parathyroid hormone (1–34)) with alendronate in postmenopausal women with osteoporosis. *J Clin Endocrinol Metab* 2002; **87**: 4528–4535.

26. Lindsay R, Nieves J, Formica C et al. Randomised controlled study of effect of parathyroid hormone on vertebral-bone mass and fracture incidence among postmenopausal women on oestrogen with osteoporosis. *Lancet* 1997; **350**: 550–555.

27. Cosman F, Nieves J, Woelfert L et al. Parathyroid hormone added to established hormone therapy: effects on vertebral fracture and maintenance of bone mass after parathyroid hormone withdrawal. *J Bone Miner Res* 2001; **16**: 925–931.

28. Lane NE, Sanchez S, Modin GW et al. Parathyroid hormone treatment can reverse corticosteroid-induced osteoporosis. *J Clin Invest* 1998; **102**: 1627–1633.

29. Lane NE, Sanchez S, Modin GW et al. Bone mass continues to increase at the hip after parathyroid hormone treatment is discontinued in glucocorticoid-induced osteoporosis: results of a randomized controlled clinical trial. *J Bone Miner Res* 2000; **15**: 944–951.

30. Hesch RD, Busch U, Prokop M et al. Increase of vertebral density by combination therapy with pulsatile 1–38hPTH and sequential addition of calcitonin nasal spray in osteoporotic patients. *Calcif Tissue Int* 1989; **44**: 176–180.

31. Hodsman AB, Fraher LJ, Watson PH et al. A randomized controlled trial to compare the efficacy of cyclical parathyroid hormone versus cyclical parathyroid hormone and sequential calcitonin to improve bone mass in postmenopausal women with osteoporosis. *J Clin Endocrinol Metab* 1997; **82**: 620–628.

32. Reeve J, Bradbeer JN, Arlot M et al. hPTH 1–34 treatment of osteoporosis with added hormone replacement therapy: biochemical, kinetic and histological responses. *Osteoporosis Int* 1991; **1**: 162–170.

33. Bradbeer JN, Arlot ME, Meunier PJ et al. Treatment of osteoporosis with parathyroid peptide (hPTH 1–34) and oestrogen: increase in volumetric density of iliac cancellous bone may depend on reduced trabecular spacing as well as increased thickness of packets of newly formed bone. *Clin Endocrinol* 1992; **37**: 282–289.

34. Black DM, Greenspan SL, Ensrud KE et al. The effects of parathyroid hormone and alendronate alone or in combination in postmenopausal osteoporosis. *N Engl J Med* 2003; **349**: 1207–1215.

35. Finkelstein JS, Hayes A, Hunzelman JL et al. The effects of parathyroid hormone, alendronate, or both in men with osteoporosis. *N Engl J Med* 2003; **349**: 1216–1226.

36. Khosla S. Parathyroid hormone plus alendronate – a combination that does not add up. *N Engl J Med* 2003; **349**: 1277–1279.

37. Nielson BP. The biological role of strontium. *Bone* 2004; **35**: 583–588.

38. Canalis E, Hott M, Deloffre P et al. The divalent strontium salt S12911 enhances bone cell replication and bone formation in vitro. *Bone* 1996; **16**: 517–523.

39. Barbara A, Delannoy P, Denis BG et al. Normal matrix mineralization induced by strontium ranelate in MC3T3-E1 osteogenic cells. *Metabolism* 2004; **53**: 532–537.

40. Takahashi N, Sasaki, Tsouderos Y et al. S12911-2 inhibits osteoclastic bone resorption in vitro. *J Bone Miner Res* 2003; **18**: 1082–1087.

41. Baron R & Tsouderos Y. In vitro effects of S12911-2 on osteoclast function and bone marrow macrophage differentiation. *Eur J Pharmacol* 2002; **450**: 11–17.

42. Henrotin Y, Labasse A, Zheng SX et al. Strontium ranelate increases cartilage matrix formation. *J Bone Miner Res* 2001; **16**: 299–308.

43. Ammann P, Shen V, Robin B et al. Strontium ranelate improves bone resistance by increasing bone mass and improving architecture in intact females rats. *J Bone Miner Res* 2004; **12**: 2012–2020.

44. Meunier PJ & Reginster JY. Design and methodology of the phase 3 trials for the clinical development of strontium ranelate in the treatment of women with postmenopausal osteoporosis. *Osteoporosis Int* 2003; **14**: S66–S76.

45. Meunier PJ, Roux C, Seeman E et al. The effects of strontium ranelate on the risk of vertebral fracture in women with postmenopausal osteoporosis. *N Engl J Med* 2004; **350**: 459–468.

46. Reginster JY, Seeman E, De Vernejoul MC et al. Strontium ranelate reduces the risk of nonvertebral fractures in postmenopausal women with osteoporosis: TROPOS study. *JCEM* 2005; first published online, 22 February.

Chapter 18

The cost-effectiveness of interventions for the prevention and treatment of osteoporosis

Rachael L. Fleurence, Cynthia P. Iglesias and David J. Torgerson

BACKGROUND

Economic evaluations are being widely used by decision-makers to evaluate the cost-effectiveness of treatments. This is important as all resources are scarce and economic evaluations seek to advise in an explicit manner the optimum use of scarce health resources.

The importance of economic evaluations has been recognized in the licensing process of new pharmaceuticals in many countries. In Australia and in the Canadian province of Ontario, for example, it is now mandatory to include some form of economic appraisal in the licensing process.[1] The National Institute for Clinical Excellence (NICE), in the UK, also requires an economic evaluation as part of its submission procedures for the appraisal of all new technologies, including devices and pharmaceuticals (www.nice.org.uk).[2] The UK approach also includes economic evaluations within a clinical guideline process, so that not only are individual drugs or therapies evaluated for their cost-effectiveness, but a 'package' of care may also be economically evaluated. Even in the USA there are moves to implement more widely the use of economic evidence in health policy decision-making. The Academy for Managed Care Pharmacy (AMCP) has developed submission guidelines that recommend including evidence of cost-effectiveness of new treatments for the inclusion on pharmacy formularies (www.amcp.org).[3]

A number of economic evaluations have been conducted in the field of osteoporosis in a variety of settings and study populations. These economic models investigate a range of interventions that are available to prevent and treat osteoporosis.[4,5] Recommendations for treatment and prevention of osteoporosis have changed radically in the last few years. Until the late 1990s hormone replacement therapy (HRT) was widely considered to be the 'gold standard' method of preventing postmenopausal osteoporotic fractures. This view was overturned, particularly by the 2002 publication of the Women's Health Initiative trial, which was stopped early because of the excess risk in cardiovascular events among women taking combined oestrogen and progestin treatment.[6,7] The oestrogen-alone trial was also stopped early, in 2004, due to the increase in observed strokes.[8] Both studies, however, confirmed a beneficial effect of HRT on hip and non-hip fractures. Nevertheless, treatment with HRT for long-term prevention is no longer recommended as it is perceived that the risks of treatment outweigh the benefits to bone.

There are alternatives to the use of HRT for fracture prevention. Therapies such as bisphosphonates, parathyroid hormone (PTH), strontium renalate and raloxifene have been shown to be effective in clinical trials for fracture prevention (although for raloxifene this only applies to vertebral fractures). Calcium and vitamin D supplementation widely used for primary and secondary fracture prevention has been found to be ineffective among generally healthy community-dwelling older people. Similarly, hip protectors have also been found to be ineffective for hip fracture prevention.[9-12]

Research into the economic consequences of preventing osteoporosis reflects the clinical research in this period of rapid change involving the introduction of new therapies or evidence for the ineffectiveness of established treatments. In this chapter, we have undertaken an overview of the economic literature. This review is based on a recent systematic review of the economic literature.[13]

In the following section of the chapter we look at the economic methods used for evaluating healthcare technologies.

ECONOMIC EVALUATION METHODS

The purpose of economic evaluations is to help decision-makers determine whether the extra cost of an intervention that is more effective than current practice can be justified given the limited resources available for healthcare programmes. In the UK, it is generally assumed that cost-effective interventions are valued approximately at £30,000 pounds per quality-adjusted life year (QALY) based on an analysis of the decisions taken by the National Institute of Clinical Excellence.[14] The following section briefly outlines the three different types of economic evaluations that can be found in the literature: cost-effectiveness, cost-utility and cost-benefit analyses.[15]

Cost-effectiveness

A cost-effectiveness analysis compares the differences in costs and effectiveness of two or more interventions. In this type of economic evaluation, effectiveness is measured in natural units. In the field of osteoporosis prevention, possible natural units are the number of fractures avoided or the quality-of-life scores obtained using specific instruments from fracture patients. Obviously, cost-effectiveness studies can only provide comparative information on interventions measured in the same units. So cost-effectiveness analyses can usefully compare different interventions aimed at preventing osteoporosis, but such analyses would not help to determine whether these interventions were cost-effective compared to a treatment for heart disease, for example. One way to overcome this shortcoming is to use life years gained as the measure of effectiveness, which allows for comparisons across diseases. However, the use of life years gained does not account for the impact on quality of life of the treatment. In determining which type of economic evaluation is best suited to the intervention under consideration, it is important to determine beforehand whether the impact of mortality is sufficient or whether quality-of-life considerations should also be included.

Costs to be accounted for in an economic evaluation should ideally include all costs incurred by society, ranging from the health service costs to the out-of-pocket payments made by the patient and losses of productivity due to the condition. However, in practice, few economic evaluations include indirect costs and many tend to adopt the perspective of the health system. This may underestimate the cost-effectiveness of a treatment for the prevention of osteoporosis if these are associated with time lost from work. This issue also highlights the difficulty of valuing productivity losses in elderly populations such as those at risk for osteoporosis, where these populations may no longer be in regular paid work. Some issues remain unresolved on the question of whether future costs incurred due to increased life expectancy should be included.[16] In the case of treatments to prevent osteoporosis, the costs of treatments and any costs incurred by the health service from side-effects of the treatment would need to be included. The issues surrounding the calculation and the nature of costs are the same for the three types of analysis.

Cost-utility

Probably the most useful technique for assessing the economic value of treatments for the prevention of osteoporosis is cost-utility analysis. A cost-utility analysis compares the costs and the utilities of two or more interventions. A utility is the measure of the preference or value placed upon a health state and is a number between 0 (representing death) and 1 (perfect health) so, for example, a woman with a hip fracture may value her present quality of life at 0.7. If she suffered the hip fracture 10 years ago, she will have lived 7 QALYs (quality-adjusted life years) compared to a woman in perfect health for 10 years, who will have lived 10 QALYs, assuming that her valuation of her quality of life has remained constant over that period.

The issue of who should value health states is still unresolved, yet this is an important issue, because different sources can provide widely varying utilities.[17] In practice, these values are generally elicited from the patients but sometimes have to be determined by health professionals or significant family members. Several methods have been proposed to elicit these utility values. The simplest is the rating scale method, which asks the respondent to mark, on a straight line with grid marks, a number corresponding to her perceived quality of life. However, economic theory would suggest that this method is the weakest in terms of deriving an estimate of the true utility value of a respondent. Theoretically superior, but more difficult for the respondent to understand, are the standard gamble and the time trade-off methods. These techniques elicit utility preferences from respondents by presenting them with successive choices between health states (or time spent in health states) to which different probabilities are attached. Other methods to calculate utilities use generic health state questionnaires such as the Euroqol or the Health State Utilities Index, that provide utilities for health states on the basis of the responses of the subject.[15] Once these utilities have been obtained, it is possible to calculate QALYs.

One of the advantages of using QALYs is that they allow for comparisons between interventions across different conditions, so unlike cost-effectiveness studies, a comparison between a treatment for cholesterol reduction to prevent heart disease and a preventive treatment for osteoporosis can be conducted. By using QALYs, it is possible to evaluate interventions that impact on the quality as well as the length of life. For example, in studies looking at HRT, benefits such as reduction in fracture risk and alleviation of menopausal symptoms can be incorporated alongside potential risks such as breast cancer or endometrial cancer, as well as cardiovascular disease.

A number of economic evaluations have used estimates for utilities in different health states associated with osteoporosis (for example, references 18 and 19). While estimates are acceptable when no empirical data are available, empirically elicited utilities should be preferred. A systematic review of empirical utility estimates for health states associated with osteoporosis has been published.[20] A comparison with commonly used assumptions in economic evaluation showed significant differences with the empirical estimates and also found there to be a wide variation between estimates for the same state (for example, the utility ranged from 0.32 to 0.80 for vertebral fracture states). The study concluded that while this variation could be partly explained by the valuation technique, health state description and the background and perspective of respondent, the wide differences may remain problematic and could affect the validity of the conclusions in economic evaluations. The review recommended a set of health state values as part of a 'reference case' for use in economic models. An example of the use of this reference case can be found in a cost-effectiveness model of hip protectors and vitamin D and calcium supplements.[21] In that study, health state values for the general population obtained using EQ-5D were used as baseline values for non-fracture patients. These were as follows: 0.747, 0.731, 0.699 and 0.676 for ages 70–74, 75–79, 80–85 and 85+ respectively. To obtain the health state utility after the occurrence of a hip fracture, these baseline values were adjusted using a multiplier of 0.797, to account for the proportionate effect of a fracture on the health state utility in the first year. This multiplier was obtained from an empirical study conducted in the UK using the time trade-off method.[22]

Cost-benefit

A cost-benefit evaluation explicitly places a monetary valuation on the outcomes of healthcare and seeks to determine whether a health technology provides an overall net gain to society, in the sense where the benefits outweigh the costs. So, for example, a cost-benefit analysis would seek to put a monetary value on the number of hip fractures avoided, or the number of QALYs gained, through the implementation of a preventive programme. Several approaches have been used in cost-benefit analyses in healthcare, although many problems remain in practice.[23] Nonetheless, there has recently been considerable interest in techniques such as contingent valuation, which elicit monetary valuations by asking people for their stated preferences among specified choices in monetary terms. This so-called willingness-to-pay approach asks people how much they would be prepared to pay to obtain the benefits of an intervention or avoid the costs of illness. Applications of cost-benefit analyses in healthcare have been relatively rare, partly due to the difficulty in eliciting reliable willingness-to-pay measures and partly due to the resistance, particularly amongst health professionals, in placing a monetary valuation on health benefits. To date, no cost-benefit evaluations have been conducted in the field of osteoporosis.

COST-EFFECTIVENESS STUDIES IN OSTEOPOROSIS TREATMENT AND PREVENTION

A number of economic evaluations have been developed in the field of osteoporosis. A recent structured review identified 42 studies published between 1980 and 2004.[13] The early economic evaluations tended to be focused mainly around HRT or oestrogen replacement theory (ERT). In particular, one research group led by Weinstein and Tosteson in the USA undertook a number of economic evaluations investigating the use of ERT and HRT in women with and without hysterectomy. The assumptions for these models were derived from observational data, which we now know were incorrect. The cost-effectiveness of bone mineral density (BMD) measurements followed by HRT compared with universal HRT treatment was also investigated by this group.[18,19,24–27] From a European perspective, a

model developed by a Swedish group of health economists has been employed a number of times to investigate various hypothetical interventions, at different costs, effectiveness and offset times.[28–30]

In line with the change, or improvement, in the evidence base of effective therapies, other economic models have been developed to look at non-HRT treatments: in particular, the cost-effectiveness of bisphosphonates and raloxifene following the results of clinical trials published in that area (FIT and MORE).[31,32] Models have also been published investigating interventions such as vitamin D and calcium, and hip protectors (for example, references 21, 33–36).

The following section describes important aspects in economic models, with examples of how these issues have been approached in practice.

Interventions

Among the 42 economic models published in the field of osteoporosis since 1980, the main intervention investigated was HRT (in which we include ERT), with 17 studies investigating its cost-effectiveness.[18,19,24–27,30,37–46] HRT was followed by bisphosphonates (11),[31,40,43,45,47–53] calcium and/or vitamin D (10),[21,36,42,43,47,47,53–55] calcitonin (six),[40,43,46,47,56,57] hypothetical interventions (five),[28,29,51,58,59] hip protectors (five),[21,33,35,60,61] raloxifene (four),[32,43,54,62] exercise, steroids and other (two each).[42,43,46,63] The majority of HRT/ERT studies were conducted before 1994, reflecting the shift away from HRT as the 'gold standard' treatment for osteoporosis. Bisphosphonates, such as alendronate, etidronate and risedronate, and raloxifene have been investigated following the results of large clinical trials.[64–68] Less expensive therapies with fewer side-effects have also been investigated – vitamin D with or without calcium and hip protectors – although following the results of recent clinical trials these economic evaluations will need to be updated in light of these data.[9–11]

Level of intervention

Different levels of interventions are available in the treatment and prevention of osteoporosis. Sculpher et al.[69] differentiate between primary, secondary prevention and treatment in their review, and provide the following definitions for these levels. Primary prevention is used for asymptomatic populations with no apparent osteoporosis or elevated risk of the condition, to reduce their risk of onset in later life. Secondary prevention is used for asymptomatic patients who have been shown to have BMD sufficiently low to place them at elevated risk of fracture, to slow down the decline (or restore) BMD and hence reduce the risk of fracture. Treatment is used for patients known to have osteoporosis and who have already experienced one or more fractures, to reduce their risk of further fractures. In existing economic evaluations, most studies (13) have looked at primary prevention.[19,24,27,29,33,37,38,42,46,54,58,60,61] For example, Segui-Gomez et al.[33] investigated the use of hip protectors in men and women aged 65+ at average risk of fracture. Secondary prevention was investigated in seven studies.[35,39,43–45,59,63] For example, Fleurence[21] studied a cohort of 3645 peri-menopausal women who had a BMD measurement with recommendation to use HRT if low BMD was present. Treatment was modelled in eight studies.[31,40,48,50,51,53,56,62] Johnell et al.[51] studied women aged 71 and over with low bone mass and at least one previous spine fracture. Finally, 14 studies investigated a combination of intervention levels.[18,21,25,26,28,30,32,36,41,47,49,52,55,57] For example, Kanis et al.[32] modelled the UK female population aged 50 or more with low BMD (secondary prevention) or with a previous vertebral fracture (treatment).

Perspectives and settings

The UK is the setting with the most economic evaluations to date, with 12 studies.[21,32,37–41,43,46,50,52,55] It is followed by the USA and Sweden, with nine studies conducted in each of these countries.[18,19,25–31,33,34,36,51,54,58–60,63] These three countries are associated with 71% of the economic evaluations reflecting the concern over the large burden of osteoporosis in their countries. Other countries where economic evaluations have been conducted are Canada (three), Australia, Germany and Spain (two each), and Italy, Japan and Denmark with one each.[24,35,42,44,45,47–49,53,56,57,62] The perspective of these studies is mostly the national health system of the country where the study is being carried out, except for the USA, where the perspective is the third-party payer.

Populations investigated

The majority of economic evaluations in the field of osteoporosis investigate female populations only, whether perimenopausal or post-menopausal (37 studies). It has been reported that actually one-third of hip fractures will occur in men and some studies have also included males in their analysis.[70] The interest in male osteoporosis has only recently been reflected in economic evaluations, as these all date from 2003 and 2004. This marks a shift in interest from investigating post-menopausal women only, to also investigating the cost-effectiveness of treatments in elderly men. Two studies investigated male and female populations.[21,33] One study investigated alendronate in men only.[31] Two studies did not investigate men and women separately, although this is not advisable since hip fracture rates are known to be different in these populations.[60,61]

Type of fracture

There has been a wide variation in the types of fractures used as outcomes in economic evaluations. Sixteen studies were conducted where hip fractures were the only fracture outcome.[25–29,33,36,42,44,46,53,55,57,58,60,61] 12 studies investigated hip, wrist and vertebral fractures,[31,35,37,38,41,47,50–52,54,56,63] seven studies included hip, wrist, vertebral and other fractures,[21,30,39,43,48,59,62] and three analysed hip and wrist fractures.[18,19,24] A clear majority of economic evaluations include hip fractures, reflecting the significant financial cost and quality-of-life burden to the patient of this type of fracture. For example, it has been shown that the mortality risk increases in the year following a hip fracture.[71,72] Three studies modelled vertebral fractures alone.[32,40,45] The inclusion of vertebral fractures in economic models is challeng-

ing, as a majority of these fractures are under-reported.[73] For example, a survey in Rochester (USA) suggested that 8% of patients with vertebral fractures came to medical attention.[74] While it can be assumed that the costs to the health system of vertebral fractures will be reflected in hospital admission data, for example, the effects of vertebral fractures on quality of life may be substantially underestimated.

Types of models

Economic evaluations can be conducted alongside clinical trials, where economic data are collected at the same time as clinical data. Often, however, economic evaluations are conducted using models that explicitly combine available information in a formal framework. These models enable the combination of evidence from a variety of sources in order to explore scenarios which for different reasons have not been empirically tested. For example, results from studies with relatively short follow-up periods can be extrapolated to longer time periods that are more relevant to policy-makers. Economic models can also explore the long-term effectiveness and cost-effectiveness of treatments in populations at different risk. The use of models is indicated in conditions such as osteoporosis because of the need to model long-term costs and effects that are not always available from trial or even observational data. In the absence of available data, decision-makers need formal frameworks on which to base their decisions and such models can provide such a basis when they are well conducted, transparent and explicit.[75] For example, a key issue with respect to pharmaceutical osteoporosis treatments is the issue of 'offset'. This is the period of activity a treatment will have after cessation of therapy. The length of this period is crucial to the cost-effectiveness of treatment, as offset provides benefit for no extra cost. PTH, for example, has provided evidence for quite a long offset period, with fracture reductions being maintained for a number of years after treatment cessation. In contrast, there is little evidence for other treatments, such as bisphosphonates, as to how long offset will be maintained. Economic models can use various assumptions of offset to ascertain whether, given reasonable assumptions based on clinical knowledge and bone biology, a treatment that is borderline in cost-effectiveness could be cost-effective with some offset. Alternatively, a treatment may not be cost-effective whatever offset time is assumed.

In the field of osteoporosis, despite the variety of interventions and populations considered, all but one of the reviewed studies employed cost-effectiveness models. The exception was an observational study on the likely cost-effectiveness of HRT for fracture prevention among young post-menopausal women.[39] In this study, Fleurence et al. analysed the data from a cohort of 3645 peri-menopausal women who had a BMD measurement with recommendation to use HRT if low BMD was present. The number and type of fractures for each patient were recorded and the cost of treating these fractures was obtained from the hospital in the area where the study was conducted. The study describes the cost per averted fracture for different treatment options. Ideally, future fracture prevention trials should collect individual patient data to allow trial-based evaluations.

Quality of models

The quality of models in the field has been shown elsewhere to be variable.[69,76] For example, some of the earlier studies made questionable use of cost-effectiveness decision rules. However, the quality of the methodology and the reporting in publications is on average increasing, reflecting the availability of structured guidelines for developing and reporting cost-effectiveness models.[77] Most studies are explicit about the inputs and structure of the model. A number of models now include vertebral and wrist fractures as well as hip fractures. Some studies also include other fractures, sometimes represented by shoulder fractures. Recently, much effort has been devoted to validating the models, by providing explicit internal and external validity checks.[78] In addition, Zethraeus et al.[76] have proposed making their model available to researchers in the field, in order to build and improve on current models rather than starting each modelling exercise anew.

Uncertainty

With the large number of assumptions that such models rely on, quantifying the uncertainty associated with the estimates is essential for the validity of the models. Although single- and multi-way sensitivity analysis may be used to investigate the effect of different model parameters, only full probabilistic models allow the exploration of the interaction of different sources of uncertainty present within a model.[77] In these models, each input parameter is assigned an appropriate statistical distribution and a 95% confidence interval, representing a range of plausible values obtained from the literature.[79] A Monte-Carlo simulation is then run to obtain a large number of iterations of the model. These results are used to obtain cost-effectiveness acceptability curves that show the probability that an intervention is cost-effective as a function of the decision-maker's ceiling cost-effectiveness ratio (this ceiling will vary according to the resources available for healthcare and is generally unknown to the analyst). An increasing number of economic evaluations are using probabilistic sensitivity analyses and cost-effectiveness acceptability curves to investigate uncertainty in the model parameters and to present this to decision-makers (for example, references 21, 31, 32, 39, 50 and 52).

For example, Fleurence[21] reported two cost-effectiveness acceptability curves from a model evaluating the cost-effectiveness of fracture prevention treatments (vitamin D/calcium and hip protectors) in male and female populations over 70 in the UK. Figure 18.1 reports the cost-effectiveness acceptability curve in the general female population aged 70+, who had not previously incurred a fracture, for daily supplements of vitamin D and calcium combined with the use of hip protectors (worn daily) compared to no treatment. The figure shows that at a ceiling ratio of $20,000/QALY, the probability that vitamin D and calcium with hip pads is cost-effective is 51%, compared to 49% for no treatment. At $30,000/QALY, the probabilities are 63% and 37% respectively. This type of analysis reflects the uncertainty surrounding the treatment recommendation and can help determine the need for further research.[80]

CONCLUSION

This chapter has described different methodologies used in economic evaluations (cost-effectiveness, cost-utility and cost-benefit analyses) and has provided a discussion of several key issues in economic evaluations in the field of osteoporosis, with examples illustrating how these issues have been approached in practice.

There have been major developments in the treatment of osteoporosis in the last few years, with the publication of the results of the Women's Health Initiative on ERT and HRT, but also a number of clinical trials of other treatments for osteoporosis, such as bisphosphonates, raloxifene, vitamin D/calcium and hip protectors. While the reduction in fractures following HRT use has been established through trials,[81] in earlier economic evaluations a number of assumptions were made on the potential protective effect of HRT from cardiovascular disease. Because of the high absolute risk of coronary heart disease (CHD), such assumptions had a large impact on the results. However, the results of the Women's Health Initiative trial have radically challenged this approach.[7,8,82] With the current guidelines recommending that HRT be used only for the short-term relief of menopausal symptoms, and the decrease in prescription and use of HRT,[83] the long-term use of HRT for the

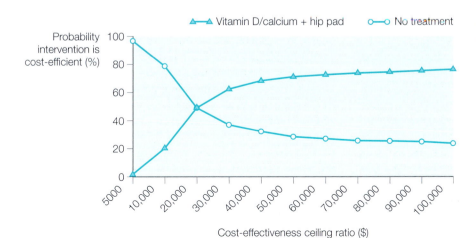

Figure 18.1. Example of cost-effectiveness acceptability curve.

prevention of fractures is no longer recommended.[84] Reflecting this major shift, no economic evaluations analysing HRT have been published since 2002.

This shift of focus in treatments is reflected in published cost-effectiveness models in the field. While a number of particular assumptions, such as the potential protective effect of HRT from cardiovascular disease, in these models may be obsolete, this does not make the models themselves obsolete. Methodological developments, such as the use of probabilistic sensitivity analysis and cost-effectiveness acceptability curves,

have also taken place. Such changes are reflected in more recent economic evaluations. The development of economic evaluations should follow an iterative process that incorporates new information, whether clinical or methodological, as it becomes available.

Future developments of economic evaluations in this field should include trial-based evaluations, as this is the only way to obtain unbiased estimates of costs as well as effects. In addition to measuring the effectiveness of therapies on fractures, it is also important that trialists collect quality-of-life data within the trial population in order to inform estimates of QALY gain (and loss) due to therapy.

PRACTICE POINTS

- Cost-effectiveness analyses of treatments for the prevention of osteoporosis provide decision-makers with criteria to allocate healthcare resources in an efficient and equitable way.

- A number of such evaluations have been developed for osteoporosis treatments.

- These evaluations need to be updated as new clinical and economic information becomes available and should follow best practice guidelines in technology assessment.

RESEARCH AGENDA

- Future clinical trials should collect economic information to inform the cost-effectiveness analysis of osteoporosis interventions.

- Quality-of-life data should also be collected in trials in order to inform estimates of QALY gain (and loss) due to therapy.

REFERENCES

1. Taylor RS, Drummond MF, Salkeld G et al. Inclusion of cost effectiveness in licensing requirements of new drugs: the fourth hurdle. *BMJ* 2004; **329**: 972–975.

2. Claxton K, Sculpher M & Drummond M. A rational framework for decision making by the National Institute for Clinical Excellence (NICE). *Lancet* 2002; **360**: 711–715.

3. Neumann PJ. Evidence-based and value-based formulary guidelines. *Health Aff (Millwood)* 2004; **23**: 124–134.

4. Fleurence R, Iglesias CP & Torgerson D. Cost-effectiveness of nutritional supplements for the treatment of osteoporosis. In: Bonjour JP & New S, eds. *Nutritional Aspects of Bone Health*. Royal Society of Chemistry, 2003.

5. Fleurence R, Iglesias CP & Torgerson D. Economic aspects of osteoporosis treatment. In: Cooper C & Lindsay R, eds. *The Prevention and Treatment of Osteoporosis in the High-risk Patient*. Martin Dunitz, 2005.

6. Rossouw JE, Anderson GL, Prentice RL et al. Risks and benefits of estrogen plus progestin in healthy postmenopausal women: principal results from the Women's Health Initiative randomized controlled trial. *JAMA* 2002; **288**: 321–333.

7. Wassertheil-Smoller S, Hendrix SL, Limacher M et al. Effect of estrogen plus progestin on stroke in postmenopausal women: the Women's Health Initiative: a randomized trial. *JAMA* 2003; **289**: 2673–2684.

8. Anderson GL, Limacher M, Assaf AR et al. Effects of conjugated equine estrogen in postmenopausal women with hysterectomy: the Women's Health Initiative randomized controlled trial. *JAMA* 2004; **291**: 1701–1712.

9. Birks YF, Porthouse J, Addie C et al. Randomized controlled trial of hip protectors among women living in the community. *Osteoporosis Int* 2004; **15**: 701–706.

10. Grant AM, Avenell A, Campbell MK et al. Oral vitamin D3 and calcium for secondary prevention of low-trauma fractures in elderly people (Randomised Evaluation of Calcium Or vitamin D, RECORD): a randomised placebo-controlled trial. *Lancet* 2005; **365**: 1621–1628.

11. Porthouse J, Cockayne S, King C et al. Randomised controlled trial of calcium and supplementation with cholecalciferol (vitamin D3) for prevention of fractures in primary care. *BMJ* 2005; **330**: 1003.

12. Trivedi DP, Doll R & Khaw KT. Effect of four monthly oral vitamin D3 (cholecalciferol) supplementation on fractures and mortality in men and women living in the community: randomised double blind controlled trial. *BMJ* 2003; **326**: 469.

13. Fleurence RL, Iglesias CP & Torgerson DJ. Economic evaluations of interventions for the prevention and treatment of osteoporosis: a structured review of the literature. *Osteoporos Int* 2006; **17**(1): 29–40.

14. Raftery J. NICE: faster access to modern treatments? Analysis of guidance on health technologies. *BMJ* 2001; **323**: 1300–1303.

15. Drummond MF, Torrance GW & Stoddart GL. *Methods for the Economic Evaluation of Health Care Programmes*. Oxford: Oxford University Press, 1995.

16. Meltzer D. Accounting for future costs in medical cost-effectiveness analysis. *J Health Econ* 1997; **16**: 33–64.

17. Gold MR, Siegel JE, Russell LB et al. *Cost-effectiveness in Health and Medicine*. New York: Oxford University Press, 1996.

18. Weinstein MC. Estrogen use in postmenopausal women – costs, risks, and benefits. *N Engl J Med* 1980; **303**: 308–316.

19. Weinstein MC & Schiff I. Cost-effectiveness of hormone replacement therapy in the menopause. *Obstet Gynecol Surv* 1983; **38**: 445–455.

20. Brazier JE, Green C & Kanis JA. A systematic review of health state utility values for osteoporosis-related conditions. *Osteoporosis Int* 2002; **13**: 768–776.

21. Fleurence RL. Cost-effectiveness of fracture prevention treatments in the elderly. *Int J Technol Assess Health Care* 2004; **20**: 184–191.

22. Brazier JE, Kohler B & Walters S. *A prospective study of the health related quality of life impact of hip fractures*. Sheffield: Scharr, University of Sheffield, 2000.

23. Robinson R. Cost-benefit analysis. *BMJ* 1993; **307**: 924–926.

24. Cheung AP & Wren BG. A cost-effectiveness analysis of hormone replacement therapy in the menopause. *Med J Aust* 1992; **156**: 312–316.

25. Tosteson AN, Rosenthal DI, Melton LJ III et al. Cost effectiveness of screening perimenopausal white women for osteoporosis: bone densitometry and hormone replacement therapy. *Ann Intern Med* 1990; **113**: 594–603.

26. Tosteson AN & Weinstein MC. Cost-effectiveness of hormone replacement therapy after the menopause. *Bailliere's Clin Obstet Gynaecol* 1991; **5**: 943–959.

27. Weinstein MC & Tosteson AN. Cost-effectiveness of hormone replacement. *Ann N Y Acad Sci* 1990; **592**: 162–172.

28. Jonsson B, Kanis J, Dawson A et al. Effect and offset of effect of treatments for hip fracture on health outcomes. *Osteoporosis Int* 1999; **10**: 193–199.

29. Kanis JA, Dawson A, Oden A et al. Cost-effectiveness of preventing hip fracture in the general female population. *Osteoporosis Int* 2001; **12**: 356–361.

30. Zethraeus N, Johannesson M & Jonsson B. A computer model to analyze the cost-effectiveness of hormone replacement therapy. *Int J Technol Assess Health Care* 1999; **15**: 352–365.

31. Borgstrom F, Johnell O, Jonsson B et al. Cost effectiveness of alendronate for the treatment of male osteoporosis in Sweden. *Bone* 2004; **34**: 1064–1071.

32. Kanis JA, Borgstrom F, Johnell O et al. Cost-effectiveness of raloxifene in the UK: an economic evaluation based on the MORE study. *Osteoporosis Int* 2005; **16**(1): 15–25.

33. Segui-Gomez M, Keuffel E & Frick KD. Cost and effectiveness of hip protectors among the elderly. *Int J Technol Assess Health Care* 2002; **18**: 55–66.

34. Singh S, Sun H & Anis AH. Cost-effectiveness of hip protectors in the prevention of osteoporosis related hip fractures in elderly nursing home residents. *J Rheumatol* 2004; **31**: 1607–1613.

35. Waldegger L, Cranney A, Man-Son-Hing M et al. Cost-effectiveness of hip protectors in institutional dwelling elderly. *Osteoporosis Int* 2003; **14**: 243–250.

36. Willis MS. The health economics of calcium and vitamin D3 for the prevention of osteoporotic hip fractures in Sweden. *Int J Technol Assess Health Care* 2002; **18**: 791–807.

37. Daly E, Roche M, Barlow D et al. HRT: an analysis of benefits, risks and costs. *Br Med Bull* 1992; **48**: 368–400.

38. Daly E, Vessey MP, Barlow D et al. Hormone replacement therapy in a risk-benefit perspective. *Maturitas* 1996; **23**: 247–259.

39. Fleurence R, Torgerson DJ & Reid DM. Cost-effectiveness of hormone replacement therapy for fracture prevention in young postmenopausal women: an economic analysis based on a prospective cohort study. *Osteoporosis Int* 2002; **13**: 637–643.

40. Francis RM, Anderson FH & Torgerson DJ. A comparison of the effectiveness and cost of treatment for vertebral fractures in women. *Br J Rheumatol* 1995; **34**: 1167–1171.

41. Garton MJ, Cooper C & Reid D. Perimenopausal bone density screening – will it help prevent osteoporosis? *Maturitas* 1997; **26**: 35–43.

42. Geelhoed E, Harris A & Prince R. Cost-effectiveness analysis of hormone replacement therapy and lifestyle intervention for hip fracture. *Aust J Public Health* 1994; **18**: 153–160.

43. Kanis JA, Brazier JE, Stevenson M et al. Treatment of established osteoporosis: a systematic review and cost-utility analysis. *Health Technol Assess* 2002; **6**: 1–146.

44. Nagata-Kobayashi S, Shimbo T & Fukui T. Cost-effectiveness analysis of screening for osteoporosis in postmenopausal Japanese women. *J Bone Miner Metab* 2002; **20**: 350–357.

45. Rosner AJ, Grima DT, Torrance GW et al. Cost effectiveness of multi-therapy treatment strategies in the prevention of vertebral fractures in postmenopausal women with osteoporosis. *Pharmacoeconomics* 1998; **14**: 559–573.

46. Torgerson DJ, Donaldson C & Reid D. Using economics to prioritize research: a case study of randomized trials for the prevention of hip fractures due to osteoporosis. *J Health Serv Res Policy* 1996; **1**: 141–146.

47. Ankjaer-Jensen A & Johnell O. Prevention of osteoporosis: cost-effectiveness of different pharmaceutical treatments. *Osteoporosis Int* 1996; **6**: 265–275.

48. Brecht JG, Kruse HP, Felsenberg D et al. Pharmacoeconomic analysis of osteoporosis treatment with risedronate. *Int J Clin Pharmacol Res* 2003; **23**: 93–105.

49. Hart WM, Rubio-Terres C, Burrell A et al. Pharmacoeconomic analysis of the treatment of postmenopausal osteoporosis with risedronate or alendronate. *Rev Espanola Enferm Metab Oseas* 2002; **11**: 97–104.

50. Iglesias CP, Torgerson DJ, Bearne A et al. The cost utility of bisphosphonate treatment in established osteoporosis. *Q J Med* 2002; **95**: 305–311.

51. Johnell O, Jonsson B, Jonsson L et al. Cost effectiveness of alendronate (fosamax) for the treatment of osteoporosis and prevention of fractures. *Pharmacoeconomics* 2003; **21**: 305–314.

52. Kanis JA, Borgstrom F, Johnell O et al. Cost-effectiveness of risedronate for the treatment of osteoporosis and prevention of fractures in postmenopausal women. *Osteoporosis Int* 2004; **15**: 862–871.

53. Rodriguez EC, Fidalgo Garcia ML & Rubio CS. A cost-effectiveness analysis of alendronate compared to placebo in the prevention of hip fracture. *Aten Primaria* 1999; **24**: 390–396.

54. Armstrong K, Chen TM, Albert D et al. Cost-effectiveness of raloxifene and hormone replacement therapy in postmenopausal women: impact of breast cancer risk. *Obstet Gynecol* 2001; **98**: 996–1003.

55. Torgerson DJ & Kanis JA. Cost-effectiveness of preventing hip fractures in the elderly population using vitamin D and calcium. *Q J Med* 1995; **88**: 135–139.

56. Coyle D, Cranney A & Lee KM. Cost effectiveness of nasal calcitonin in postmenopausal women: use of Cochrane Collaboration methods for meta-analysis within economic evaluation. *Pharmacoeconomics* 2001; **19**: 565–575.

57. Visentin P, Ciravegna R & Fabris F. Estimating the cost per avoided hip fracture by osteoporosis treatment in Italy. *Maturitas* 1997; **26**: 185–192.

58. Jonsson B. Targeting high-risk populations. *Osteoporosis Int* 1998; **8**(Suppl. 1): S13–S16.

59. Jonsson B, Christiansen C, Johnell O et al. Cost-effectiveness of fracture prevention in established osteoporosis. *Osteoporosis Int* 1995; **5**: 136–142.

60. Colon-Emeric CS, Biggs DP, Schenck AP et al. Risk factors for hip fracture in skilled nursing facilities: who should be evaluated? *Osteoporosis Int* 2003; **14**: 484–489.

61. Singh S, Sun H & Anis AH. Cost-effectiveness of hip protectors in the prevention of osteoporosis related hip fractures in elderly nursing home residents. *J Rheumatol* 2004; **31**: 1607–1613.

62. Brecht JG, Kruse HP, Mohrke W et al. Health-economic comparison of three recommended drugs for the treatment of osteoporosis. *Int J Clin Pharmacol Res* 2004; **24**: 1–10.

63. Willis M, Odegaard K, Persson U et al. A cost-effectiveness model of tibolone as treatment for the prevention of osteoporosis fractures in postmenopausal women in Sweden. *Clin Drug Invest* 2001; **21**: 115–127.

64. Black DM, Cummings SR, Karpf DB et al. Randomised trial of effect of alendronate on risk of fracture in women with existing vertebral fractures. Fracture Intervention Trial Research Group. *Lancet* 1996; **348**:1535–1541.

65. Cummings SR, Eckert S, Krueger KA et al. The effect of raloxifene on risk of breast cancer in postmenopausal women: results from the MORE randomized trial. Multiple Outcomes of Raloxifene Evaluation. *JAMA* 1999; **281**: 2189–2197.

66. Ettinger B, Black DM, Mitlak BH et al. Reduction of vertebral fracture risk in postmenopausal women with osteoporosis treated with raloxifene: results from a 3-year randomized clinical trial. Multiple Outcomes of Raloxifene Evaluation (MORE) Investigators. *JAMA* 1999; **282**: 637–645.

67. Levis S, Quandt SA, Thompson D et al. Alendronate reduces the risk of multiple symptomatic fractures: results from the fracture intervention trial. *J Am Geriatr Soc* 2002; **50**: 409–415.

68. Reginster J, Minne HW, Sorensen OH et al. Randomized trial of the effects of risedronate on vertebral fractures in women with established postmenopausal osteoporosis. Vertebral Efficacy with Risedronate Therapy (VERT) Study Group. *Osteoporosis Int* 2000; **11**: 83–91.

69. Sculpher M, Torgerson D, Goeree R et al. A critical structured review of economic evaluations of interventions for the prevention and treatment of osteoporosis. Discussion Paper, 1999.

70. Johnell O, Kanis J & Gullberg G. Mortality, morbidity, and assessment of fracture risk in male osteoporosis. *Calcif Tissue Int* 2001; **69**: 182–184.

71. Cooper C, Atkinson EJ, Jacobsen SJ et al. Population-based study of survival after osteoporotic fractures. *Am J Epidemiol* 1993; **137**: 1001–1005.

72. Van Staa TP, Dennison EM, Leufkens HG et al. Epidemiology of fractures in England and Wales. *Bone* 2001; **29**: 517–522.

73. Kanis JA & Pitt FA. Epidemiology of osteoporosis. *Bone* 1992; **13**(Suppl. 1): S7–15.

74. Cooper C. Epidemiology and public health impact of osteoporosis. *Baillieres Clin Rheumatol* 1993; **7**: 459–477.

75. Buxton MJ, Drummond MF, Van Hout BA et al. Modelling in economic evaluation: an unavoidable fact of life. *Health Econ* 1997; **6**: 217–227.

76. Zethraeus N, Ben Sedrine W, Caulin F et al. Models for assessing the cost-effectiveness of the treatment and prevention of osteoporosis. *Osteoporosis Int* 2002; **13**: 841–857.

77. Sculpher M, Fenwick E & Claxton K. Assessing quality in decision analytic cost-effectiveness models. A suggested framework and example of application. *Pharmacoeconomics* 2000; **17**: 461–477.

78. Tosteson AN, Jonsson B, Grima DT et al. Challenges for model-based economic evaluations of postmenopausal osteoporosis interventions. *Osteoporosis Int* 2001; **12**: 849–857.

79. Claxton K, Neumann PJ & Araki SS. The value of information: an application to a policy model of Alzheimer's disease. *Int J Technol Assess Health Care* 2001; **17**: 38–55.

80. Claxton K, Ginnelly L, Sculpher M et al. A pilot study on the use of decision theory and value of information analysis as part of the NHS Health Technology Assessment programme. *Health Technol Assess* 2004; **8**: 1–103, iii.

81. Torgerson DJ & Bell-Syer SE. Hormone replacement therapy and prevention of nonvertebral fractures: a meta-analysis of randomized trials. *JAMA* 2001; **285**: 2891–2897.

82. Manson JE, Hsia J, Johnson KC et al. Estrogen plus progestin and the risk of coronary heart disease. *N Engl J Med* 2003; **349**: 523–534.

83. Majumdar SR, Almasi EA & Stafford RS. Promotion and prescribing of hormone therapy after report of harm by the Women's Health Initiative. *JAMA* 2004; **292**: 1983–1988.

84. Grady D. Postmenopausal hormones – therapy for symptoms only. *N Engl J Med* 2003; **348**: 1835–1837.

Chapter 19
Risk assessment in osteoporosis

Olof Johnell

It is well known that the clinical manifestation of osteoporosis, the osteoporotic fracture, has a high prevalence.[1] The lifetime risk of a fracture at the age of 50 in women in the UK[2] is 53% and in men 21%, in Sweden[3] 46% and 22% respectively, and in the USA[4] 40% versus 13%. It has also been shown that osteoporotic fractures are associated with a high morbidity and mortality.[5] Thus, osteoporosis is an important healthcare problem. Furthermore, there has been a development of treatment of proven efficacy and this will increase the demand for management of patients with osteoporosis. Measurement of bone mineral density (BMD) is a central component in the international description of osteoporosis: a systematic disease characterized by low bone mass and microarchitectural deterioration of bone mass, with a consequent increase in bone fragility and susceptibility to fracture.[6] The diagnosis, according to the WHO group, is based on a BMD measurement.[7]

The clinical significance of osteoporosis is the fracture that occurs. BMD is an important component of the risk of fracture, but other abnormalities in the skeleton also contribute to fragility. Several non-skeletal factors, such as liability to fall and force of impact, contribute to fracture risk. Since BMD is one component of fracture risk, the accurate assessment of fracture risk should ideally take into account other readily measured indices of fracture risk that add further information to that provided by BMD.[8] The strategy for identifying patients for an intervention in a case-finding strategy has focused on identifying clinical risk factors for low BMD, and those with risk factors will be referred for BMD measurement and thereafter an intervention will be offered if the BMD falls below a given threshold, in some countries below a T-score of ≤2.5 SD. These kinds of guidelines have been presented by the European Foundation for Osteoporosis,[9] where risk factors were identified that could provide an indication for the diagnostic use of BMD. The risk factors were, for example, presence of oestrogen deficiency, glucocorticoid therapy, maternal family history of hip fracture, low body mass index (<19), other disorders associated with osteoporosis, radiographic evidence of osteopoenia and/or vertebral deformity, previous fragility fracture (particularly hip, spine or wrist), loss of height and thoracic kyphosis. In the USA the National Osteoporosis Foundation (NOF) have published similar guidelines,[10] *Physicians Guide to Prevention and Treatment of Osteoporosis* (http://www.nof.org). The US guidelines have a similar approach and try to identify the highest risk, but in the USA a BMD measurement could be offered to all women >65 years of age and for women ≤65 years of age depending on whether they had a major risk factor, such as a history of fracture as an adult, a history of fragility fracture in a first-degree relative, low body weight (<127 lb), current smoking or use of oral glucocorticoid therapy for >3 months. Also, they have some additional risk factors in their algorithm. The decision on intervention was then based on the BMD measurement in combination with the risk factors (with the exception of some previous fractures, where treatment can be started without a BMD measurement).

Only using a T-score value has some limitations,[8,11] e.g. that the majority of fractures will occur in those individuals never assessed and besides, a T-score is only defined for dual-energy X-ray absorptiometry (DEXA). For exactly the same T-score the absolute 10-year risk is different for different ages and T-scores are different for different techniques. A growing view is that assessment of fracture risk should encompass all aspects of risk and that intervention should not be guided solely based on BMD value, but also on the absolute fracture risk. Thus, there is a distinction to be made between the diagnosis of osteoporosis and assessment of fracture risk.

FRACTURE PROBABILITY

Fracture risk is commonly expressed as a relative risk, but has a different meaning in different contexts. In the case of BMD gradients of risk are used,[11] e.g. 2.6-fold increase in hip fracture risk for each SD in BMD shown in a meta-analysis. For clinical risk factors, risk is commonly expressed as the risk in the individuals with a risk factor compared with the risk in those without a risk factor or, sometimes, as the risk compared with the general population. To be able to compare risks, risk estimates need to be expressed in a standardized manner, e.g. as the relative risk to a population risk or as the gradient of risk.[8,11] Nevertheless, the use of the relative risk can be problematic; for a given BMD value the relative risk with fracture decreases with age, whereas the absolute risk increases with age.[11] This is confusing for clinicians. Thus, there has been debate whether it is more appropriate to present the risk in absolute terms, i.e. the probability or likelihood of fracture over a given period of time. The absolute risk of fracture depends on age and life expectancy, as well as the current relative risk. Previously, calculations have been done on lifetime risk. But this also has some disadvantages; treatments are usually not given for a lifetime or data show low compliance. Furthermore, the feasibility of lifelong interventions has never been tested, and the predictive value of BMD and some other risk factors for fracture risk may attenuate over time. Over a long time span, other diseases may occur and influence the fracture risk. For these reasons, the IOF[9] and NOF[10] have recommended that the risk of fracture should be expressed as a fixed-term absolute risk, e.g. probability over a 10-year period.

A period of 10 years covers the likely duration of treatment and any benefit that may continue once the treatment is finished. An important advantage of using the fracture probability – absolute risk – in risk assessment is that it can standardize the output from multiple techniques and sites used for assessment and also combine risk factors.[11]

OPTIMIZATION OF A CASE-FINDING STRATEGY

It is evident from these findings that consideration of multiple risk factors improves risk stratification of individuals and thereby better identifies the high-risk patients. A new strategy can be envisaged and the first step is the assessment of fracture probability based only on clinical risk factors. This will identify three groups of individuals.[8] The first group is those with a very high risk above the threshold in whom a BMD test would not alter their classification. These patients can be offered treatment irrespective of BMD as in the NOF guidelines with the presence of some fractures. For the remainder, ideally a BMD measurement could be made in all individuals. But these patients may also be split into two groups; in one group the absolute risk based on the clinical risk factors has a very low probability of an osteoporotic fracture so that the estimate of BMD measurement would not alter the classification to be above the given level of risk for an intervention. Then we are left with an intermediate group in whom fracture probability is close to the intervention threshold, where the probability is high and the BMD test might re-categorize individuals at high risk to low risk and vice versa. This strategy differs from the previous ones in that fracture risk is an indication for an intervention and BMD is considered in those who had intermediate risk where its value would lead to a change of category for the patient.

ETHNIC AND GEOGRAPHIC APPLICABILITY

It is important to take into account all osteoporotic fractures, not only hip fractures. But the problem is that most data available worldwide are on hip fractures.[12] We created an algorithm for countries where the fracture pattern, i.e. the relationship between the different osteoporotic fractures, was known.[13] Thus, we can use the hip fracture risk and recalculate to encompass all osteoporotic fractures. There is a worldwide variation to be taken into account on hip fractures and that will also be included in a case-finding strategy.

RISK FACTOR ASSESSMENT

BMD alone is not an adequate measurement to provide an instrument for population screening, as there are many other risk factors that contribute to fracture risk. There are several considerations in the selection of risk factors for use in fracture prediction. They need to be:[11]

- valid in multiple populations;
- adjusted for age, sex and type of fracture;
- readily assessable by primary care physicians;
- contributory factors to a risk that is amenable to the therapeutic manipulation intended;
- intuitive rather than contra-intuitive to medical care.

Age

The most important risk factor. A woman aged 50 with a T-score of −2 has an absolute 10-year risk of 1.7% and a woman with exactly the same T-score aged 80 has a 10-year risk of 11.5%[14] – a greater than six-fold difference with exactly the same BMD value.

Gender

As pointed out earlier, women have a higher incidence of osteoporotic fractures than men. In Sweden the lifetime risk for an osteoporotic fracture is 46% for women and 22% for men.[3] This is only partly dependent on the shorter life expectancy in men.

BMD

BMD is one of the most important risk factors for osteoporotic fractures and the ability to predict fracture is comparable to the use of blood pressure to predict stroke and substantially better than cholesterol in predicting myocardial infarction. In a previous meta-analysis it has been shown that predicting hip fractures with measurement at the femoral neck has an increased risk of 2.6.[15] In a new meta-analysis[16] based on data on individuals in 12 large international cohorts with a total follow-up of almost 170,000 person-years, the gradient of risk for BMD and fractures was examined and it was shown that the predictive effect was dependent on age, with a significantly higher gradient of risk at the age of 50 than at the age of 80 for hip fractures; the gradient of risk with BMD measured at the femoral neck was higher with lower BMD.

Data from ultrasound and peripheral measurements were also used[16] and the predictive ability of these devices was somewhat less than that of DEXA at the femoral neck. Thus, BMD is a risk factor that can be used in an international setting and the variation in predictive value with age and BMD should be taken into account.

In the large international cohort study, other risk factors have also been identified that apply globally.

Previous fracture

A previous fracture is a well-documented risk factor for future fracture. In a meta-analysis of worldwide cohorts,[17] a previous fracture was associated with a significantly increased risk of any fracture (relative risk (RR): 1.9; 95% CI: 1.8–2.9) with similar results for osteoporotic fracture for hip fractures. The results were similar for men and women. The risk ratio was only marginally adjusted downwards when BMD was taken into account. For hip fracture the risk ratio was higher at younger ages. Thus, previous fracture can also be used for case-finding in an international setting.

Use of glucocorticoids

This risk factor has also been found in several studies. In an international worldwide cohort study,[18] the relative risk for hip fractures ranged from 4.4 at the age of 50 years to 2.5 at the age of 85, and there was no significant difference between men and women. The risk was only marginally changed when BMD was included in the model. This is also a risk factor that can be used in case-finding in an international setting.

Low body mass index

This is a well-documented risk factor found in several studies. In an international cohort study,[19] the risk ratio per unit higher body mass index was 0.93 for hip fractures (95% CI: 0.91–0.94), with no difference between men and women. After adjusting for BMD, the relative risk was only significant for BMD in women, 0.94 per unit higher body mass index. The contribution to fracture risk was much more marked at lower values of body mass index than values above the mean. Thus, those with low body mass index should be used in risk assessment.

Family history of fracture

This has been established in several epidemiological and genetic studies. In an international cohort study,[20] the effects of a family history of osteoporotic or hip fractures in a first-degree relative were studied. A family history of hip fracture in parents was associated with a high risk of osteoporotic fracture in women (RR: 1.6; 95% CI: 1.3–2.0) and of hip fractures (RR: 2.5; 95% CI: 1.5–3.9). This risk was not significantly changed when BMD was added to the model and this risk factor can be used in case-finding in an international setting.

Secondary osteoporosis

Secondary osteoporosis is a well-recognized risk factor for osteoporosis shown by several studies.

Smoking

This is another risk factor used in several guidelines. In an international worldwide cohort,[21] smoking was significantly associated with an increased risk of hip fractures (RR: 1.8; 95% CI: 1.5–2.2) and somewhat lower when adjusted for BMD (RR: 1.6; 95% CI: 1.3–2.2).

Low BMD accounted for only 23% of smoking-related risk of fractures. Thus, smoking is also a risk factor that can be used in a case-finding strategy in an international setting.

Alcohol intake

There has been a discussion whether moderate alcohol intake has any negative effect; the possibility of a positive effect has also been discussed. But excessive alcohol intake is a well-recognized risk factor for osteoporosis and an international worldwide cohort[22] showed that there was a 7% increase for each unit of alcohol above 1 unit daily and when the risk of hip fracture was compared with more than 2 units per day the risk was 1.7 (95% CI: 1.2–2.4). After adjustment for BMD the relative risk was little affected. There was a slight reduction after adjusting for smoking (RR: 1.5; 95% CI: 1.1–2.2). Thus, also alcohol intake is an important risk factor and can be used in a case-finding strategy, but as for smoking it can also be used in a public health approach.

There are several risk factors that have been validated in international cohorts and that can be used for case-finding strategies.[8] Most of them are independent of BMD; they add to the fracture risk when considered together with BMD.

In this discussion of risk assessment, important risk factors for public health, e.g. falling, nutrition and physical exercise, are not considered as they are discussed in other parts of the book.

There are several other risk factors that are currently being tested in an international setting, such as biochemical markers of bone turnover, ultrasound measurements and imminently genetic testing.

Another important consideration is that there are interactions between risk factors.[8] We found such an interaction between BMD and age, in that BMD has a higher predictive value at younger ages.[16] There is also a similar association between some of the risk factors. This has to be taken into account in a final model with all risk factors. Such a model has to be created and when this is achieved, treatment can be based on absolute fracture risk. This is being carried out in a WHO project, which will soon give algorithms for those who could be offered an intervention based on absolute risk.

INTERVENTION THRESHOLDS

Previously, intervention thresholds have been determined only on the T-score of BMD, but the field is moving towards absolute risk and with this the cost-effectiveness can be calculated.[8] There have been several models created to calculate cost-effectiveness based on absolute risk. In the WHO project intervention thresholds have been calculated, for Sweden and the UK, based on all fractures and expressed as absolute 10-year hip fracture risks, since hip fracture risk is the only available fracture risk in most countries. But the intervention thresholds depend not only on cost-effectiveness that incorporates the efficacy and side-effects, but also on who pays, the wealth of the country, the healthcare budget of the country and its healthcare priorities.

CONCLUSIONS

The diagnosis of osteoporosis is based on BMD measurement at the hip using DEXA. However, other sites and techniques have been shown to be able to predict fractures. Also, clinical risk factors contribute to fracture risk that, at least in part, is independent of BMD. The risk factors are age, gender, previous fragility fracture, a family history of fracture, use of oral glucocorticoids, smoking, secondary osteoporosis, alcohol intake and low body mass index. These risk factors can be used in combinations and together with BMD to enhance the prediction of fractures for identification of high-risk groups. In the future we should use fracture probability as an intervention threshold like 10-year probability of fracture, and the threshold can be calculated from cost-effectiveness. A WHO project is now finalized encompassing all these aspects, and hopefully will make it easier to find the high-risk patients and treat the right patients.

PRACTICE POINTS

- Clinical risk factors and bone mineral density can be utilized to predict 10-year absolute risk of osteoporotic fractures.
- These 10-year risks are critical to the development of thresholds at which pharmacotherapy in osteoporosis can be targeted most effectively.

RESEARCH AGENDA

- Establish intervention thresholds in several countries or regions.
- Intervention trials based on high risk.

REFERENCES

1. Johnell O & Kanis J. Epidemiology of osteoporotic fractures. *Osteoporosis Int* 2005; **16**(Suppl. 2): S3–S7.
2. Van Staa TP, Dennison EM, Leufkens HG et al. Epidemiology of fractures in England and Wales. *Bone* 2001; **29**: 517–522.
3. Kanis JA, Johnell O, Odén A et al. Long-term risk of osteoporotic fracture in Malmö. *Osteoporosis Int* 2000; **11**: 669–674.
4. Melton LJ III, Chriscilles EA, Cooper C et al. Perspective: how many women have osteoporosis? *J Bone Miner Res* 1992; **7**: 1005–1010.
5. Johnell O, Kanis JA, Odén A et al. Mortality after osteoporotic fractures. *Osteoporosis Int* 2004; **15**(1): 38–42.
6. Consensus Development Conference. Prophylaxis and treatment of osteoporosis. *Am J Med* 1991; **90**: 107–110.
7. World Health Organization. Assessment of fracture risk and its application to screening for postmenopausal osteoporosis. *Technical Report Series*. Geneva: WHO, 1994.
8. Kanis JA, Borgström F, De Laet C et al. Assessment of fracture risk. *Osteoporosis Int* 2005; **16**: 581–589.
9. Kanis JA, Delmas P, Burckhardt P et al. Guidelines for diagnosis and management of osteoporosis. *Osteoporosis Int* 1997; **7**: 390–406.
10. National Osteoporosis Foundation. *Physician's Guide to Prevention and Treatment of Osteoporosis*. http://www.nof.org.
11. Kanis JA, Black D, Cooper C et al. A new approach to the development of assessment guidelines for osteoporosis. *Osteoporosis Int* 2002; **13**: 527–536.
12. Kanis JA, Johnell O, de Laet C et al. International variations in hip fracture probabilities: implications for risk assessment. *J Bone Miner Res* 2002; **17**(7): 1237–1244.
13. Kanis JA, Odén A, Johnell O et al. The burden of osteoporotic fractures: a method for setting intervention thresholds. *Osteoporosis Int* 2001; **12**: 417–427.
14. Kanis JA, Johnell O, Odén A et al. Ten year probabilities of osteoporotic fractures according to BMD and diagnostic thresholds. *Osteoporosis Int* 2001; **12**: 989–995.
15. Marshall D, Johnell O & Wedel H. Meta-analysis of how well measures of bone mineral density predict occurrence of osteoporotic fractures. *BMJ* 1996; **18**: 1254–1259.
16. Johnell O, Kanis JA, Odén A et al. Predict value of BMD for hip and other fractures. *J Bone Miner Res* 2005; **20**: 1185–1194.
17. Kanis JA, Johnell O, De Laet C et al. A meta-analysis of previous fracture and subsequent fracture risk. *Bone* 2004; **35**: 375–382.
18. Kanis JA, Johansson H, Odén A et al. A meta-analysis of prior corticosteroid use and fracture risk. *Osteoporosis Int* 2004; **19**: 893–896.
19. De Laet C, Kanis JA, Odén A et al. Body mass index as a predictor of fracture risk: a meta-analysis. *Osteoporosis Int* 2005; **16**(11): 1330–1338.
20. Kanis JA, Johansson H, Odén A et al. A family history of fracture and fracture risk: a meta-analysis. *Bone* 2004; **35**: 1029–1037.
21. Kanis JA, Johnell O, Odén A et al. Smoking and fracture risk: a meta-analysis. *Osteoporosis Int* 2005; **16**: 155–162.
22. Kanis JA, Johansson H, Johnell O et al. Alcohol intake as a risk factor for fracture. *Osteoporosis Int* 2005; **16**(7): 737–742.

Notes   Page numbers ending in 'b,' 'f,' and 't' denote boxes, figures and tables respectively. Please note that as the main subject of this book is osteoporosis, all entries refer to this subject unless otherwise stated.

Abbreviations   BMS = bone mineral density; PBM = peak bone mass; SERMs = selective oestrogen receptor-modulating drugs.